ACUTE RENAL DISORDERS AND RENAL EMERGENCIES

DEVELOPMENTS IN NEPHROLOGY

Cheigh JS, Stenzel KH, Rubin AL eds: Manual of clinical nephrology of the Rogosin Kidney Center. 1981. ISBN 90-247-2397-3.

Nolph KD ed: Peritoneal dialysis. 1981. ISBN 90-247-2477-5.

Gruskin AB, Norman ME eds: Pediatric nephrology. 1981. ISBN 90-247-2514-3.

Schück O ed: Examination of the kidney function. 1981. ISBN 0-89838-565-2.

Strauss J Ed: Hypertension, fluid-electrolytes and tubulopathies in pediatric nephrology. 1981. ISBN 90-247-2633-6.

Strauss J ed: Neonatal Kidney and Fluid-Electrolytes. 1983. ISBN 0-89838-575-x.

Acute Renal Disorders and Renal Emergencies

Proceedings of Pediatric Nephrology
Seminar X held at Bal Harbour,
Florida, January 30 - February 3, 1983

edited by

JOSÉ STRAUSS, MD
Division of Pediatric Nephrology
University of Miami
School of Medicine
Miami, Florida, USA

with the assistance of

LOUISE STRAUSS, MS, MA

1984/ **MARTINUS NIJHOFF PUBLISHING**
a member of the KLUWER ACADEMIC PUBLISHERS GROUP
BOSTON / THE HAGUE / DORDRECHT / LANCASTER

Distributors

for the United States and Canada: Kluwer Boston, Inc., 190 Old Derby Street, Hingham, MA 02043, USA
for all other countries: Kluwer Academic Publishers Group, Distribution Center, P.O. Box 322, 3300 AH Dordrecht, The Netherlands

Pediatric Nephrology Seminar (10th : 1983 : Bal Harbour, Fla.)
Acute renal disorders and renal emergencies.

(Developments in nephrology)
Includes bibliographical references and indexes.
1. Renal insufficiency, Acute, in children--Congresses. 2. Hemolytic-uremic syndrome--Congresses. 3. Pediatric nephrology--Congresses. 4. Pediatric emergencies--Congresses. I. Strauss, José. II. Strauss, Louise. III. Title. IV. Series: Developments in nephrology (1983) [DNLM: 1. Hemolytic-Uremic Syndrome--in infancy & childhood--Congresses. 2. Kidney Failure, Acute--in infancy & childhood--congresses. W1 DE998EB / WS 320 P373 1983a]
RJ476.R46P43 1983 618.92'61 84-10742

ISBN-13: 978-1-4613-3824-6 e-ISBN-13: 978-1-4613-3822-2
DOI: 10.1007/978-1-4613-3822-2

DEDICATION

To the Department Chairmen

who accepted me as I was, and helped me become

what I am -

Edward Fischel
Richard Day
Rustin McIntosh
Robert Ward
William Cleveland

In the arena of life,
be fair to others; demand fairness of others.
-JS

FOREWORD

My thoughts about the Hemolytic Uremic Syndrome (HUS) got started in 1961 along with my attempt to return to Argentina. As I sought my way in Buenos Aires, I visited Carlos Gianantonio whom I had met in Caracas the year before during the Pan American pediatric meetings. At that time he was actively working on HUS which had become an epidemic in Buenos Aires and other parts of Argentina. I was impressed by the team effort and devotion of his group to such heavy demands. They obviously were meeting the challenge at an amazingly high level under a very crippling physical situation with shortages of space, laboratories and equipment. His group together with Dr. Becu, at the time the pathologist at the Children's Hospital of Buenos Aires (we had met through his mother who was instrumental in arranging my return to Buenos Aires), wrote some of the classic papers on HUS. Through the years as Dr. Gianantonio became more involved in general pediatrics, the administrative aspects and its orientation in Latin America, he became known for his deep philosophical questions as to what we are doing and where we are going. His questions have obvious implications regarding an agressive approach to our pediatric nephrology patients.

Among the many who greatly admire Dr. Gianantonio and have learned from him is Bernard Kaplan. In 1978 at the International Pediatric Nephrology Symposium, Dr. Kaplan verbalized his thoughts about the need to have an international exchange of views and data on HUS. He thought that our Seminar was uniquely suited for this purpose and wondered whether HUS might be a subject I would like to consider. As with most things that Dr. Kaplan says, this suggestion had obvious merit and was warmly received by other pediatric nephrologists.

As a result, at this Seminar we have had the unique opportunity to analyze the implications of the term "Hemolytic Uremic Syndrome", the possibility that it may actually comprise more than one entity, and the newer diagnostic and therapeutic modalities that have become available. In the process we have been exposed to Dr. Kaplan's keen mind, clear expositions, probing questions, and constructive suggestions. He was an extremely generous participant during the Seminar and for this volume. So was Alan Gruskin, as is expected by those who know him and follow this series. Dr. John Byrnes brought his original research on the hematological aspects of HUS and some of the work on which our group is collaborating. (We are most excited about his ideas and the preliminary results being obtained with our patients).

The general subject this year, acute renal diseases and renal emergencies, (the result of a discussion with Dr. McVicar in preparation of the Seminar's topics) turned out to be a good one - in contraposition to chronic and progressive diseases which we plan to discuss in 1985. For example, questions asked about mineral metabolism probably would not have come up if we had not gone into the acute renal problem approach. There was a unity in the total since the subjects touched - with the unstinting participation of Drs. Gruskin, Eichenwald, McVicar, Kaplan, Gianantonio and our University of Miami Faculty - had as a common thread their acute clinical presentation. This vantage point brought out questions not usually considered when the approach is histological or physiological.

From another point of view, the highlight of this year's seminar was that it was the tenth. Our experience in planning and managing ten has strengthened our commitment to the format we follow in terms of subjects and time use. Our aim has developed into a focus on current questions put together with a selection of problems which have a common theme - not as loosely as the first two seminars, not as restrictive as another in emphasizing just one disease - as we easily could have done with HUS, but a fit which incorporates the practical with esoteric questions in a mix of various components (papers, discussions, workshops, and self-teaching sessions) and encourages complete involvement of faculty and registrants. By keeping the total number of participants relatively small, we have not been bound by a rigid schedule; self-pacing and time for genuine exchange remain possible. Also, by moderating all of the day sessions myself - a choice questioned by some the first years-the interrelationships of presentations and discussions fuse and create a unity of direction and accomplishment, many tell me now.

Whatever the judgement of others, I myself have grown with these ten efforts - all related but each unique. I enjoy the challenge your continued interest and support give me to go on with another year and I appreciate the opportunity to create this sharing experience annually.

Jose Strauss

CONTENTS

ACKNOWLEDGEMENTS

Can you believe that not one person is paid for his/her contribution to this Seminar or volume? Faculty expenses are met by registrants fees and pharmaceutical company support but all else is done without financial remuneration. The faculty - guest and local - say that they are rewarded by the opportunity for such exchange. Perhaps this attitude is the source of the Seminar's success year after year.

These are the companies who helped this time:

Abbott Laboratories
American McGaw
Armour Pharmaceutical Co.
Beach Products, Inc.
Burroughs Wellcome Company
Ciba Pharmaceutical Company
Cordis Dow Corporation
Cutter Medical
Drake Willock
Hoechst-Roussel Pharmaceuticals, Inc.
Hoffman-LaRoche
Lifemed
Mead Johnson Nutritional Division
Norwich-Eaton Pharmaceuticals
Merck, Sharp & Dohme
Ross Laboratories
Schering Corporation
Smith, Kline & French Laboratories
E.R. Squibb & Sons, Inc.
Travenol Laboratories, Inc.
Upjohn Company
Willen Drug Company
William R. Rorer, Inc.
Wyeth Laboratories

Since this volume is printed from the camera-ready pages submitted by each author, I would like to acknowledge the authors' contribution of this technical effort in addition to the actual writing of the papers. All not prepared by the authors' assistants was done by Estela Garcia in her usual careful, constructive way, and Isadore Glassman. Pearl Seidler came through again as the one responsible for tying ends together for the Seminar. All members of our Division cooperated as needed, filled in for each other, and shared in the problems as well as the rewards of this effort. Each author assumes complete responsibility for the content of his/her paper. Variations in format and type have been accepted to minimize the total time and effort required to complete publication details.

Finally, I call your attention to the appreciated continued moral support of Dr. Bernard Fogel, Vice President for Medical Affairs and Dean of the School of Medicine of the University of Miami, and Dr. William Cleveland, Chairman of the Department of Pediatrics.

José Strauss

TENTH ANNIVERSARY STATEMENT

February 3, 1983

1983 MARKS THE TENTH YEAR THAT DR. JOSE STRAUSS AND HIS VERY CAPABLE STAFF HAVE ORGANIZED THE SEMINARS IN PEDIATRIC NEPHROLOGY.

THE VALUE OF THIS FORUM TO THE DEVELOPMENT OF PEDIATRIC NEPHROLOGY CAN READILY BE APPRECIATED WHEN ONE REVIEWS THE BROAD RANGE OF TOPICS AND LONG LIST OF INTERNATIONALLY PROMINENT GUEST LECTURERS AND PARTICIPANTS.

TRUE TO HIS COMMITMENT TO MAKING THE SEMINARS RESPONSIVE TO THE NEEDS OF THE PARTICIPANTS, DR. STRAUSS HAS CONDUCTED A PROGRAM WHICH IS AT ONCE OF THE HIGHEST QUALITY AND WHICH ALSO PROVIDES THE GREATEST OPPORTUNITY FOR BOTH FORMAL AND INFORMAL EXCHANGE.

IT IS WITH GREAT RESPECT AND GRATITUDE THAT WE THE INVITED LECTURERS OF THIS 1983 SEMINAR, ON BEHALF OF ALL THE PREVIOUS AND CURRENT PARTICIPANTS, PRESENT YOU WITH AN INSCRIBED PLACQUE TO HONOR THE TENTH ANNIVERSARY OF YOUR OUTSTANDING ACHIEVEMENT.

THIS AWARD
IS PRESENTED TO

JOSE STRAUSS, M.D.

BY HIS COLLEAGUES

in recognition of his outstanding contribution to the development of Pediatric Nephrology

TENTH ANNUAL PEDIATRIC NEPHROLOGY SEMINAR
BAL HARBOUR, FLORIDA, FEBRUARY 3, 1983

Guest Lecturers
1983

Heinz F. Eichenwald
Carlos A. Gianantonio
Alan Gruskin
Bernard S. Kaplan
Melinda McVicar

Guest Lecturers
1974-82

Guiseppe A. Andres
Anita Aperia
Sonia Balsan
Lewis Barness
T.M. Barratt
Jay Bernstein
Sidney Blumenthal
Michael Broyer

Ronald J. Kallen
Carl M. Kjellstrand
Barbara Korsch
John E. Lewy
George McCracken
Wallace W. McCrory
Rawle M. McIntosh
Jack Metcoff
Alfred F. Michael

Philip L Calcagno
Luis Callis
J. Stewart Cameron
Jorge de la Cruz
Salha Daniel
Harriet Dustan
Chester M. Edelman, Jr.
Richard Fine

Bernard Mirkin
Eddie Moore
Felipe Mota-H.
Ricardo Munoz-A.
Antonia C. Novello
William Oh
Keith Peters
Donald E. Potter
George A. Richard

Robert Good
Gustavo Gordillo
Ira Greifer
José Grunberg
Jean-Pierre Guignard
Renée Habib
Robert H. Heptinstall
John C. Hodson

Juan Rodriguez-Soriano
Robert W. Schrier
Eduardo Slatopolski
Adrian Spitzer
Robert C. Tarazi
Robert Vernier
Margarita Vitacco
Dixon Walker
Richard Weil III

I

HEMOLYTIC UREMIC SYNDROME

THE HEMOLYTIC-UREMIC SYNDROMES: THE MOST IMPORTANT CAUSE OF ACUTE RENAL FAILURE IN INFANTS AND CHILDREN

Bernard S. Kaplan, M.B., B.Ch., F.C.P.(S.A.), Paul R. Goodyer, M.D., Jack S.C. Fong, M.D., C.M., F.R.C.P.(C) and Peter D. Thomson, M.B., B.Ch., F.C.P.(S.A.)

Dr. M.A. Kibel, thundering like the Victoria Falls when the Zambezi River is in full flood, wrote in the Year Book of Pediatrics (1966-1967) that "there are still a few skeptics who would doubt the existence of a malady...affecting young children...(which is) characterized by hemolytic anemia and nephropathy of varying degrees." "There is no doubt," quoth he, "that this fascinating syndrome has not engendered the interest it deserves, presumably because the Great Seats of Learning, other than Johannesburg and Buenos Aires, have not experienced outbreaks. So, put an end to this torpor, Mr. Editor, sir. Step out and proclaim an International Conference of Gasser's Syndrome!" Dr. Gellis gave one of his clasical replies: "(That Kibel is a gasser. - Ed.)" (1).

A decade before, in 1955, Gasser et al. (2) had described the hemolytic-uremic syndromes (Hamolytich-urämische syndrome). Since then, thousands of cases have been reported from many parts of the world (3,4), but especially from Argentina (5). HUS has now become the most important cause of acute renal failure in pediatric patients in terms of prevalence, mortality, morbidity and, in some countries, long-term sequelae (6). Many of our concepts have changed, much has been learned (and unlearned), and above all, the death rate in the acute phase has been reduced dramatically (5,6). In addition, Dr. José Strauss has organized the first symposium in North America on HUS.

CLASSIFICATION OF HUS

The HUS can be classified in a number of different ways in order to account for its many possibilities (Figure 1). One must always remember that any classification is full of problems (Figure 2).

1. HUS may be one among others of a community of syndromes with endothelial cell damage (9). (Others include thrombotic thrombocytopenic purpura, malignant hypertension.)
2. Epidemiology

HUS may occur epidemically, endemically or sporadically. HUS seems to occur more frequently in some parts of the world than others: Argentina, the Netherlands, California, and the Witwatersrand of South Africa are regions of frequent occurrence. Small epidemics have

---

This is publication number 00000 of The McGill University-Montreal Children's Hospital Research Institute

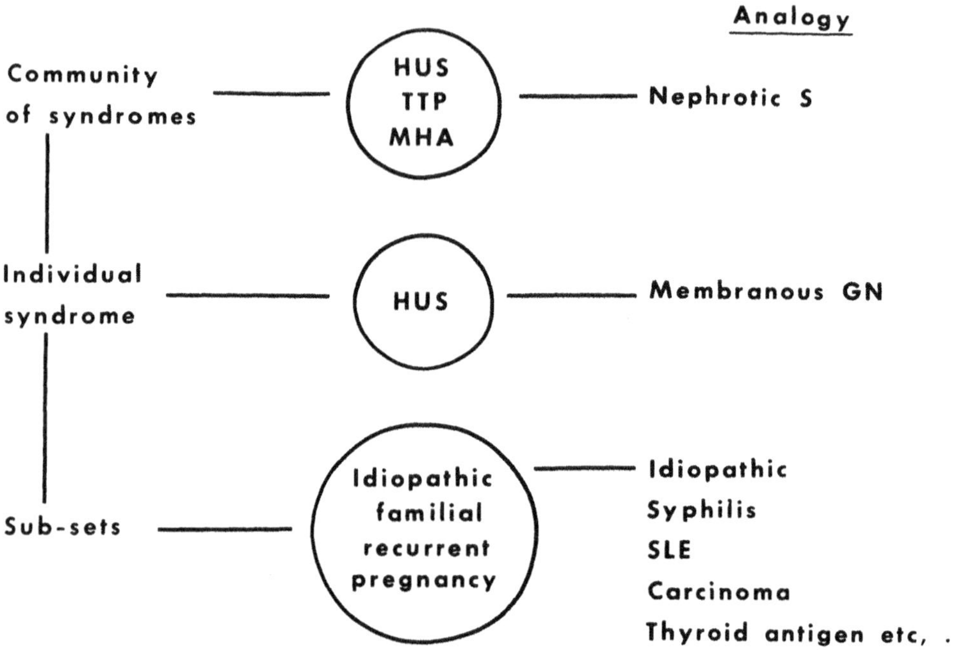

Figure 1. "There are advantages to be gained from surveying a scene from the highest peak. However, there are times when one must also look at the details. Both approaches to these syndromes are important, especially in those that are complex and poorly understood. By constructing groups of syndromes one may achieve better understanding of their pathogenesis, and by looking at subsets an attempt can be made to compare the results of treatment and offer a more accurate prognosis." (8)

occurred in a number of places including Quebec, Edmonton, and Toronto. The age of onset ranges from the neonatal period to adulthood but tends to be mainly in children between 6 months and 4 years of age. Blacks seem to be much less frequently affected than Whites.

3. Classification of Causes of HUS

Many 'agents' or situations have been identified in association with HUS.

Viruses - Echo, coxsackie, (infectious mononucleosis)
Microtatobiote?
Bacteria - Shigella(10), salmonella, yersinia, pneumococcus, campylobacter
Endotoxin (10)
Mycoplasma pneumoniae
Genetic predisposition (autosomal recessive, autosomal dominant)
Chemicals - Pyran copolymer, oral contraceptives, penicillin/ampicillin (11)

Pregnancy - intra, and post-partum
Metabolic defect - Prostacyclin, α-tocopherol
Radiation

4. Classification of Pathogenesis of HUS

There are a number of theories, some of which may prove to be correct, some of which may overlap and others which may be mutually exclusive. These include:

Disseminated intravascular coagulation - there is no evidence that this occurs in most patients with HUS, although data supportive of low-grade intravascular coagulation have been reported by Monnens *et al.* (12).

Local intravascular coagulation seems to occur at the onset of the disease, but rarely thereafter. As a consequence, fibrin strands within the microvessels of the kidney damage erythrocytes which are then removed by the spleen (13). Platelets may be damaged and removed in the same way (14).

Intrarenal platelet aggregation - Intrarenal aggregation of platelets may have a role in the pathogenesis of HUS (15,16).

Reduction of local fibrinolysis is an attractive, but as yet unproven possibility. A dialysable plasma inhibitor of glomerular fibrinolysis has been identified, but its role has not been determined (17).

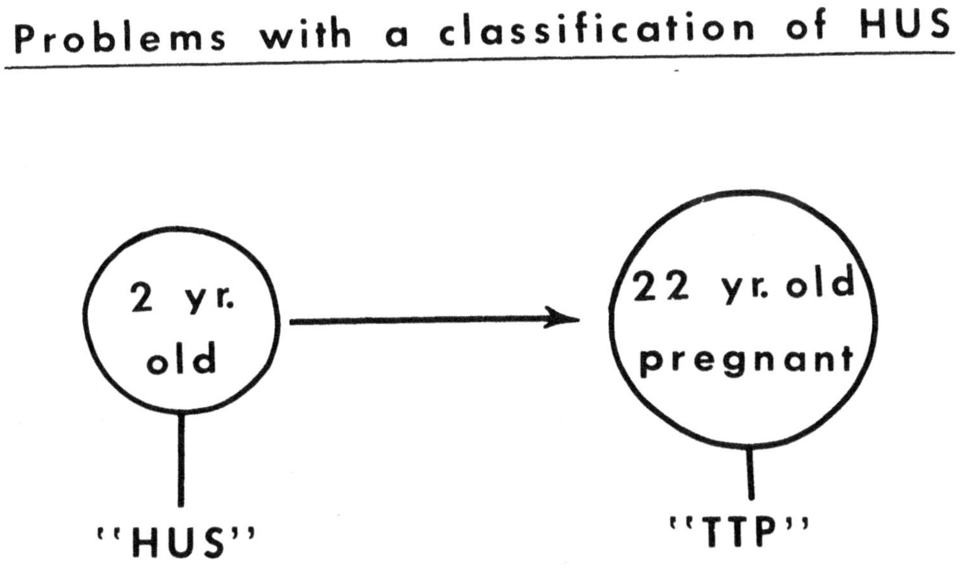

Figure 2. This patient's case history was described by Mettler (Case 3 FL) (7). At 2 years of age, she had what in retrospect was thought to be HUS. During a pregnancy at 22 years of age, a clinical and histological diagnosis of TTP was made. Following deterioration of liver and kidney function, she died. Did she have HUS and then TTP? Or recurrent HUS? Or recurrent TTP?

Immunologic mechanisms have been invoked but most observations do not point to a direct role for complement or immunoglobulins as important pathogenetic mechanisms. Persistent intravascular activation of C3 has been documented in a number of cases (18).

Prostacyclin - Reduced activity of prostacyclin has been well documented but the precise roles of prostacyclin and thromboxane in the pathogenesis of the renal lesions remain to be determined (19).

The role of neuraminidase in revealing the Thomson-Friedenreich antigen on red cells with consequent agglutination is an exciting avenue currently being explored (20). Neuraminidase is produced by pneumococci. HUS associated with pneumococcal infection has a poor outcome.

The central event, however, seems to be injury to the endothelial cells by some agent. All the important renal events that follow may be the result of damage to this important cell. Endothelial cells produce prostacyclin, factor VIII, and fibrinolytic factors, and are covered on their luminal surfaces by α_2-macroglobulin, an antithrombotic agent. The glomerular, and often arteriolar endothelial cells, are swollen and become separated from the underlying glomerular basement membrane. The space thus formed is filled with lipid, fibrin and cell fragments.

5. Classification and Severity of Clinical Features

The prodrome consists of an episode of gastroenteritis days to weeks before the onset of HUS. This can be mild or severe. The prodrome may occasionally be an upper respiratory infection, or a childhood illness.

The syndrome may be mild or severe. Mildly affected cases have HUS without a period of anuria. Severely affected cases have more than 24 hours of anuria. Convulsions, hypertension and oliguria, when they all occur in the same patient tend to be indicative of a more progressive form of the illness.

Central nervous system, gastrointestinal, cardiac and liver involvement may occur in varying combinations and degrees of severity.

Relapses can occur during the course of the illness and, after the patient has recovered, one to 20 recurrences can occur. Fortunately, recurrent episodes of HUS are uncommon.

A diagnosis of HUS should be suspected in every infant and child who presents with combinations of pallor, petechiae, seizures, hypertension, oliguria, or anuria, after an episode of gastroenteritis or an upper respiratory tract infection.

Laboratory Findings - Whenever HUS is suspected, the following tests are mandatory: urinalysis, hemoglobin, platelet count, examination of the peripheral smear, BUN concentration, serum sodium, potassium and chloride concentrations.

A diagnosis can be made in every case on the basis of these studies, although, occasionally, some of these investigations may need to be repeated a few times.

Some patients present with features of acute abdomen (21,22) that may mimic acute appendicitis, intussusception or peritonitis. If the above tests are done and interpreted before surgery, needless operations can be avoided.

6. Summary of Laboratory Findings

Urine: Volume may be normal, increased, or reduced; or, the patient may be anuric; hematuria, proteinuria, casts

Hemogram: Low hemoglobin 3-10 g/dl, leukocytosis up to 30,000/cmm, thrombocytopenia 5,000-140,000/cmm;anisocytes, poikilocytes, fragmented erythrocytes.

Chemistry: Elevated BUN, creatinine, uric acid, phosphate, hydrogen ion, and lipid concentrations; reduced concentration of sodium, calcium, albumin bicarbonate; potassium concentrations may be increased or decreased.

ATYPICAL FORMS OF HUS

HUS with Recurrent Episodes

A number of patients have been reported in whom more than one discrete episode of HUS occurred (23). Some cases have been confused with thrombotic thrombocytopenic purpura and others have had recurrences in association with pregnancy. This subset which has been defined by recurrences of HUS is clearly not a discrete entity, but an uncommon, albeit important and interesting, atypical form (or forms) of HUS.

The prognosis for patients with recurrent episodes tends to be worse than that for patients with the more typical form of HUS.

HUS with an Inherited Predisposition (Table 1)

An analysis of familial cases of HUS suggested that there is, in some families, an autosomal recessive predisposition to develop HUS (24) (Figure 3). In these families, affected siblings develop HUS one to many years apart and the prognosis has been poor with an overall mortality rate of close to 70%.

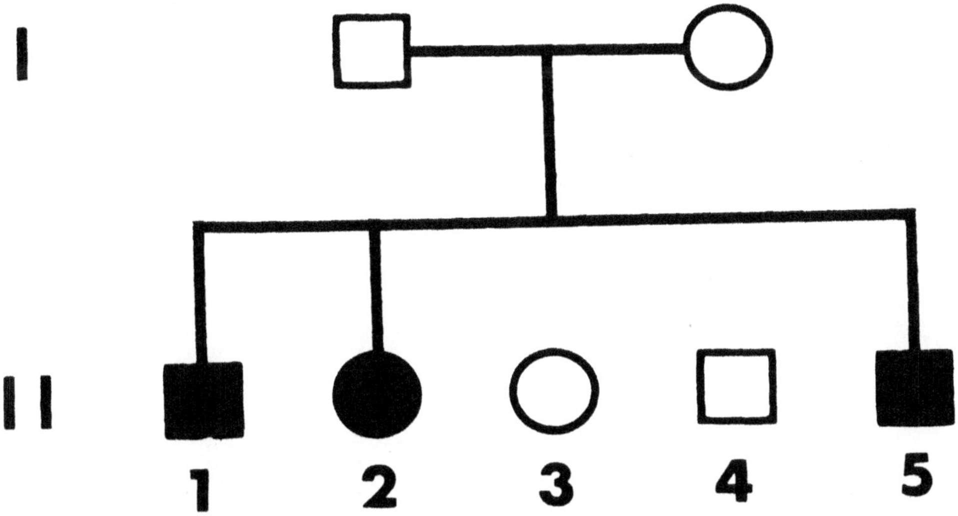

Figure 3. Pedigree of the C family (24). Case 1 died in 1967 at 9 months, Case 2 died at 8 months in 1969 and Case 3 died in 1974 at 7 months all from HUS. The children II3 and II4 were adopted; neither has had HUS.

Table 1. HUS in Families.

	Group	Interval Between Onset In Each Case	Age of Onset	Etiology	Relapses	Prognosis
A	"Epidemic"	< 3 weeks	childhood (usually)	? viral, bacterial		Good
B	"Recessive"	> 1 year	childhood (usually)	may have no prodrome	can occur	Poor
C	"Dominant"	> 1 year	young adults (usually)	can be associated with pregnancy		Very poor

There are also a few families in which HUS appears to have been inherited by an autosomal dominant mode. Affected members tended to be adolescents or young adults and the mortality rate has been 70%. An additional 23% developed end-stage renal failure.

Recent studies have suggested that a deficiency in prostacyclin activity associated with HUS in the proband can be demonstrated in a few families as though it were behaving in either an autosomal recessive (24) or dominant (25,26) mode. These studies lend credence to the suggestion that the predisposition to develop HUS may be genetically determined in a small subset of patients with this syndrome.

HUS with a Progressive Course

Some patients have an inexorable course. They tend to present in a relatively mild fashion and develop progressive renal insufficiency without necessarily being anuric, have recurrent episodes of hemolysis and thrombocytopenia, and often have neurologic and other extrarenal organ involvement. Most of these patients do poorly irrespective of the manner in which they have been treated. They behave in many ways like the familial cases (recessive or dominant), but have not been included in that subset because none of their siblings have had HUS. A brief case report of one of our recent cases of HUS with progressive involvement is included in this review because many of the problems encountered in the treatment of such patients were present in this case.

Case DB: HUS with a Progressive Course

D.B. (age 5½ years) was admitted to The Montreal Children's Hospital in December 1981, following three days of diarrhea, fever, occasional vomiting and a slight cough. One day prior to admission, he became lethargic and complained of abdominal pain. His stools began to be tinged with blood.

On admission, he was well-nourished, alert and responsive. He had a fever (38.8°C p.o.) and mild elevation of the diastolic blood pressure (110/80-85 mmHg). The only positive findings on physical examination were left lower quadrant abdominal tenderness with slight rebound and mild bilateral costo-vertebral angle tenderness.

Within twenty-four hours of admission, he developed gross hematuria and the initial laboratory data were suggestive of the hemolytic-uremic syndrome. The hemoglobin concentration fell from 15.7 g/dl to 13.9 g/dl; fragmentation and crenation of erythrocytes were seen on the peripheral blood smear. The platelet count was $24{,}000 \times 10^6$/L and the white blood cell count was $28{,}700 \times 10^9$/L with marked toxic granulation. Urine output remained about 300 ml/day. Urinalysis revealed 4+ proteinuria with many erythrocytes in the sediment. Serum creatinine rose from 0.6 mg/dl to 1.2 mg/dl. Cultures of blood, urine, stool and throat were all negative.

During the second hospital day, his abdominal pain worsened and he developed clinical and radiologic signs of an acute abdomen. A laparatomy demonstrated scattered petechial hemorrhages throughout the mesentery and full-thickness necrosis of the left colon in the entire distribution of the left colic artery. This 27 cm segment of colon was removed and a colostomy was performed. Post-operatively, he began to bleed from the wound and at venipuncture sites despite normal prothrombin and partial thromboplastin times. The bleeding appeared to improve after infusion of fresh-frozen plasma (20 cc/kg) and platelets (5 units).

During the third and fourth hospital days, hemolysis, thrombocytopenia and non-oliguric renal failure persisted. In addition, he became progressively disoriented and had several generalized tonic-clonic convulsions. During this period, blood pressure remained at 110/70-80 mmHg. Seizures were controlled with dilantin and an electroencephalogram showed a severe diffuse encephalopathy without lateralizing features or epileptiform abnormalities.

On the sixth hospital day, a pericardial friction rub and rising diastolic blood pressure (115/90-95 mmHg) were noted. A large posterior pericardial effusion was demonstrated by an ultrasound examination. Serum creatinine had risen to 5.6 mg/dl and intermittent peritoneal dialysis was instituted.

On the seventh hospital day, plasmapheresis was attempted after infusion of fresh frozen plasma (15 cc/kg). During the second pass, he had a cardiac arrest, but was resuscitated; 90 cc of serous fluid were aspirated from the pericardial sac. Shortly thereafter, he had a second cardiac arrest and could not be resuscitated.

Post mortem examination revealed extreme fibrin thrombi in the kidneys and choroid plexus; focal fibrin thrombi in the epicardium, myocardium, adrenal cortex and lungs; focal acinar necrosis of the pancreas; serosal hemorrhages in the mesentery; fibrinoid change of one splenic arteriole; stress involution of the thymus; depletion of T and B zones of lymph nodes; an hypercellular bone marrow with left shift of the granulocytic cell line, normoblastic erythropoiesis and normal megakaryocytes.

SUMMARY

Hemolytic-uremic syndrome (HUS) is probably the most common and important cause of acute renal failure in infants and children. The diagnosis must be suspected in any infant or child who has combinations of pallor, petechiae, seizures, hypertension, hematuria, oliguria and anuria that have occurred within a few days to several weeks after an episode of gastroenteritis or an upper respiratory tract infection. The hallmarks are hemolytic anemia with fragmentation of red blood cells, thrombocytopenia and acute nephropathy.

There are probably many causes and it is likely that there are several pathogenetic mechanisms. Notable causes include shigella, pneumococci and oral contraceptives. Possible mechanisms may involve local intravascular coagulation, neuraminidase induced agglutination, and reduction of prostacyclin activity. Endothelial cell injury may be the central event.

Atypical cases include those with recurrent episodes; patients with inherited predisposition to develop HUS; patients with an inexorable course.

REFERENCES

1. Kibel, M.A.: Year Book of Pediatrics 1966-1967. Gellis, S.S. (ed.). Chicago, Year Book Medical Publishers, 1967, p. 301.
2. Gasser, C., Gauthier, E., Steck, A., et al.: Hämolytisch-urämische Syndrome: Bilaterale Nierenrindennekrosen bei akuten erworbenen Hämolytischen Anämien. Schweiz Med Wochensch 38:905,1955.

3. Van Wierengen, P.M.V., Monnens, L.A.H., and Schretlen, E.D.A.M.: Haemolytic-uraemic syndrome. Epidemiological and clinical study. Arch Dis Child 49:432, 1974.
4. Raghupathy, P., Date, A., Shastry, J.C.M., et al.: Haemolytic-uraemic syndrome complicating shigella dysentery in South Indian children. Br Med J 2:1518, 1978.
5. Gianantonio, C.A., Vitacco, M., Mendilaharzu, F., et al.: The hemolytic-uremic syndrome. Nephron 11:174, 1973.
6. Gianantonio, C.A., Vitacco, M., Mendilaharzu, F., et al.: The hemolytic-uremic syndrome. J Pediatr 64:478, 1964.
7. Mettler, N.E.: Isolation of a microtatobiote from patients with hemolytic-uremic syndrome and thrombotic thrombocytopenic purpura and from mites in the United States. N Engl J Med 281:1023, 1969.
8. Kaplan, B.S., and de Chadarevian, J-P.: Hemolytic-uremic syndrome. Canad Med Assoc J 117:1246, 1977.
9. Lieberman, E.: Hemolytic-uremic syndrome. J Pediatr 80:1, 1972.
10. Koster, F., Levin, J., Walker, L., et al.: Hemolytic-uremic syndrome after shigellosis: Relation to endotoxemia and circulating immune complexes. N Engl J Med 298:927, 1978.
11. Brandslund, I., Petersen, P.H., Strunge, P., et al.: Haemolytic uraemic syndrome and accumulation of haemoglobin-haptoglobin complexes in plasma in serum sickness caused by penicillin drugs. Haemostasis 9:193, 1980.
12. Monnens, L., van Aken, W., and De Jong, M.: "Active" intravascular coagulation in the epidemic form of hemolytic-uremic syndrome. Clin Nephrol 17:284, 1982.
13. Brain, M.C.: The haemolytic-uraemic syndrome. Semin Hematol 6: 162, 1969.
14. Katz, J., Krawitz, S., Sacks, D.V., et al.: Platelet, erythrocyte, and fibrinogen kinetics in the hemolytic-uremic syndrome of infancy. J Pediatr 83:739, 1973.
15. Courtecuisse, V., Habib, R., and Mornier, C.: Nonlethal hemolytic and uremic syndromes in children: An electron-microscope study of renal biopsies from six cases. Exp Mol Pathol 7:327, 1967.
16. Miller, K., Dresner, I.G., and Michael, A.F.: Localization of platelet antigens in human kidney disease. Kidney Int 18:472, 1980.
17. Bergstein, J.M., Kuederli, U., Bang, N.U.: Plasma inhibitor of glomerular fibrinolysis in the hemolytic-uremic syndrome. Am J Med 73:322, 1982.
18. Kourilsky, O., Vandewalle, A., Smith, M.D., et al.: Persistent intravascular C3 activation after bilateral nephrectomy in patients with thrombotic microangiopathy. Clin nephrol 6:417, 1976.
19. Remuzzi, G., Livio, M., Mecca, G., et al.: Prostacyclin and kidney disease: Focus on uremia and thrombotic microangiopathy. In Lewis, P.J., and O'Grady, J. (eds.): Clinical Pharmacology of Prostacyclin. New York, Raven Press, 1981.
20. Poschmann, A.: Neuraminidase-indzwierte Hamolyse. Mschr Kinderheilk 124:15, 1976.
21. Smith, C.D., Schuster, S.R., Gruppe, W.E., et al.: Hemolytic-uremic syndrome: A diagnostic and therapeutic dilemma for the surgeon. J Pediatr Surg 13:597, 1978.
22. Whitington, P.F., Friedman, A.L., and Chesney, R.W.: Gastrointestinal disease in the hemolytic-uremic syndrome. Gastroenterology 76: 728, 1979.

23. Kaplan, B.S. Hemolytic uremic syndrome with recurrent episodes: An important subset. Clin Nephrol 8:495, 1977.
24. Kaplan, B.S., Chesney, R.W., and Drummond, K.N.: Hemolytic uremic syndrome in families. N Engl J Med 292:1090, 1975.
25. Karlsberg, R.P., Lacher, J.W., and Bartecchi, C.E.: Adult hemolytic-uremic syndrome. Arch Intern Med 137:1155, 1977.
26. Hogewind, B.L., de la Riviere, G.B., van Es, L.A., et al.: Familial occurrence of the haemolytic uraemic syndrome. Acta Med Scand 207: 73, 1980.

PAST AND PRESENT OF THE HEMOLYTIC UREMIC SYNDROME IN ARGENTINA

Carlos A. Gianantonio, M.D.

The first descriptions of the Hemolytic Uremic Syndrome (HUS) in Argentina date from 1957. Twenty-eight infants were diagnosed from 1957 to 1962 (1), with 13 deaths. At that time the complexity of the management of acute renal failure in small patients was only being discovered and there was no experience with dialytic procedures in infants.

Most of the fatalities were due to toxic hyperkalemia and/or hospital acquired infections. Hypervolemia present on admission led to congestive circulatory failure in some children and was managed conservatively or with blood exchange transfusions. Other lethal complications were extreme and recurrent acidosis related usually to secondary infections, progressive malnutrition and deterioration after days or weeks of oliguria with the consequent reduction in caloric intake, multiple medical aggressions and emotional impairment.

As can be seen in Tables 1 and 2, there was a constant decline in the mortality rate from 15% in 1965 to 4.79% in 1981. Although these data were obtained from 8 (1965/76) and 14 (1977/81) pediatric nephrology services, the basic criteria for treatment were grossly similar. This reduction in the mortality of HUS was related to several factors: better knowledge of the disease, earlier diagnosis, and most of all, the increasing performance of peritoneal dialysis as a standard and safe pediatric procedure (2,3).

The abrupt downward trend in the mortality rate observed from 1969 to 1970 is in all probability mainly due to the introduction of early peritoneal dialysis. With our present policy, which includes peritoneal dialysis in all the severe cases immediately after admission and during the first 48 hours in the average infant with oliguria, the mortality rate has dropped practically to zero (Table 3). The number of cases has shown a steady increase, year after year, beginning in 1957 and up to 1976, when a plateau was reached with slightly above 200 patients a year. This number

Table 1. Incidence of HUS in Argentina

Period	1965/1976	1977/1981	1965/1981
No. of cases	1456	1078	2534
Patients/year	121.3	215.6	149
Age ($\bar{x}$, months)	12.1	13.05	12.5
Mortality rate (%)	5.9	4.67	5.38

Data compiled from 8 (1965-76) and 14 (1977-81) pediatric nephrology services.

Table 2. HUS in Argentina - Incidence and Mortality

Year	No. Cases	Mortality(%)	Year	No. Cases	Mortality(%)
1965	34	15.0	1974	165	4.7
1966	37	10.02	1975	185	4.2
1967	100	9.3	1976	197	4.3
1968	98	9.2	1977	193	7.02
1969	104	8.04	1978	208	3.78
1970	123	6.0	1979	242	4.28
1971	122	5.8	1980	222	3.5
1972	148	5.2	1981	213	4.79
1973	148	5.0			

does not represent the total number of patients because the data were obtained from pediatric nephrology services. For obvious reasons, the patients coming to such units have clear signs of renal compromise, so that the mildest cases with predominant hemolytic anemia are not included in this report.

It is also likely that some patients may die, even now, without diagnosis, notwithstanding the fact that the Argentinian pediatricians are well aware of the clinical manifestations of the syndrome. It is our belief that the great number of patients that are being treated does not reflect an increased incidence of the syndrome but is the consequence of the early diagnosis and the prompt referral of the patients by the primary care pediatricians (Table 4).

Table 3. HUS - Acute Stage

Year	No of patients	Age - $\bar{x}$ (months)	Deceased
1977	3	13.3	0
1978	13	13.1	1 (1 hour after admission)
1979	18	14.6	0
1980	19	18.3	1 (10 years old; fatal arrythmia)
1981	17	14.2	0
1982	18	11.9	0
Total	88	14.2	2

Department of Pediatrics - Hospital Italiano

Table 4. HUS - Changing Patterns of the Acute Phase

	1962/66	1976/82
Age (months: $\bar{x}$)	12.2	14.2
Mortality (%)	15	2.2
Oliguric period (days: $\bar{x}$)	12	7
Peritoneal dialysis (% of cases)	30	53
Early peritoneal dialysis (< 48 hours: %)	40	70
Number of dialyses	6	6
Severe CNS signs (%)	50	25
Arterial hypertension (%)	35	6

Hospital de Niños and Hospital Italiano

We have clinical and pathological evidences of the presence of HUS in the Buenos Aires area as far back as 1950. The seasonal incidence of HUS describes an endemo-epidemic pattern, with a wide peak that includes the summer and early autumn months of the southern hemisphere. The male/female ratio is about one; this ratio and the mean age of the patients have not changed significantly (12.1 months during 1965/76; 13.05 in 1977/81).

When the severity of the acute stage is related to the subsequent occurrence of chronic renal failure, it becomes apparent that the pattern has not changed over the years (Tables 5 and 6)(3,4). The patients with prolonged oliguria or anuria may not recover a normal renal function,

Table 5. Clinical Grading of Severity

Severity	Mild	Moderate	Severe
Oliguria (days)	< 7	7-14	> 14
Anuria (days)		< 7	> 7
CNS symptoms	0 to +	0 to +++	++ to +++
Arterial Hypertension	0 to +	0 to ++	+ to +++
G.I. bleeding	0 to +	0 to ++	++ to +++
Anemia	+ to +++	0 to +++	0 to +++
Mortality (%)	1	2	25
Chronic renal disease (%)*	2	15	60

*Estimated rate

and persist in chronic renal failure until they die, months after the initial phase of HUS. Since the most severe forms of HUS are less frequent now than in our previous experience, the consequences of extensive renal cortical necrosis are not often seen. However, 30% of a randomly selected group

Table 6. Chronic Renal Failure (1965/76)

Etiology	No.	Percent
Glomerular nephropathies	230	35.7
Hereditary nephropathies	60	9.3
Renal hypoplasia and dysplasia	56	8.7
Urologic disease	196	30.4
Vascular nephropathies (HUS)	73	11.3
Miscellaneous	29	4.5
TOTAL	644	100

Latin American Survey 1976

of patients have diminished glomerular filtration rate and persistent proteinuria and/or arterial hypertension, one year after the acute phase (Table 7). In our experience, these are signs that imply a guarded prognosis, as some of these children will end up in chronic renal failure near puberty.

Table 7. Patients followed more than one year after initial illness. Acute Phase.

		No. of patients
TOTAL		24
No Renal Abnormalities	A - 10	
	B - 4	16
	C - 2	
Renal Abnormalities	A - 1	
	B - 3	8
	C - 4	
Decreased GFR		3
Proteinuria (400-800 mg/24 hr)		7
Arterial Hypertension		2

Department of Pediatrics - Hospital Italiano

Discussion

The dramatic decrease in the mortality rate during the acute phase of HUS, coupled with the less severe course of the illness (Table 4) (shortened oliguric period, less hypertensive patients and a substantial reduction of severe central nervous system dysfunctions) does not have a single explanation. We have not been using heparin, aspirin or dipyridamole in the standard management of these infants, after our failure to prove the beneficial effects of anticoagulation (5,6). We have only limited experience with plasma infusions and with fibrinolytic agents.

It is not reasonable to propose a change in the syndrome itself as the cause of this improved situation. We believe that better standards of general care of these critically ill infants, coupled with less medical aggressions to the patients, the avoidance of unnecessary procedures and the prevention of hospital acquired infections, are part of the explanation. However, it is our thinking that the early performance of peritoneal dialysis is the most likely reason for the improved results.

The rapid regression of the hemodynamic complications of the syndrome, together with the improved metabolic complications and nutrition of the patient (in both caloric and nitrogen intakes during the oliguric period), are the most important benefits of early peritoneal dialysis. Other effects of dialysis, such as the extraction of some deleterious substance mediator or metabolite, are unproven.

The practical point is that in Argentina, a substantial reduction in the fatality rate of HUS has resulted in the salvage of many lives (a few hundred in fact).

In a survey in several Latin American countries, HUS was responsible for 65% of all cases of acute renal failure in infants and children (7) (Table 8) due to the high prevalence of HUS in Argentina. Unfortunately HUS in Argentina is a frequent cause of terminal renal failure in childhood, as can be seen in Table 6, from the previously mentioned Latin American Survey (7), where the HUS cases were provided nearly exclusively by the Argentinan Pediatric Nephrology Centers (8,9). It is obvious that in Argentina the future efforts must be concentrated in prevention of the syndrome, once its epidemiology is unveiled.

Table 8. Acute renal failure in infants and children (1975/1976).

	No.	%	Age ($\bar{x}$) Months	Mortality (%)
A - Glomerular nephropathies	142	21.58	97	16
B - Tubulo-interstitial	20	3.04	61.7	53.9
C - Vascular (includes HUS)	428	65.05	11.3	11.9
D - Functional	68	10.33	52.7	36.5
TOTAL	658	100	35.8	15.9

Our present and most discouraging problem is the high incidence of kidney scarring with early uremia, and the late development of progressive glomerular damage, in a significant proportion of the patients. Our experience with infusions of fresh frozen plasma or plasma exchange is too limited and recent to be analyzed, especially in relation to its eventual influence on the late consequences of HUS. Finally, it should be stressed that although we understand that it is right and convenient to assign on a world-wide basis the qualification of "syndrome" to the particular association of clinical and biological phemomena we are discussing, we have no doubt that in our country we are facing a clear cut disease, whose etiology, as in many other diseases, is still unknown.

References

1. Gianantonio, C.A., Vitacco, M., Mendilaharzu, J., et al: Acute renal failure in infancy and childhood. J. Pediat. 61:660, 1962.

2. Gianantonio, C.A., Vitacco, M., Mendilaharzu, F., et al: The hemolytic-uremic syndrome. J. Pediat. 64:478, 1964.

3. Gianantonio, C., Vitacco, M., Mendilaharzu, F., et al: The hemolytic-uremic syndrome. Nephron 11:174,1973.

4. Gianantonio, C.A., Vitacco, M., Mendilaharzu, F., et al: The hemolytic-uremic syndrome - renal status of 76 patients at long term follow-up. J. Pediat. 72:757, 1968.

5. Avalos, J.S., Vitacco, M., Molina, F., et al: Coagulation studies in the hemolytic-uremic syndrome. J. Pediat. 75:538, 1970.

6. Vitacco, M., Sanchez Alvalos, J., and Gianantonio, C.A.: Heparin therapy in the hemolytic-uremic syndrome. J. Pediat. 82:271, 1973.

7. Gianantonio, C.A.: Epidemiology and prevention of kidney disease (South America). Abstracts; Fourth Meeting, International Pediatric Nephrology Association. Helsinki - Finland, 1977.

8. Campiano, C.A., Iotti, R., Beraldi, M.V., et al: Sindrome uremico hemolitico. Controles a distancia a traves de la biopsia. Arch. Argentinos de Pediat. 77:36, 1979.

9. Cossio, P.M., Laguens, R.P., Pantin, D.J., et al: Persistent glomerular nephritis following the hemolytic uremic syndrome. Immuno-pathological and morphological studies. Clin. Exper. Immunol. 29:361, 1977.

I wish to thank the following colleagues for their contribution to the data of Tables 1 and 2:

Drs. M.E. Canz, J.C. Andia, Fernando Mendilaharzu, R. Martini, A.M. Lubetkin, L.E. Voyer, Fran. Spizzirri, N. Rossi, H. Repetto, M. Palá, E.S. de Miodovsky, R.A. Exeni, M. Lahoz Garcia and José Ramirez.

THROMBOCYTOPENIA IN HEMOLYTIC-UREMIC SYNDROME

Jack S.C. Fong, M.D., M.Sc., F.R.C.P.(C) and Bernard S. Kaplan, M.B., B.Ch., F.C.P.(S.A.)

Thrombocytopenia, unlike acute hemolysis and acute nephropathy, does not occur in every patient with hemolytic uremic syndrome (HUS). The mechanism whereby thrombocytopenia occurs is not known, the pathogenetic role of platelets in HUS has not been clearly defined, the duration of thrombocytopenia is variable and the level to which the platelets fall has no prognostic value (1-3). Thrombocytopenia, however, is such a dramatic laboratory observation that much attention has been directed at this finding and, although the role of platelets in the pathogenesis of HUS has been unclear, a variety of therapeutic agents has been advocated on the assumption that normalization of the platelet count may be beneficial. None. unfortunately, has of value and enthusiasm has waned for the use of heparin, aspirin and dipyridamol (4-11).

The demonstration of a deficiency in prostacyclin, and normalization in some patients of the platelet count following infusions of fresh frozen plasma, or plasmapheresis, have renewed interest in the role of platelets in HUS. (12-15)

THROMBOCYTOPENIA IN HUS

As stated above, not all patients with HUS have platelet counts below 140,000/cmm. However, we now believe that it is not only the absolute count to which attention must be paid, but also the decrement. For example, demonstration of a fall from 500,000 to 200,000/cmm may be as important as an initial level of 130,000/cmm. In most cases, the platelet count returns to normal by 7 to 10 days after the onset. The return to normal is usually very sudden, occurring in 2 to 3 days whereupon the value may exceed 500,000/cmm. The count may fluctuate in some patients and recurrence of thrombocytopenia may be associated with a relapse in the patient's condition.

PATHOGENESIS OF THROMBOCYTOPENIA

A number of mechanisms may account for the occurrence of the thrombocytopenia; none is mutually exclusive. That the thrombocytopenia is primarily caused by peripheral factors is suggested by demonstration of normal bone marrow activity. A variety of peripheral factors could cause platelet consumption and/or destruction. Evidence favouring consumption includes the reduced life-span of infused platelets (2,16); sequestration of labelled platelets in the spleen, liver and to a lesser extent, kidneys (1,2) (this could also favour the concept of platelet destruction in the kidneys and removal by spleen and liver); the demonstration of platelet antigen in glomeruli (17) (this was shown a rather long time after onset); and, in some patients, prompt normalization following bilateral nephrectomy (18,19) (this could also favour the idea that the platelets are damaged in the kidneys). Thus a careful analysis of the above observations cannot dissect out clearly the separate roles of consumption and destruction. A need to do so is of more than academic interest because consumption might imply a more active role in the production of nephropathy than would destruction.

PLATELET MORPHOLOGY

Despite marked interest in the role of platelets in HUS, it is surprising that so little has been written about the morphology of circulating platelets in different stages of the illness. We are aware of only one reference to platelet morphology studied by electron microscopy (20). In that study, there are no details of the number of patients studie d the times at which they were looked at or their platelet counts. Three types of platelets were found: giant forms (5%), normal platelets (60%) and those with dense cytoplasm (35%) (20).

We have examined circulating platelets by electron microscopy in 9 cases in the acute and convalescent phases and have found markedly abnormal platelets in the first few days of the illness. Platelets studied a week later have a more normal appearance.

ACTIVATION OF PLATELETS

As we shall show below, there is good evidence that platelets have been activated. The most logical triggering event for platelet activation in HUS is a microangiopathy in which there is damage to, and possibly detachment of, endothelial cells. Endothelial cell trauma may lead to release of their contents including factors which may influence platelet function; factor VIII levels are elevated in HUS (21-24). Prostacyclin (PGI_2) is produced by endothelium and it has an important anti-aggregating role. A balance between PGI_2 and thromboxane A_2 (TXA_2; produced mainly in platelets; has potent aggregating activity) is crucial in maintaining normal platelet reactivity (25). Although research has focused mainly on the demonstration of PGI_2 inhibitors in HUS, it is also possible that endothelial cell damage could result in reduced PGI_2 production. The presence of inhibitors and/or decreased PGI_2 production shifts the balance in favour of TXA_2 activity which is not decreased in HUS. Denudation of endothelium results in exposure of subendothelial components that can activate platelets (26-27).

Hemolysis may also stimulate platelet reactivities through the release of cytoplasmic contents including serotonin, adenosine diphosphate and hemoglobin (28). Both cytosol and erythrocyte stroma have thromboplastic activities that may trigger intravascular coagulation with the generation of thrombin which then acts on platelets.

In general, the process of localized intravascular coagulation in HUS is well substantiated by laboratory data, whereas the occurrence of disseminated intravascular coagulation has been demonstrated in only a few patients (29-31). Nevertheless, the generation of thrombin as a result of any coagulation event will activate platelets as well. The overall activity of thrombin is normally modified by antithrombins, the most important of which is antithrombin-III (AT-III). A patient with post-partum HUS had low levels of AT-III which, upon replacement of this protein, appeared to be associated with normalization of circulating platelet level and clinical improvement (32). We have demonstrated mild to modest reductions in the levels of AT-III in HUS patients (4). In view of this, there is potential risk of inducing a hypercoagulable state in some patients with low AT-III levels by treatment with heparin (33).

Whereas damaged endothelium may account in part for the reduced levels of PGI_2 in the acute phase of the HUS (13,15,34),this cannot explain the persistence of decreased levels of PGI2 in some patients during remission (14). Failure to demonstrate that plasma from these patients supports the *in vitro* production of PGI_2 by rat aortic rings suggests that a plasma factor(s) may be lacking (13,14,35). This contention is supported by the demonstration of a similar defect in unaffected family members who have low levels of PGI_2.

PLASMA ANTIOXIDANTS

The nature of the specific plasma factor(s) that may be causing the reduction of PGI_2 is unknown, yet it is worth noting that prostaglandins are oxidation products of arachidonic acid and it is therefore tempting to speculate on the role of plasma antioxidants which include alpha-tocopherol, haptoglobin, ceruloplasmin and transferrin (36). It is well established that alpha-tocopherol interferes with prostaglandin metabolism and that it inhibits platelet aggregation (37-39). Both alpha-tocopherol deficiency and evidence of a peroxidation process have been found in HUS patients (40). Since peroxidation of arachidonic acid results in the generation of various prostaglandin metabolites, reduced alpha-tocopherol or other antioxidants may play a role in the increased platelet TXA_2 generation that has been shown in two patients with HUS during their acute illness (34). Metabolic perturbations, in particular azotemia and hypocalcemia, may also reduce platelet aggregation (41,42).

FRESH FROZEN PLASMA

Awareness of deficits in humoral factors that influence platelet reactivities in HUS has led to the use of plasma infusions and/or plasmapheresis with, in some cases, apparent success (12,43,56). Plasma factors thus furnished may include stimulatory factor(s) for prostacyclin production, antioxidants, AT-III and others not yet identified. It is reasonable to speculate that other factor(s) may be present; for example, a deficiency of "platelet aggregation inhibitor factor" has been demonstrated in patients with thrombotic thrombocytopenic purpura - which is closely related to HUS (44). However, attempts to find a platelet aggregating factor in HUS have not been successful (13,35). Plasma transfusion has also been effective in correcting thrombocytopenia in a patient with microangiopathic hemolytic anemia and thrombocytopenia (45). Lack of response to fresh frozen plasma can be expected if these patients are not capable of generating sufficient PGI_2 because of extensive endothelial damage (26,27). A recent study showed that, even with a sufficient amount of PGI_2, thrombin-induced platelet adherence to the subendothelial components is not inhibited by PGI_2 (46). Net balance between the opposing influences of agonistic and antagonistic factors may vary among different patients, and during the course of the patient's illness.

PLATELET EXHAUSTION

Despite the numerous possible variations of factors that may influence platelet function, we believe there is good evidence to conclude that platelet activation takes place during the acute phase. Stimulated platelets normally respond by actively secreting their contents of B-thromboglobulin (BTG) and platelet factor 4 (PF4). Elevated levels of these platelet specific proteins are found during the acute illness in HUS patients (27,47-49). Reduced glomerular filtration can account only in part for the elevated levels (50). Human BTG has been shown to bind to bovine aortic endothelial cells and inhibit PGI_2 production (51). Some of the activated platelets may fail to aggregate and stay on in the circulation; others may aggregate and return to the circulation later through the process of deaggregation. During the acute phase in HUS, platelets in circulation are shown to be in a biochemically "exhausted" state with reduced contents of BTG and serotonin and, from a functional aspect, have a characteristic pattern of impaired aggregation responses (49,52-55). These include no response to epinephrine, a slight response to ADP and a modest response to collagen (49). It is unlikely that this absence of normal aggregability is solely the consequence of azotemia because these abnormal responses improve despite continuing poor renal function. One important conclusion derived from these studies on platelet aggregation is the futility of treating patients with drugs that affect platelet aggregation. The inability of ASA and dipyridamole to increase the platelet count has been demonstrated in a study which was unfortunately flawed by the use of doses of ASA that were larger than appropriate (7).

HUS FOLLOWED BY IDIOPATHIC THROMBOCYTOPENIC PURPURA (ITP)

Two children have developed ITP several weeks to 13 months after recovery from HUS. The occurrence of two conditions in which there is peripheral destruction of platelets raises many unanswered questions. It is of interest that the infusion of 250 ml of fresh frozen plasma produced a transient 5 fold increase in the platelet count of our patient during his episode of ITP (57).

SUMMARY

There is much evidence in favour of the concept that platelet activation, consumption, destruction and exhaustion occur in hemolytic uremic syndrome (HUS). Most patients have counts below 140,000/cmm; the count returns to normal usually between 7 to 10 days. Several mechanisms may be involved in the production of the thrombocytopenia: these include consumption in platelet thrombi and peripheral destruction. Ultrastructural examination reveals markedly abnormal circulating platelets during the first few days of the illness. There is good evidence for platelet activation: platelet beta-thromboglobulin content is reduced and platelet aggregation is markedly impaired. A number of factors can activate platelets in HUS: microangiopathy, reduced prostacyclin activity, hemolysis by releasing serotonin, ADP, hemoglobin. A reduction in plasma antioxidants may play a role in the reduction of prostacyclin activity. No drug regimen has been proven to be of value in returning the platelet count to normal, but fresh frozen plasma can produce a rapid increase in the platelet count.

REFERENCES

1. Katz, J., Krawitz, S., Sacks, D.V., _et al._: Platelet, erythrocyte, and fibrinogen kinetics in the hemolytic-uremic syndrome of infancy. J. Pediatr., 83: 739, 1973.
2. Metz, J.: Observations on the mechanisms of the haematological changes in the haemolytic uraemic syndrome of infancy. Br. J. Haematol., 23(Suppl.): 53, 1972.

3. Rossi, E.C., Carone, F.A., and del Greco, F.: Platelets and the hemolytic uremic syndrome. Ann. Clin. Lab. Sci., 11: 269, 1981.
4. Fong, J.S.C., de Chadarevian, J-P., and Kaplan, B.S.: Hemolytic-uremic syndrome: Current concepts and management. Ped. Clin. N. Amer., 29: 835, 1982.
5. Proesmans, W., ki Muaka, B., Van Damme, B., et al.: The use of heparin in childhood hemolytic-uremic syndrome. In Remuzzi, G., Mecca, G., and de Gaetano, G. (eds.): Hemostasis,Prostaglandins and Renal Disease, New York, Raven Press, 1980.
6. Monnens, L., van Collenburg, J., de Jog, M., et al.: Treatment of the hemolytic-uremic syndrome. Helv. Paediatr. Acta, 33: 321, 1978.
7. O'Regan, S., Chesney, R.W., Mongeau, J-G., et al.: Aspirin and dipyridamole therapy in the hemolytic-uremic syndrome. J. Pediatr., 97: 473, 1980.
8. Vitacco, M., Avalos, J.S., and Gianantonio, C.A.: Heparin therapy in the hemolytic-uremic syndrome. J. Pediatr., 83: 271, 1973.
9. Thorsen, C.A., Rossi, E.C., Green, D., and Carone, F.A.: The treatment of the hemolytic-uremic syndrome with inhibitors of platelet function. Am. J. Med., 66: 711, 1979.
10. Powell, H.R., and Ekert, H.: Streptokinase and anti-thrombotic therapy in the hemolytic-uremic syndrome. J. Pediatr., 84: 345, 1974.
11. Stuart, J., Winterborn, M.H., White, R.H.R., and Flinn, R.M.: Thrombolytic therapy in haemolytic-uraemic syndrome. Br. Med. J., 3: 217, 1974.
12. Remuzzi, G., Misiani, R., Marchesi, D., et al.: Treatment of the hemolytic-uremic syndrome with plasma. Clin. Nephrol., 12: 279, 1979.
13. Remuzzi, G., Misiani, R., Marchesi, D., et al.: Haemolytic-uraemic syndrome: Deficiency of plasma factor(s) regulating prostacyclin activity? Lancet, ii: 871, 1978.
14. Remuzzi, G., Marchesi, D., Misiani, R., et al.: Familial deficiency of a plasma factor stimulating vascular prostacyclin activity. Thromb. Res., 16: 517, 1979.
15. Defreyn, G., Proesmans, W., Machin, S.J., Lemmens, F., and Vermylen, J.: Abnormal prostacyclin metabolism in the hemolytic uremic syndrome: equivocal effect of prostacyclin infusions. Clin. Nephrol., 18: 43, 1982.
16. Harker, L.A., and Slichter, S.J.: Platelet and fibrinogen

consumption in man. N. Engl. J. Med., 287: 999, 1972.

17. Miller, K., Dresner, I.G., and Michael, A.F.: Localization of platelet antigens in human kidney disease. Kidney Int., 18: 472, 1980.
18. Calvert, G.D.: Post-partum haemolytic uraemic syndrome: Case report and brief review. J. Obstet. Gynaecol. Br. Commonw., 79: 244, 1972.
19. Hall, G.H., Caldwell, R.A., and Shaldon, C.: Heparin-treated haemolytic-uraemic syndrome Simulating Fabry's disease. Br. Med. J., 2: 317, 1971.
20. van Wieringen, P.M.V.: Het Haemolytisch-Uraemisch Syndroom op de Kinderleeftijd. Thesis., 1977. Drukkerij van Mameren B.V. - Nijmegen.
21. Hoyer, J.R., Michael, A.F., and Hoyer, L.W.: Immunofluorescent localization of antihemophilic factor antigen and fibrinogen in human renal disease. J. Clin. Invest., 53: 1375, 1974.
22. Jaffe, E.A.: Endothelial cells and the biology of factor VIII. N. Engl. J. Med., 296: 377, 1977.
23. Ekberg, M., Nilsson, J.M., and Denneberg, T.: Coagulation studies in hemolytic uremic syndrome and thrombotic thrombocytopenic purpura. Acta Med. Scand., 196: 373, 1974.
24. Appiani, A.C., Edefonti, A., Bettinelli, A., Cossu, M.M., Paracchini, M.L., and Rossi, E.: The relationship between plasma levels of the factor VIII complex and platelet release products (B-thromboglobulin and platelet factor 4) in children with hemolytic-uremic syndrome. Clin. Nephrol., 17: 195, 1982.
25. Moncada, S., and Amezcua, J.L.: Prostacyclin, thromboxane A_2 interactions in haemostasis and thrombosis. Haemostasis, 8: 252, 1979.
26. Gingrich, R.D., and Hoak, J.C.: Platelet-endothelial cell interactions. Sem. Hemat., 16: 208, 1979.
27. Harker, L.A., Ross, R., and Glosmet, J.A.: The role of endothelial cell injury and platelet response in atherogenesis. Thrombos. Haemostas., 39: 312, 1978.
28. Born, G.V.R., and Wehmeier, A.: Inhibition of platelet thrombus formation by chlorpromazine acting to diminish haemolysis. Nature, 282: 212, 1979.
29. Avalos, J.S., Vitacco, M., Penalver, J., et al.: Coagulation studies

in the hemolytic-uremic syndrome. J. Pediatr., 76: 538, 1970.

30. Montgomery, R.R., and Hathaway, W.E.: The hemolytic-uremic syndrome. In McIntosh, R.M., Guggenheim, S.J., and Schrier, R.W. (eds.): Kidney Disease: Hematologic and Vascular Problems, New York, John Wiley and Sons, 1977.

31. Monnens, L., van Aken, W., and de Jong, M.: "Active" intravascular coagulation in the epidemic form of hemolytic-uremic syndrome. Clin. Nephrol., 17: 284, 1982.

32. Brandt, P., Jespersen, J., and Gregersen, G.: Post-partum haemolytic-uraemic syndrome treated with antithrombin-III. Nephron, 27: 15, 1981.

33. Wessler, S., and Gitel, S.N.: Heparin: New concepts relevant to clinical use. Blood, 53: 525, 1979.

34. Remuzzi, G., Livio, M., Mecca, G., et al.: Prostacyclin and kidney disease: Focus on uremia and thrombotic microangiopathy. In Lewis, P.J., and O'Grady, J. (eds.): Clinical Pharmacology of Prostacyclin, New York, Raven Press, 1981.

35. Wiles, P.G., Solomon, L.R., Lawler, W., and Mallick, N.P.: Inherited plasma factor deficiency in haemolytic-uraemic syndrome. Lancet, i: 1105, 1981.

36. Dormandy, T.L.: Free-radical oxidation and antioxidants. Lancet, i: 647, 1978.

37. Ali, M., Gudbranson, C.G., and McDonald, W.D.: Inhibition of human cyclooxygenase by alpha-tocopherol. Postaglandins Med., 4: 79, 1980.

38. Fong, J.S.C.: Alpha-tocopherol: Its inhibition on human platelet aggregation. Experientia, 32: 639, 1976.

39. Panganamala, R.V., Miller, J.S., Gwebu, E.T., et al.: Differential inhibitory effects of vitamin E and other antioxidants on prostaglandin synthetase, platelet aggregation and lipoxidase. Prostaglandins, 14: 261, 1977.

40. O'Regan, S., Chesney, R.W., Kaplan, B.S., et al.: Red cell membrane abnormalities in the hemolytic-uremic syndrome. Clin. Nephrol. 15: 14, 1980.

41. Horowitz, H.T., Stein, I.M., Cohen, B.D., and White, J.G.: Further studies on the platelet inhibitory effect of guanidinosuccinic acid and its role in uremic bleeding. Am. J. Med., 49: 336, 1970.

42. Rabiner, S.F., and Molinas, F.: The role of phenol and phenolic

acids on the thrombocytopathy and defective platelet aggregation of patients with renal failure. Am. J. Med., 49: 346, 1970.

43. Beattie, T.J., Murphy, A.V., Willoughby, M.L.N., et al.: Plasmapheresis in the haemolytic-uraemic syndrome in children. Br. Med. J., 282: 1667, 1981.

44. Lian, E.C., Harkness, D.R., Byrnes, J.J., Wallach, H., and Nunez, R.: Presence of a platelet aggregating factor in the plasma of patients with thrombotic thrombocytopenic purpura (TTP) and its inhibition by normal plasma. Blood, 53: 333, 1979.

45. Upshaw, Jr., J.D.: Congenital deficiency of a factor in normal plasma that reverses microangiopathic hemolysis and thrombocytopenia. N. Engl. J. Med., 298: 1350, 1978.

46. Fry, G.L., Czervionke, R.L., Hoak, J.L., Smith, J.B., and Haycraft, D.L.: Platelet adherence to cultured vascular cells: influence of prostacyclin (PGI_2). Blood, 55: 271, 1980.

47. Edenfonti, A., Tentori, F., Bertinelli, A., et al.: Pattern of platelet serontonin (5HT), plasma beta-thromboglobulin (BTG) and platelet factor 4 (PF4) in hemolytic uremic syndrome (HUS) in children. Int. J. Pediatr. Nephrol., 2: 149, 1981.

48. Beattie, T.J., Murphy, A.V., and Arneil, G.C.: Studies on prostaglandin metabolism in hemolytic-uremic syndrome. Int. J. Pediatr. Nephrol., 2: 130, 1981.

49. Fong, J.S.C., and Kaplan, B.S.: Impairment of platelet aggregation in hemolytic uremic syndrome: Evidence for platelet "exhaustion". Blood, 60: 564, 1982.

50. Green, D., Santhanam, S., Krumlovsky, F.A., et al.: Elevated B-thromboglobulin in patients with chronic renal failure: Effect of hemodialysis. J. Lab. Clin. Med., 95: 679, 1980.

51. Hope, W., Martin, T.J., Chesterman, C.N., and Morgan, F.J.: Human B-thromboglobulin inhibits PGI_2 production and binds to a specific site in bovine aortic endothelial cells. Nature, 282: 210, 1979.

52. Parbtani, A., and Cameron, J.S.: Platelet and plasma serotonin concentrations in glomerulonephritis I. Thromb. Res., 15: 109, 1979.

53. Pareti, F.I., Capitanio, A., Mannucci, L., et al.: Acquired dysfunction due to the circulation of "exhausted" platelets. Am. J. Med., 69: 235, 1980.

54. Kaplan, B.S., and Fong, J.S.C.: Platelet aggregation in haemolytic

uraemic syndrome. Lancet, 1: 46, 1980.

55. Kaplan, B.S., and Fong, J.S.C.: Reduced platelet aggregation in the hemolytic uremic syndrome. Thromb. Haemost., 43: 154, 1980.

56. Mendoza,S.A.,Sellers, B.B., and Griswold, W.R.: Hemolytic uremic syndrome and idiopathic thrombocytopenic purpura in a single patient. J. Pediatr., 91: 851, 1977.

57. Kaplan, B.S.: Hemolytic-uremic syndrome followed by idiopathic thrombocytopenic purpura. Int. J. Pediatr. Nephrol. 2: 97, 1981.

This is publication number 00000 of The McGill University-Montreal Children's Hospital Research Institute.

Acknowledgement

We thank Mrs. Sharon MacMillan for secretarial assistance.

URIC ACID PERTURBATIONS IN THE HEMOLYTIC UREMIC SYNDROME

Alan B. Gruskin, J. Lawrence Naiman, Martin S. Polinsky, Michael Mellon, H. Jorge Baluarte, Bruce A. Kaiser, Sharon A. Perlman and Bruce Z. Morgenstern

Although hyperuricemia has been found in a large number of disorders,(1) its occurrence in the hemolytic uremic syndrome (HUS) is not generally appreciated. (2,3) In 1969, while performing studies of the transperitoneal movement of solute (4) (including uric acid) in children undergoing their initial dialysis, we observed marked hyperuricemia disproportionate to the degree of renal failure in two infants with HUS. We have subsequently confirmed these observations in a series of 26 children with HUS and have performed studies in rabbits in an effort to identify the mechanism(s) leading to hyperuricemia. This report has four objectives: 1) to review our experience with and interpretation of uric acid metabolism in patients with HUS, 2) to present data which provide information on possible mechanisms for the hyperuricemia, 3) to consider uric acid metabolism in experimental models of hemolysis and acute and chronic renal failure, and 4) to review available literature on the subject of uric acid metabolism in renal failure.

Clinical Data in Children with HUS

We reviewed data from 26 children with HUS between 1968 and 1983; their ages ranged from 2 months to 12 2/12 years. There were 16 males and 10 females. Interestingly, despite our institution's location in a large urban setting, none of the children was black. Seventeen of the 26 children had neurologic manifestations, ranging from irritability to seizures and prolonged coma. Nineteen children received dialysis, and twenty children received one or more transfusions. All had nephropathy, the characteristic microangiopathic hemolytic anemia, and 25 of 26 had thrombocytopenia. The mean BUN and serum creatinine values in our patients were 88.1 and 3.8 mg/dl respectively and were elevated in all 26 children; the mean BUN/creatinine ratio was 26.6. The initial values of serum uric acid obtained within a few days of the onset of symptoms ranged from 3.6 to 30 mg/dl, with a mean of 12.9 $\pm$ 4.7 (SD). Because concentrations of serum uric acid increase with age, changes in these concentrations need to be interpreted accordingly. (5,6). Normal values in young children are approximately 50% of those found in adults. Uric acid levels were clearly elevated (>8.0 mg/dl) in 22 of the 26 children. In 3 of the 4 remaining children, serum uric acid levels were above normal for age. These data confirm the finding of hyperuricemia in 18 children with HUS reported by Kaplan and Thomson.(3)

Positive correlations were found between serum uric acid and the initial serum creatinine ($p < 0.001$). There was a positive correlation between uric acid levels and BUN ($p < 0.03$) only in those children with uric acid concentrations above 8.0 mg/dl. In an attempt to ascertain whether or not the elevated uric acid level reflected pre-renal azotemia (defined as BUN/creatinine > 20), comparisons were made between uric acid levels and the BUN/creatinine ratio. No correlation was found between these values, either when all the uric acid values were examined or when only those values which exceeded 8.0 mg/dl were considered. Similar concentrations of serum uric acid were found in the 12 children with a BUN/creatinine ratio greater than 20 and in the 10 children whose BUN/creatinine ratio was less than 20. In summary we were unable to establish a clear relationship between serum concentration of uric acid and pre-renal azotemia, but did find an inverse correlation between the level of GFR (calculated from the serum creatinine) and serum uric acid levels.

Experimental Studies

In order to explore possible mechanisms by which hyperuricemia occurs in HUS two sets of laboratory studies were performed. The first consisted of in vitro experiments comparing the uric acid content of red cells, white cells and platelets. Centrifugally separated red cells, white cells and platelets were each suspended in a balanced uric acid-free salt solution and spun into a pellet. Uric acid was measured before and after freeze lysis of the cells. Significant quantities of uric acid were released from both red and white cells but not from platelets.

In order to assess the relative contributions of hemolysis and renal insufficiency to hyperuricemia, a second group of studies was performed in rabbits. Changes in the uric acid/BUN ratio associated with various forms of hemolysis and renal insufficiency were examined. Three groups of three rabbits each were studied: 1) pure chronic renal failure induced by bilateral ureteral ligation; 2) pure hemolysis induced by phenylhydrazine (7) and 3) a mixed hemolytic-uremic syndrome model induced by infusing thrombin into thorotrast-pretreated animals. (8) This latter group developed disseminated intravascular coagulation and bilateral cortical necrosis, demonstrated on post-mortem examination.

The values of uric acid and BUN, as well as the uric acid/BUN ratio, were compared in the three groups. Although serum uric acid levels increased in all three groups, both the rate of increase and peak values varied among the groups: hyperuricemia disproportionate to the degree of renal failure occurred only in the group with the induced hemolytic uremic like syndrome. Serum uric acid levels increased more rapidly than did BUN; the uric acid/BUN ratio increased from 0.2 to 0.25 within 8 hours. In the pure hemolysis group, both the serum uric acid levels and BUN increased somewhat; the uric acid/BUN ratio increased minimally over a period of four days. In the group with pure renal failure the uric acid/BUN ratio fell progressively over eight days, although serum levels of both uric acid and BUN increased significantly.

Etiology of Hyperuricemia in the Hemolytic Uremic Syndrome

Increases in serum uric acid levels result from one or more perturbations of uric acid metabolism: 1) increased intake of precursors, 2) increased production due to either a block in catabolism or an increase in nucleic acid turnover (as in leukemia); and 3) a decrease in renal excretion. In regard to the latter, the renal handling of uric acid is a complex process involving four steps (9,10,11): 1) glomerular filtration; 2) active reabsorption in the early proximal tubule; 3) secretion in the distal proximal tubule; and 4) post secretory reabsorption. Net excretion of uric acid is approximately 6-10% of its filtered load. Because most of the filtered load of uric acid is reabsorbed, it is the quantity secreted and subsequently reabsorbed which determines the quantity excreted.

The available data suggest that multiple alterations in uric acid metabolism occur in children with HUS. Probable mechanisms for the increase in serum uric acid include release from cells (hemolysis) into the extracellular compartment, increased production, and decreased excretion due to decreased GFR or alterations in tubular transport.

Increased delivery of uric acid into the extracellular compartment may arise from a number of sources in the child with HUS. Since the concentration of uric acid within red cells is approximately 55% that of plasma, (12,13) rapid ongoing hemolysis can "dump" uric acid into plasma. Leukocytosis in some patients may lead to a rapid turnover of white cells (catabolism of nucleotides to uric acid); also, intracellular stores of uric acid may be released into the extracellular compartment. In addition to uric acid release from destruction of red and white cells and from white cell turnover, other mechanisms may contribute to the development of hyperuricemia by providing uric acid precursors. Hypercatabolic disorders such as HUS are associated with an increased rate of cellular breakdown and increased uric acid production. Extensive and rapid tissue breakdown in some of the involved extrarenal organ systems (liver, muscle, bone, etc,) (14) with its concomitant increase in nucleic acid turnover may lead to an increase in production of uric acid. Hyperuricemia may also be seen in association with fever (15), starvation (16), and status epilepticus. (17)

Alterations in renal function may contribute to the development of hyperuricemia in HUS through different mechanisms. A rapidly falling GFR combined with an increasing extracellular concentration of uric acid are probably the most important mechanisms leading to hyperuricemia in children with HUS. Children below 1 year of age may be at increased risk of developing higher levels of serum uric acid because they have a lower GFR per unit of body surface area, and also a higher metabolic rate. The rate of fall in GFR, in addition to reflecting the intrinsic insult to the renal vascular endothelium, may be hastened by concomitant dehydration (15), intraluminal uric acid deposition (18, 19), and changes in circulating levels of catecholamine and angiotensin II. (20)

Another renal mechanism may be related to the effect of volume depletion on net uric acid excretion. Many children with HUS experience some degree of volume depletion because of losses of gastrointestinal contents and anorexia. Both clinical and experimental studies have shown that extracellular volume depletion and diminished proximal tubular flow rates are associated with alterations in proximal tubular function that lead to a decreased rate of excretion of uric acid. (21,22)

Hyperuricemia has been observed in 80% of a series of children with acute diarrhea and dehydration. (15) In that series, serum uric acid levels ranged from normal to as high as 39 mg/dl, and a positive correlation was observed between serum uric acid concentration and BUN on admission. We were unable to demonstrate a correlation between serum uric acid levels and either the BUN or

BUN/creatinine ratio in our patients with HUS. However, we were able to demonstrate a positive correlation between serum uric acid and serum creatinine concentrations. The absence of a relationship between uric acid and BUN may be due to the simultaneous influence of the multiple factors leading to hyperuricemia (such as hemolysis) as well as the effects of extrarenal processes on the BUN, including decreases in extracellular volume and increases in tissue catabolism.

The final renal mechanism which may contribute to hyperuricemia is diminished tubular secretion of uric acid independent of volume related factors. Uric acid is transported across the luminal membrane by the organic anion system. Competitive transport of uric acid by a number of agents such as aspirin and lactate has been demonstrated. (23-26) Lactic acid has been reported to be high in one child with HUS, (3) and could result from volume depletion and secondary hypoperfusion. In addition, children with HUS are commonly given aspirin to treat fever. Drugs used during the course of treating HUS may also influence uric acid metabolism. Thiazide (22) and loop diuretics (25) are commonly associated with the development of hyperuricemia. Uremic serum has also been shown to inhibit urate uptake by isolated rabbit tubules; (27) furthermore, the inhibitory factor could be removed by dialysis.

Hyperuricemia in association with acute renal failure is not limited to patients with HUS. Concentrations of serum uric acid in patients with other forms of acute renal failure, as well as those with HUS, are substantially higher than values observed in patients with chronic renal failure. (28,29) Similar reasons can be offered for the development of hyperuricemia in other forms of acute renal failure.

Uric acid metabolism in patients with chronic renal failure differs from that in acute renal failure. Serum uric acid levels rarely exceed 10 mg/dl in adult patients with chronic renal insufficiency. A number of factors may limit the degree of hyperuricemia in such patients, including an increased fractional excretion of urate, enhanced tubular secretion of uric acid, and possibly an increased accumulation of endogenous uricosuric substances. (27) The net result of these changes is that the fractional excretion of urate may increase to as high as 50% of its filtered load (30-32), and help maintain lower serum concentrations. In such patients, uric acid is also removed by increased intestinal secretion of urate and by intestinal uricolysis. (33)

Hyperuricemia may also occur as part of the hypertensive process (34-37) This has been reported in children (1, 35) and adults (36, 37) with essential and secondary forms of hypertension. The incidence of hyperuricemia in patients with cystic kidney disease and chronic renal failure was significantly higher among those who were hypertensive than those who were normotensive. (38) The mechanism of hyperuricemia in hypertensive patients is unclear but may reflect alterations in renal hemodynamics (39), including changes in filtration fraction or redistribution of renal blood flow. In hypertensive patients, plasma renin activity has been observed to correlate with serum uric acid levels. (39) Hyperreninemia commonly occurs in children with HUS. (40) The mechanism by which serum uric acid levels increase may be related to renin mediated changes in renal hemodynamics.

It is not clear whether the elevated serum levels of uric acid in HUS are directly nephrotoxic. Acute uric acid nephropathy in children with lymphoproliferative disorders has occurred with serum uric acid levels similar to those observed in children with HUS. (41) Hyperuricemia may cause renal damage by two mechanisms. (18,19) Firstly, uric acid may precipitate intraluminally, especially when urine flow rates and pH are low. Uric acid nephrolithiasis is a theoretical possibility. Secondly, monosodium urate crystals can deposit in the renal interstitium giving rise to an interstitial nephritis.

Hyperuricemia may also increase thrombogenicity by altering platelet function. (42, 43) It has been reported that the deposition of fibrin thrombi in afferent arterioles and glomerular capillaries seen in rats with experimentally induced DIC and hyperuricemia can be significantly reduced by the administration of allopurinol. (44) Although tubular and interstitial changes similar to those reported in experimental uric acid nephropathy have been noted (3, 45, 46), a clear-cut relationship between hyperuricemia and renal damage in children with HUS has not yet been demonstrated.

In summary, hyperuricemia is a common biochemical perturbation in children with HUS. Its origin is most likely multifactorial reflecting changes in the production of uric acid and its input into the extracellular compartment, as well as a series of alterations in renal function including changes in its filtered load and possibly the tubular handling of uric acid. The development of hyperuricemia in children with HUS may have diagnostic, pathophysiologic, and therapeutic implications.

References

1. Prebis, J.W., Gruskin, A.B., Polinsky, M.S. and Baluarte, H.J.: Uric acid in childhood essential hypertension. Proc. Fifth Int. Ped. Neph. Symp., Martinus Nijhoff, pp. 122-126, ed. Gruskin, A.B. and Norman, M.E., 1980.

2. Naiman, J.L., Mellon, M. and Gruskin, A.B.: Disproportionate hyperuricemia in hemolysis associated with renal failure. Abst. Soc. Pediatr. Res. May, 1970.

3. Kaplan, B.S., and Thomson, P.D.: Hyperuricemia in the hemolytic-uremic syndrome. Am J Dis Child., 130: 854, 1976.

4. Gruskin, A.B., and Cote, M.L.: Kinetics of Peritoneal Dialysis in Children. Abst. Soc. Ped. Res. 1970, p. 44.

5 Stapleton, F.B., Linshaw, M.A., Hassanein, K. and Gruskin, A.B.: Uric acid excretion in normal children. J. Pediatr. 92: 911, 1978.

6. Harkness, R.A. and Nicol, A.D.: Plasma uric acid levels in children. Arch. Dis. Child., 44: 773, 1969.

7. Ponder, E.: Hemolysis and Related Phenomena. Grune and Stratton 1948; p. 362.

8. Seller, R.A., Forman, E.N., Bolger, J.F., Abildgaard, C.F., and Schulmann, I.: Induction of intravascular coagulation and renal cortical necrosis in rabbits by simultaneous injection of thorotrast and endotoxin. Brit J Haemat., 16; 501, 1969.

9. Steele, T.H.: Control of uric acid excretion. N Engl J Med., 284: 1193, 1971.

10. Steele, T.H. and Rieselbach: The renal mechanism for urate homeostasis in normal man. Am J Med., 43: 868, 1967.

11. Francoise, R-R., and Weiner, I.M.: Renal excretion of urate: Factors determining the action of drugs. Kidney Int., 18: 665, 1980.

12. Jorgensen, S. and Nielsen, A.A.: Uric acid in human blood corpuscles and plasma. Scand. J. Lab. & CLin. Med. 8: 108, 1956.

13. Bishop, C., Rankine, D.M. and Talbott, H.J.: The nucleotides in normal human blood. J. Biol. Chem. 234: 1233, 1959.

14. Fong, J.S.C., de Chadarevian, J-P, and Kaplan, B.S.: Hemolytic Uremic Syndrome. Pediatr Clin. N. Amer. 29: 835, 1982.

15. Adler, R., Robinson, R., Pazdral, P., and Grushkin, C.: Hyperuricemia in diarrheal dehydration. Am J Dis Child., 136: 211, 1982.

16. Alderman, M.H., Davis, R.P.: Hyperuricemia in starvation. Proc. Soc. Exp. Biol. Med., 118: 790, 1965.

17. Warren, D.J.: Hyperuricemic acute renal failure after epileptic seizures. Lancet 2: 385, 1975.

18. Klinenberg, J.R., Kippen, I., and Bluestone, R.: Hyperuricemic nephropathy: Pathologic features and factors influencing urate deposition. Nephron 14: 88,1975.

19. Kjellstrand, C.M., Campbell, D.C.,II., von Hartizsch, H.B. and Buselmeier, T.J.: Hyperuricemic acute renal failure. Arch. Intern. Med. 133: 349, 1974.

20. Ferris, T.F. and Gorden, P.: Effect of angiotensin and norepinephrine upon urate clearance in man. Am.J.Med., 44: 359, 1968.

21. Senekjian, H.O., Knight, T.F., Sansom, S.C. and Weinman, E.J.: Effect of flow rate and the extracellular fluid volume on proximal urate and water absorption. Kidney Int. 17: 155, 1980.

22. Steele, T.H., Oppenheimer, S.: Factors affecting urate excretion following diuretic administration in man. Am. J. Med. 47: 564, 1969.

23. Yu, T.F., Sirota, J.H., Berger, L., et al.: Effect of sodium lactate infusion on urate clearance in man. Proc. Soc. Exp. Biol. Med. 96: 809, 1957.

24. Goldfinger, S., Klinenberg, J.R. and Seegmiller, J.E.: Renal retention of uric acid induced by infusion of beta-hydroxybutyrate and acetoacetate. N. Engl. J. Med. 272: 351, 1965.

25. Chennavasin, P., Seiwell, R., Brater, D.C. and Liang, W.M.: Pharmacodynamic analysis of the furosemide-probenecid interaction in man. Kidney Int. 16: 187, 1979.

26. Oliva, P.B.: Lactic acidosis. Am. J. Med. 48: 209, 1970.

27. Orringer, E.P., Weiss, F.R. and Preuss, H.G.: Azotemic inhibition of organic anion transport in the kidney of the rat: mechanisms and characteristics. Clin. Sci. 40: 159, 1971.

28. Steele, T.H., and Rieselbach, R.E.: The contribution of residual nephrons within the chronically diseased kidney to urate homeostasis in man. Am.J. Med., 43: 876, 1967.

29. McPhaul, J.J., Jr.: Hyperuricemia and urate excretion in chronic renal disease. Metabolism, 17: 430, 1968.

30. Diamond, H. and Meisel, A.: Influence of volume expansion, serum sodium, and fractional excretion of sodium on urate excretion. Pfluegers Arch. 356: 47, 1975.

31. Steele, T.H.: Evidence of altered renal urate reabsorption during changes in volume of the extracellular fluid. J. Lab. Clin. Med. 74: 288, 1969.

32. Weinman, E.J., Eknoyan, G. and Suki, W.N.: The influence of extracellular fluid volume on the tubular reabsorption of uric acid. J. Clin. Invest. 55: 283, 1975.

33. Sorensen, L.B.: Role of the intestinal tract in the elimination of uric acid. Arthritis Rheum. 8: 695, 1965.

34. Cannon, P.J., Svahn, D.S., Demartini, F.E.: The influence of hypertonic saline infusions upon the fractional reabsorption of urate and other ions in normal and hypertensive man. Circulation 41: 97, 1970.

35. Prebis, J.W., Gruskin, A.B., Polinsky, M.S., Baluarte, H.J.: Uric acid in childhood essential hypertension. J. Pediatr. 98: 702, 1981.

36. Dollery, C.T., Duncan, H. and Schumer, B.: Hyperuricemia related to treatment of hypertension. Brit. Med. J. 2: 832, 1960.

37. Cannon, P.J., Stason, W.B., DeMartini, F.E., et al.: Hyperuricemia in primary and renal hypertension. N. Engl. J. Med. 275: 457, 1966.

38. Chodorowski, Z., Rynkiewicz, H., and Manitius, A.: Serum uric acid levels and urinary uric acid excretion in patients with polycystic kidney disease. Clin. Res. 26: 460A, 1978.

39. Messerili, F.H., Frohlich, E.D., Dreslinski, G.R., Suarez, D.H., Artistimuno, G.G.: Serum uric acid in essential hypertension: an indicator of renal involvement. Ann.Intern.Med. 93:, 817, 1980.

40. Grunfeld, B., Gimenez, M., Liapchuc, S., et al.: Systemic hypertension and plasma renin activity in children with the hemolytic uremic syndrome. Int. J. Pediatr. Neph. 3: 211, 1982.

41. Gold, G.L. and Fritz, R.D.: Hyperuricemia associated with the treatment of acute leukemia. Ann. Intern. Med. 47: 428, 1957.

42. Viozzi, F.J., Bluhm, G.B, Riddle, J.M.: Gout and arterial thrombosis. Henry Ford Hosp. Med.J. 20: 119, 1972.

43. Bluhm, G.B., Riddle, J.M.: Platelets and vascular disease in gout. Semin. Arthritis Rheum. 2: 355, 1973.

44. Streitman, K., Boda, D., Eck, E. and Magori, A.: Pathological importance of hyperuricemia and possibility of allopurinol therapy in experimental disseminated intravascular coagulation. Int. J. Ped. Neph. 2: 136, 1981.

45. Epstein, F.H. and Pigeon, G.: Experimental urate nephropathy: Studies on the distribution of urate in renal tissue. Nephron 1: 144, 1964.

46. Smith, J.F. and Lee, Y.C.: Experimental uric acid nephritis in the rabbit. J. Exp. Med. 105, 615, 1957.

Supported in part by NIH Grants, RR75, HL23511, HL18969 and the Hoechst Roussel Corporation.

Mailing Address: A.B. Gruskin. St. Christopher's Hospital for Children, 5th & Lehigh Avenue, Philadelphia, PA. 19133.

EXTRARENAL MANIFESTATIONS OF THE HEMOLYTIC UREMIC SYNDROME

Carlos A. Gianantonio, M.D.

The hemolytic uremic syndrome (HUS), as it occurs in infants and children, in the usual clinical presentation consists of the association of acute hemolytic anemia (with fragmented erythrocytes), acute renal failure, gastrointestinal bleeding and signs of central nervous system injury (1).

Although the main interest has been concentrated in the hematological and renal manifestations of HUS, it is clear now that these are only part of a systemic disease which consists of a widespread compromise of small arteries and capillaries, associated with extensive deposition of fibrin in the vascular tree and peripheral platelet consumption (2,3).

With the exception of the renal and neurologic sequelae, the organ compromise of the acute phase of HUS appears to be self limited. The exceptional case with a progressive course or with relapses of the initial symptoms does not modify the concept of a circumscribed process.

MATERIAL AND METHODS

This presentation is based on the autopsy material of patients with acute HUS who died at the Children's Hospital of Buenos Aires (4) (Table 1) and the clinical observations of the patients admitted to that institution and to the Hospital Italiano.

Extrarenal microthrombotic lesions were observed in 27 patients of 34 (80 per cent) that were autopsied before the 10th day of illness, while only 9 of 28 patients (32 percent) who died later during the acute phase, had similar extrarenal lesions.

THE CENTRAL NERVOUS SYSTEM

The signs of central nervous system dysfunction, found in nearly every patient during the acute phase of HUS (Table 2), coincided with establishment of the renal insult and the hemolytic anemia, and when mild, they were self limited. Most of the infants with severe neurologic symptoms recovered without obvious residual handicaps, although in many of them it

Table 1. Extrarenal lesions in HUS

	No. of Cases
Autopsy material	62
Extrarenal microangiopathy	35
Colon	22
Heart	18
Brain (30 autopsies)	16
Pancreas	15
Adrenals	4
Lungs	3
Small Bowel	2
Esophagus	2
Liver, spleen, bladder	1

took many months to attain a normalcy in behavior and neurologic examination.

Table 2. Central nervous system in HUS
Clinical findings during the acute phase

Abnormality	% of patients	
Minor	90	
Irritability	60	
Somnolence	30	
Myoclonic jerks	40	
Tremor	20	
Severe	* H.I. 25	* H.de N. 50
Convulsions	20	30
Stupor	10	40
Coma	5	15
Decerebrate rigidity	2	10
Motor deficits	3	10

* Hospital Italiano and Hospital de Niños

However, the compromise of the central nervous system contributed to death in some of these infants who concurrently presented extensive renal cortical necrosis. In a few patients, permanent sequelae were important and sometimes multiple, with school and behavioral problems predominating (Table 3).

Table 3. The Central nervous system in HUS. Clinical status of 15 children with sequelae

	No. of patients
Follow up more than 10 years	15
Severe CNS dysfunction (acute stage)	15
Developmental retardation	6
Focal motor deficit	5
Recurrent convulsions	5
Learning problems	7
Language disorders	4
Cortical blindness	1
Behavioral problems	9
Abnormal EEG	13
Abnormal brain CAT scans	12

In many patients the electroencephalograms and the brain CAT scans were abnormal in disproportion to the clinical picture. Some of the CAT scans were compatible with multiple cerebral infarctions; porencephalic cavities were observed in a few of these patients during the late studies.

Intracranial hemorrhages (Table 4), observed in 19 of 30 autopsies (12 were intracerebral), were small, multiple and not coalescent as a rule. The foci of microthrombosis predominated in the choroid plexus.

Retinal hemorrhages, small and flame-shaped, were found clinically in 10 to 15 per cent of the patients with severe neurologic compromise.

THE HEART

Many patients admitted years ago were severely overhydrated and hypervolemic, with the clinical picture of congestive heart failure. The correct management of this complication very rapidly reversed the heart function and size to normal. In some infants, the severity of the anemia added to the circulatory overload which precipitated myocardial failure.

This also was true in cases of severe metabolic imbalances such as toxic hyperkalemia, extreme metabolic acidosis or sustained hypocalcemia.

Table 4. Pathology of the brain in HUS	
Number of autopsies	30
Hemorrhage	19
Intracerebral (multiple, small)	12
Subdural	4
Subarachnoid	3
Microthrombosis	11
Choroid plexus	7
Focal necrosis	4
Focal gliosis	1

Data from patients of Gallo, G., Mendilaharzu, F., Delgado, N., Sojo, E. and Gianantonio, C.

However, in a not well defined number of patients, signs of myocardial dysfunction associated with ECG suggestive of ischemia, were present during the acute phase of HUS, and contributed to the death of infants because of pump failure and/or fatal arrhythmias.

Furthermore, in exceptional instances, the cardiac abnormalities still were present when other manifestations of HUS were gone and weeks after the acute phase, precipitated cardiac emergencies not related to arterial hypertension.

As can be seen in Table 5, multiple areas of myocardial infarction were found in about one third of the autopsied patients. In some cases,

Table 5. Pathology of the Heart in HUS	
Number of autopsies	62
Arterial + capillary thrombosis + myocardial necrosis	18
Clinical and/or ECG findings	13
Immediate cause of death	5

Data from patients of Gallo, G., Mendilaharzu, F., Delgado, N., Sojo, E. and Gianantonio, Carlos A.

contractility of the myocardium appeared to be compromised because of the number of infarcted areas, while in others, the areas of necrosis coalesced up to the size of small to medium classic infarcts. We have not registered residual cardiac abnormalities in survivors checked up to the late adolescent years.

GASTROINTESTINAL TRACT

A clear cut disturbance of the gastrointestinal tract is an essential part of HUS. For convenience of description, and taking into account the period of maximal relevance, we have assigned the gastrointestinal symptoms to the prodromal phase of HUS. In practically every patient, before the appearance of anemia and oliguria, profuse and oftentimes blood-tinged vomiting, colicky abdominal pain , mucous and/or bloody diarrhea and melena were present for a few days. In most infants, afterwards the intestinal blood loss overlapped with manifestations of the acute phase. The only consequence was the limiting of oral intake of fluids and calories and an increase in the anemia and retention of nitrogen waste products.

However, in a few patients the problems were more severe (Table 6)

Table 6. Pathology of gastrointestinal tract in HUS

Number of autopsies	62
Colonic wall microthrombosis + necrosis + hemorrhage	22
Small Bowel (idem)	2
Esophagus (idem)	2
Stomach	1
Clinical correlates	
Melena; hematemesis; ileus; abdominal pain	16
Diarrhea; abdominal pain	7
Intussusception	2
Extensive colonic necrosis	2

Data from patients of Gallo, G., Mendilaharzu, F., Delgado, N., Sojo, E. and Gianantonio, Carlos A.

because the areas of microthrombosis, colonic wall necrosis and hemorrhage ended in perforation of the colon or in the development of tumor-like hematomas which sometimes led to intestinal obstruction or intussusception.

We have examples of severe annular stenosis of the colon that required surgical correction, weeks or months after the acute phase of the HUS.

When the physician is not aware of the clinical picture of HUS, gastrointestinal symptoms may be erroneously attributed to shigellosis, ulcerative colitis, intestinal intussusception, bleeding Meckel's diverticulum, intestinal lymphoma, etc.

DISCUSSION

There is no question that HUS is a disease of the microvasculature, characterized by endothelial damage and thrombosis of the involved vessels (2,4,5). Although discussion of the etiology and pathogenesis are beyond the scope of this paper, it is likely that a profound disruption of the mechanisms that protect the patency of the small arteries and capillaries, and inhibit the aggregation of platelets, is precipitated by an unknown factor (6).

Although some of the most important extrarenal manifestations of HUS are hemolytic anemia (7) and arterial hypertension (8), they have been arbitrarily excluded from this presentation, as it is intended to be a discussion of some clinico-pathologic correlations.

As was mentioned earlier, the altered function of the central nervous system is clinically irrelevant in the majority of the patients. However, since management of acute renal failure is so effective today, it is clear that the most grave manifestations of the neurologic compromise remain as a life threatening problem (2,3,9).

We have no experience in the management of these infants with the hypertherapy presently employed in many neurologic emergencies because the mechanisms underlying the brain dysfunction in HUS are far from clear (Table 7) (10). Although the cases in which there is a definite metabolic abnormality are not numerous, we have been offering peritoneal dialysis to these patients in the hope that it could be of some help. We have the impression that it is really so, although we have no explanation for the results.

It is true,however, that the finding of areas of ischemic necrosis in the patients who die early in the course of HUS, added to the recent demonstration of patterns of infarction, the initial and late brain CAT

Table 7. HUS-Acute phase. Peritoneal dialysis in the management of severe CNS dysfunction.

Number of patients	220
Dialyzed patients	42
Metabolic disturbance	
Extreme acidosis	25
Dilutional hyponatremia	10
Hypernatremia	6
Hypertensive encephalopathy	2
Drug poisoning	5

Data from patients of Vitacco, M., Gianantonio, Carlos A. et al.

scans obtained in the sickest infants, suggests that the pathogenesis of the central nervous system injury may not be different from that of the renal damage.

As in other types of acute renal failure, in HUS, the heart may present many functional abnormalities related to metabolic and hemodynamic variables. The presence of multiple small infarcts that attain clinical importance has not been adequately stressed. As was mentioned before, the myocardial lesion was a determinant of death in some patients either because of cardiac failure or arrythmia. The presence of severe arterial hypertension was an aggravating factor in some infants.

We have not found late problems related to the heart, but we have not been following a complete study protocol over the years.

It is interesting to see how in medicine, as in life, everything has the colour of the crystal we put before our eyes. HUS was initially approached by the hematologists and later on by the nephrologists. The important gastroenterologic manifestations are now being recognized as a potential source of confusion with other diseases and as an uncommon but concrete cause of grave complications such as perforation of the bowel, intussusception and colonic stenosis.

The vascular lesions (thrombosis with secondary hemorrhage) affect small arteries from the esophagus down to the rectum, although they concentrate in the colonic mucosa and sub-mucosa (11).

There is much to be learned about the consequences of the microvascular lesions in the liver, the pancreas the adrenals and the lungs. Clinically they seem unimportant after the acute phase.

Our insistence in the late development of chronic renal failure in the group of patients with greater risk, in our country points to the most relevant present problem posed by HUS.

REFERENCES

1. Gianantonio, C.A., Vitacco, M., Mendilaharzu, F., Rutty, A.H., Medilaharzu, J.: The hemolytic-uremic syndrome. J. Pediat. 64:478, 1964.

2. Gianantonio, C.A., Vitacco, M., Mendilaharzu, F., Gallo, G. and Sojo, E.T.: The hemolytic-uremic syndrome. Nephron 11:174,1973.

3. Upadhaya, K., Barwick, K., Fishaut, M., et al: The importance of non-renal involvement in hemolytic uremic syndrome. Pediatrics 65:115,1980.

4. Gallo, G.E., Mendilaharzu, F., Delgado, N. and Sojo, E.T.: Extrarenal lesions in the hemolytic uremic syndrome. Abstract, 18th Meeting Soc. Latinoamericana Invest. Pediatricas, Guaruja, Brasil, 1980.

5. Levy, M., Gagnadoux, M.F. and Habib, R.: Pathology of the hemolytic uremic syndrome. In Hemostasis, Prostaglandins and Renal Disease, New York: Raven Press, 1980, pp. 383-397.

6. Fong, J.S., de Chadarevian, J.P. and Kaplan, B.S.: Hemolytic-uremic syndrome. Pediatr. Clin. North Am. 29:835-856.

7. Brain, M.C., Dacie, J.V., et al: Microangiopathic haemolytic anemia. Brit. J. Haematol. 8:358, 1962.

8. Grunfeld, B., Gimenez, M., Mendilaharzu, F. and Gianantonio, C.A.: Systemic hypertension and plasma renin activity in children with hemolytic-uremic syndrome. Int. J. Pediat. Nephrol. 3:211, 1982.

9. Bale, J.F., Brasher, C. and Seigler, R.L.: CNS manifestation of the hemolytic uremic syndrome. Am. J. Dis. Child. 134:869, 1980.

10. Vitacco, M.: Dialisis peritoneal en Pediatria. Buenos Aires: Ed. Ergon, 1975.

11. Whitington, P.F., Friedman, A. and Chesney, R.W.: Gastrointestinal disease in the hemolytic uremic syndrome. Gastroenterology 76:728, 1979.

SIMILARITIES AND DIFFERENCES BETWEEN THE HEMOLYTIC UREMIC SYNDROME AND THROMBOTIC THROMBOCYTOPENIC PURPURA

J.J. BYRNES, M.D.

Thrombotic thrombocytopenic purpura (TTP) and the hemolytic uremic syndrome (HUS) are both defined by a constellation of clinical manifestations. Precise definition of the essence of either TTP or HUS has not yet been realized. The clinical elements that constitute the HUS are contained in those that compose TTP. Due to this overlap in clinical manifestations, the distinction between the HUS and TTP may be difficult, especially in the adult presentations. Furthermore, platelet aggregation causing microvascular occlusion is an essential component of both disorders. The pathologic tissue abnormalities are similar; only the organ distribution is different. Some would argue that TTP and the HUS are simply variations of a common process. Others emphasize the heterogeneous aspects of both disorders. Until a better understanding of the predisposing factors, the precipitating mechanisms and the pathogenetic sequence is achieved, this argument cannot be resolved. The purpose here is to review the available information pertaining to these aspects of TTP and the HUS, to compare and contrast these data, and hopefully to provide a foundation of current knowledge from which to proceed in further analysis and understanding of these two important syndromes.

Clinical and pathologic features

TTP was first recognized and described both pathologically and clinically by Moschcowitz in 1924 (1). Subsequently, there were reports variously termed Moschcowitz's disease, thrombotic acroangiothrombosis, disseminated arteriolar and capillary thrombosis and platelet thrombosis syndrome. The term thrombotic thrombocytopenic purpura has prevailed.

The pathologic lesion consists of thrombi of arterioles and capillaries by a finely granular, amorphous, eosinophilic material. There is endothelial proliferation in response to the thrombosis. The endothelialation of the intravascular thrombosis leads to subendothelial localization of the eosinophilic material. This has been a source of confusion as it was once thought to represent a "pre-thrombotic lesion" and to be evidence for a primary vascular abnormality. Microaneurysms are often found at arteriolar capillary junctions. There is an absence of inflammatory change in the involved vessels and a rather limited area of infarction. A lesion considered characteristic of TTP is the glomeruloid structure in the kidney. A microaneurysm filled with thrombotic material becomes organized and assumes a "glomeruloid" appearance. Lesions resembling TTP may occur in a number of other conditions such as burns, mercury poisoning, leukemia, malignant tumors, rickettsial diseases and others (1-4).

When the subject of TTP was reviewed in 1955 by Singer, 55 cases had been reported in the literature. At that time thrombocytopenic purpura, severe hemolytic anemia and transitory, bizarre neurologic symptoms and signs constituted a triad considered characteristic and adequate for clinical diagnosis. Fever and urinary abnormalities, although not marked, were noted to be variably present (7). In 1966, Amorosi and Ultman collated and analyzed the previously published experience of 271 patients with TTP and reported their own experience with an additional 16 patients. The age incidence varied from infancy to 77 years; however, most cases occurred between 10 and 39 years of age, with the peak incidence in the third decade. Females were more frequently affected than males (3:2). Although variable in course, the disease was usually rapidly progressive, with 75% of patients dying within 90 days. They found five outstanding and almost universal clinical features to the disease. The pentad consisted of fever; bleeding or purpura, generally with thrombocytopenia; microangiopathic hemolytic anemia; neurologic manifestations - which often were remittent; and renal disease - including proteinuria, hematuria and azotemia. This pentad continues to be considered the clinical essence of the syndrome. Less frequent manifestations included abdominal pain, in some cases secondary to pancreatitis, hepatomegaly (25%), splenomegaly (20%) and variable skin eruptions. As four of their patients were pregnant, they noted a possible association. At post-mortem examination, the characteristic microvascular occlusions were seen in virtually all organs. Most frequently involved were the heart, brain, kidneys, pancreas and adrenals, in this order (8). Studies continue to elaborate on the diffuse nature of the process and document the wide variance in clinical manifestations.

The hemolytic uremic syndrome was delineated by Gasser et al in 1955 to consist of the triad of acute nephropathy, hemolytic anemia with fragmented cells, and thrombocytopenia (9). Renal disease is a prominent feature of the HUS in contrast to TTP where it generally is not so severe. Proteinuria and hematuria are present in all patients and renal failure often requires dialysis; chronic renal failure may develop in 25-30% of patients following therapy for this syndrome (10) whereas this is uncommon in TTP. In the HUS the pathologic changes are often solely glomerular, especially in early biopsies of uncomplicated cases. The most characteristic lesion is the subendothelial presence of finely granular eosinophilic material. Platelets and leukocytes may be present in the capillaries; but actual thrombosis is not often seen but can reach massive proportions. Luminal thrombosis is more common than in the glomeruli and may be seen in vessels up to the size of arcuate arteries. A characteristic change is the formation of aneurysms similar to those seen in TTP. These are most often located at the entrance of arterioles into the glomerulus. When the aneurysm, filled with thrombotic material becomes organized it often assumes a "glomeruloid" appearance (11) as in TTP. The consequence of arterial obstruction is degeneration and infarction of a portion of the renal cortex supplied by the damaged vessels. Sometimes the whole cortex becomes necrotic. The presence of necrosis carries a poor prognosis. In some cases other organs, in addition to the kidney, may be affected by vascular thrombosis and local infarction.

The HUS encompasses several clinico-pathologic entities which are different in apparent etiology, epidemiology and clinical presentation. Although first described and most often encountered in children, it is also seen in adults. Often there is an apparent provoking event, especially viral or bacterial infections (12-15). HUS occurs in both geographical epidemic and endemic manners. HUS is also associated with pregnancy, especially the post-partum state, and with the use of oral contraceptives (16). The diverse entities encompassed by the syndrome may be tied together by a common final pathogenetic pathway responsible for the common clinical manifestations.

As the components of the HUS triad are contained within the pentad of primary manifestations of TTP, the diagnostic distinction can be difficult. Furthermore, at presentation all elements of the TTP pentad may not be present. Also, fever and neurologic disturbance may occur in the HUS. In the HUS, neurologic manifestations are reported in 50% (42) to 92% (43) of patients - generally seizures or altered states of consciousness which often are attributed to metabolic disturbance, not to microthrombi in the brain. Thus, the distinction may be all the more difficult. Due to this overlap in manifestations, some have considered HUS a variant of TTP. As will be evident in the following comparison, the similarity between TTP and the HUS extends even beyond the overlap in clinical manifestations. However, differences still remain which suggest that the distinction between TTP and HUS continues to be warranted.

Pathogenesis

Today it is generally agreed that platelet aggregates primarily constitute the intravascular thrombus of TTP and the HUS. However, the sequence of events leading to the deposition of platelet aggregates remains undetermined and a source of controversy. Some investigators believe that platelet aggregation is the initial event and that the vascular changes are consequent to vessel obstruction and release of various substances by the platelets. Others believe that the disorder is primarily a vasculopathy and that platelet aggregates form secondarily at sites of vessel wall damage.

Studies by Harker and Schlicter demonstrated selective platelet destruction in TTP. Four patients had a 3.3-fold increase in platelet destruction, and platelet survival was markedly shortened to 0.21-1.86 days. However, the fibrinogen turnover rate was normal. Similar results were also obtained in patients with HUS. In contrast, patients with disseminated intravascular coagulation (DIC) had accelerated consumption of both platelets and fibrinogen (17). Jaffe et al studied 12 patients with TTP. No coagulation abnormalities were found in six patients; minimal abnormalities were present in three and major abnormalities compatible with DIC in the other three. There was little relationship between the coagulation abnormalities and the disease course except for the extent of hemolysis. Thus, DIC is not a primary factor in the pathogenesis of TTP or HUS and the changes suggestive of DIC, when present, may result from rather than cause the hemolytic anemia (18).

Studies of vascular tissue from patients with TTP and the HUS have shown various functional abnormalities. In 1968, Kwaan et al reported studies on three patients with TTP. Of particular note was the absence of plasminogen activator in the vessels occluded by thrombi, in contrast to its presence in normal amounts in uninvolved blood vessels. The plasma clotting factors and fibrinolytic activity were normal, suggesting that the loss of plasminogen activator around the thrombi was due to a local vascular defect. No such defect was seen in intravascular thrombosis of other types. They concluded that a vascular defect associated with loss of plasminogen activator played an important role in the formation of the microthrombi in TTP (19). This study was later extended to 12 patients (20). The absence of fibrinolytic activity in the TTP lesion may be the result of primary endothelial damage in this disease, or alternatively, the lack of fibrinolysis may be due to inhibition by the rich platelet content of the thrombi, since it has been shown that the platelets themselves contain large quantities of inhibitors against both plasminogen activators and plasmin (21).

The platelet aggregation inhibitory activity released from normal vascular tissue was examined by Remuzzi et al. This substance has many characteristics in common with prostacycline, the potent natural inhibitor of platelet aggregation. The activity was absent from vascular tissues obtained from a patient with active TTP (22) and from two patients with the HUS (23). However, after successful treatment the activity was found to be normal. On the basis of this evidence, they postulate that patients developing HUS or TTP lack a factor that stimulates prostacycline activity in the vasculature, favoring the formation of platelet thrombi in the microcirculation.

An immunologic basis for TTP has been proposed by others. Recently, evidence for immunologically mediated endothelial cell damage in TTP has been presented by two groups. Plasma from patients with TTP was observed to exhibit complement dependent cytotoxicity against endothelial cells growing in culture (24,25).

Neame et al, using both light and electron microscopic techniques, concluded that TTP is a syndrome in which disseminated intravascular thrombosis of platelets is the primary abnormality. They described three different types of intravascular thrombi as representing stages in the evolution of platelet thrombi: 1) an intravascular deposit of loosely aggregated platelets; 2) a dense aggregate, sometimes rimmed with thin layers of fibrin; and 3) a variable mixture of platelets and fibrin, which sometimes consisted almost entirely of fibrin (26). Similar conclusions were reached in a clinical pathologic correlative study of a patient with TTP who expired shortly after platelet transfusions. Fresh, loosely aggregated platelets were found in the organs involved shortly before death whereas platelets, fibrin and microvascular endothelial abnormalities were found in the organs with longer standing involvement (27).

The studies of Lian et al further support the postulate that the vascular findings in TTP are consequent to disseminated intravascular platelet aggregation. Plasma from patients with TTP were shown to induce _in vitro_ aggregation of washed platelets from both normal donors and patients during remission. They have shown that platelet aggregating factor is not dialyzable nor absorbable by $Al(OH)_3$ and is not inactivated by diisopropylfluorophosphate, hirudin or heparin in the presence of normal amounts of antithrombin. Thus, it apparently is not thrombin or another serine protease (28). Antiplatelet agents such as aspirin, dipyridamole, sulfinpyrizone and prostaglandin E_1, and elimination of ADP in the reaction mixture had very little effect on the platelet aggregation (29).

Based upon Lian's observations regarding the nature of the platelet aggregating factor in TTP and similarities to von Willebrand factor mediated platelet aggregations, Moake and associates have examined von Willebrand factor in patients with TTP. They found unusually large von Willebrand factor multimers in the plasma of patients with recurrent TTP. The unusually large von Willebrand factor multimers are similar to those synthesized by endothelial cells. They conclude that there may be a defect in processing of the very large forms after synthesis and that these unusually large plasma von Willebrand multimers mediate platelet aggregation in TTP (30).

Similar studies were performed on plasma from patients with the HUS. Again, Moake and associates found evidence for von Willebrand factor mediated platelet aggregations. However, in HUS normal sized multimers of von Willebrand factor, rather than the unusually large forms in TTP, appear to be responsible for platelet aggregation (personal communication).

Acquired dysfunction of platelets has been demonstrated in patients with TTP and HUS. The bleeding time results were even longer than predicted from generally low platelet counts. Defective platelet aggregation and reduced levels of adenine nucleotides and serotonin with reduced uptake and storage of the amine have been found. The platelet functional defect resembles that observed in patients with congenital storage pool deficiency. The acquired defect is thought to be related to the continued circulation of "exhausted" platelets, following their exposure to inducers of the release reaction but escape from deposition into a thrombus (31). This finding has been seen by other investigators including our observation in a patient with chronic TTP.

Etiologic considerations

Whatever the final sequence in pathogenesis, the proximate causes of TTP and HUS are even more obscure. Reports suggesting an infectious etiology have been based on the isolation of viruses and bacteria or serologic evidence of a recent infection. A prodrome may be present for weeks to months before fulminant TTP becomes manifest. Some patients relate nonspecific symptoms in retrospect such as fatigue, abdominal pains and fever, often described as "flu-like." Amorosi and Ultman noted that 40% of patients with TTP may have a prodromal illness resembling a viral infection (8). Whether the symptomatology actually represented a viral illness or unrecognized early manifestations of TTP is unknown. Mettler reported the isolation of a microtatobiote from the blood of a patient with typical fatal TTP. The same organism was also isolated from two children with HUS (33). Berberich et al reported a four-fold increase in antibody titer to Coxsackie B viruses in two patients with TTP (34). Myers et al observed a 16-fold increase in complement fixation titer for herpes simplex in one patient with TTP (35). Reynolds et al found serologic evidence of infection with mycoplasma pneumoniae in one case of TTP (36). A case of probable TTP occurred two weeks after influenza vaccination (37) and TTP developed within 24 hours of combined triple antigen and typhoid A and B vaccination (38). The role of infection in precipitating the HUS is stronger. HUS is known to occur in epidemics and has been associated with viruses such as Coxsackie A and B (39,40). Frequently in children, a gastrointestinal disorder precedes the onset of HUS. Cases of HUS occurring consequent to shigellosis have been studied. Koster et al found that 50% of those developing HUS in association with shigellosis had a positive assay for endotoxin, whereas only 5% of those with uncomplicated shigellosis had a positive test (41). Recently 11 of 15 cases (73%) of sporadic HUS in Canada had evidence of infection by a cytotoxin producing E. coli, suggesting that there was an association between these organisms and these cases of HUS (42).

The chronic, recurrent variant of TTP may be triggered by infection. Boswell et al reported probable recurrent TTP with exacerbations over a 16 year period. Each of the three episodes followed antibiotic therapy for symptoms of a suspected infection (43). Upshaw observed 32 episodes of the TTP syndrome in a woman with chronic, recurrent TTP. Five episodes appeared to occur spontaneously, 18 were preceded by viral or bacterial infection, and the others seemed precipitated by other physiologic stress, including pregnancy (44).

A review of the experience in the literature suggested that the incidence of TTP in pregnant women is excessive. May et al found that among the 350 cases reported, including three of their own, there were 28 cases during pregnancy and two post-partum. Only five patients survived more than six months post-partum and only one for more than two years. As the placenta is subject to microvascular occlusive process, fetal death generally occurs. The fetus survived in seven antepartum cases. In only one did both the mother and fetus survive (45). Interestingly, the thrombi are found only in the maternal circulation of the placenta and not in the fetus, suggesting that the factor responsible for TTP does not cross the fetal-maternal placental barrier (46). The occurrence of TTP in two sisters, two years apart, both during late pregnancy further suggests that pregnancy may precipitate a disorder to which there is a genetic disposition (47). Piver described a patient who had two pregnancies with exacerbations of a chronic TTP syndrome, seemingly related to the pregnancies (48). TTP has been described in patients taking oral contraceptives (49,50). HUS also has an association with pregnancy and the use of oral contraceptives. The term "hemolytic uremic syndrome of young women" has been proposed for the post-partum nephrosclerosis described by Robson et al (51) and for the nephrosclerosis occurring in young women taking estrogen containing oral contraceptives, described by Brown et al (52).

A genetic susceptibility to TTP is suggested by several reports. Wallace et al described a family in which four members of a sib-ship of seven suffered from a recurrent disorder with the clinical features of TTP (53). Simultaneous occurrence of TTP in two sisters, 29 and 30 years old, sharing the same living quarters and both taking oral contraceptives, raises the possibility of several associations, including a genetic factor (54). Environmental factors are suggested by the concomitant occurrence of TTP in a young husband and wife (55). The familial occurrence of the HUS has been reported more frequently (56-60). Kaplan noted two patterns of occurrence in siblings, either simultaneously or more than a year apart, the first suggesting an environmental influence and possibly a genetic influence in the second (61).

Several conclusions seem warranted. No specific infection is responsible for either TTP or HUS. Pregnancy likewise seems to be associated with the onset of TTP or HUS in some cases. The evidence for a genetic influence implies an ongoing predisposition, as do the chronic and recurrent forms of the disorder. It may be that various challenges can precipitate TTP or HUS in susceptible individuals.

Treatment of TTP

It has been difficult to evaluate the results of the various therapeutic maneuvers in TTP. The disease is relatively rare and often rapidly fatal. Splenectomy has been associated with a remission in a number of cases; however, no clear rationale has been proposed for its use (62-71).

It has been argued that whether the pathogenetic mechanism in TTP is platelet adhesion to damaged endothelium or primary platelet aggregation, the use of agents to inhibit platelet aggregation should be of benefit. There are more than 30 patients reported in whom various combinations of antiplatelet agents appeared to be of benefit (72). However, general experience clearly shows that, by themselves, antiplatelet agents are ineffective in most cases of TTP.

The first report of the effectiveness of exchange transfusion in TTP was published by Rubenstein et al, in 1959 (73). In 1976, Bukowski et al reported their 13 year experience in the management of TTP with exchange transfusions. Exchange transfusions resulted in complete remissions in nine of their 15 patients (74). This experience led to the finding that plasma infusions are effective in treating patients with TTP. An 18 year old woman developed severe TTP in her 19th week of pregnancy; exchange transfusions were remarkably effective in producing remission. However, the remissions were transient, each lasting a week to ten days, and then another exchange transfusion would be required. However, during the ninth exchange transfusion and based on the assumption that the exchange transfusions were effective because of removal of a toxic substance, 12 units of blood were exchanged with 12 units of washed red blood cells and 3,600 ml of plasma protein fraction. Rather than sustaining the remission, a fulminant relapse occurred immediately. The platelet count plummeted. The only difference between this, the only unsuccessful exchange transfusion, and the others that were so effective was the absence of whole plasma in the reinfusate. The replacement of a factor contained in the whole plasma thus became the likely explanation for the effectiveness of the whole blood exchanges. Therefore, 12 units of whole plasma were infused.

The response, which was immediate and dramatic, confirmed that the replacement of a plasma factor was responsible for the effectiveness of the exchange transfusions (75).

We have reported the management of 18 other patients with TTP in whom plasma infusion was the primary mode of therapy. Of the 18, 13 are alive and well, but one continues to require plasma infusions on a regular basis. One patient responded well to plasma but had several sporadic recurrences and expired before treatment could be restarted. Our experience and that of others clearly indicates that plasma therapy is the most effective form of therapy. The experience with plasma infusions also indicates a wide range in amount and duration of the plasma requirement. Some patients are effectively treated by a single infusion or plasma exchange consisting of less than their plasma volume; others require much more (76).

Corticosteroid, immunosuppressive agents including vincristine and cytoxan may have an ancillary role in alleviating or terminating the plasma requirement.

Treatment of HUS

There has been considerable controversy concerning the management of patients with HUS. The variability of the disorder explains the difficulty in determining the effectiveness of any specific form of therapy. The severity of the renal involvement, reflected by the duration of oliguria, generally correlates with the rate of recovery in both adults and children. In mildly affected children in whom anuria is present for less than 24 hours, careful attention to fluid and electrolytes is generally adequate and satisfactory (12). In more severely affected children dialysis is frequently required. Early institution of dialysis and careful management have resulted in improved survival. However, because even in the best series HUS in children has a definite mortality, additional forms of therapy have been investigated, especially in the more severely affected. On a theoretical basis, the use of anticoagulants has seemed reasonable. However, there is no consensus on their value (77). Fibrinolytic therapy (78,79) and antiplatelet aggregating agents (80,81) have been employed with conflicting results reported. The management of HUS in adults has generally been similar to that in children. However, the renal impairment is more often severe in adults than in children and hemodialysis is generally required. Heparin therapy has been extensively used, especially in post-partum HUS. However, due to the variability of the disorder there has been difficulty in determining the effectiveness of any specific form of therapy.

Based upon the effectiveness of plasma therapy in TTP and the apparent similarities, plasma therapy has been employed in HUS. We have treated five patients with HUS, two children and three adults, one of whom had post-partum HUS. All survived and appeared to benefit from plasma therapy. They improved coincident with administration of plasma. Remuzzi et al initially reported success in the treatment of two patients with HUS (82) and more recently, he and his collaborators have presented a series of 17 patients treated by plasma infusion. Plasma was infused with a loading dose of 30-40 ml/kg then 15-20 ml/kg daily. All but one responded with rapid disappearance of hematological abnormalities, although 15 of the 17 were oliguric; renal function recovered completely in eight children and two adults. The patients who failed to respond to plasma infusion recovered rapidly and completely after plasmapheresis. The effectiveness of plasma infusion was particularly evident in one patient who repeatedly relapsed as soon as plasma infusion was stopped and promptly responded once treatment was restarted (83). We conclude that careful clinical trials are warranted to establish the value of plasma infusion in the treatment of HUS.

The nature of the therapeutic plasma factor

The effectiveness of plasma infusions in the treatment of patients with TTP implies deficiency of a factor in the patient's plasma. Plasma obtained from outdated blood is also effective; therefore, the factor must be rather stable. Since disseminated intravascular platelet aggregation has been suggested as a pathogenetic mechanism and since normal platelets aggregate when suspended in TTP plasma, the effect of the addition of normal plasma to TTP plasma was examined. The platelet aggregating activity was neutralized by preincubation of the TTP plasma with normal plasma (28). Thus, there was a correlation with both a proposed pathogenetic mechanism - disseminated intravascular platelet aggregation - and the clinical effectiveness of plasma infusions - the inhibition of the abnormal platelet aggregation. The factor present in normal plasma that inhibits aggregation induced by TTP plasma is currently being purified and further characterized. Studies from Lian's laboratory suggest that a form of IgG is responsible for inhibition of TTP plasma mediated platelet aggregation (84). Remussi et al propose that plasma infusion in TTP and the HUS are effective by providing a factor which stimulates vascular synthesis of prostacycline (23). Identification of the beneficial plasma factor is urgently needed as a concentrate of the factor would greatly facilitate the clinical management of these patients. Furthermore, identification of the factor or factors would probably advance our understanding of the regulation of platelet function.

Summary

The similarities and differences between the HUS and TTP are summarized in the accompanying table. The typical presentation of the HUS in a young child with oliguria following a recent gastrointestinal disturbance is readily distinguished from TTP. However, the adult presentation of the HUS may greatly resemble TTP and only the relative degree of renal dysfunction and manner of neurologic disturbance help to distinguish between them clinically. Plasma therapy is the most effective modality, often dramatically effective in TTP. In the HUS plasma therapy is promising but requires further definition in clinical trials.

Comparison of the HUS and TTP

	HUS	TTP
Clinical Manifestations		
Prodrome	Often	Occasionally
Hemolysis	Moderate	Moderate-severe
Thrombocytopenia	Moderate-severe	Severe
Renal dysfunction		
oliguria	Generally	Rare
hematuria-proteinuria	Always	Often
Neurologic dysfunction	Often but non-focal (metabolic)	Generally focal, remittent-progressive
Fever	Often	Often
Pathology		
Microthrombi	Confined to kidneys	Systemic
Epidemiology		
Epidemic occurrence	Yes	No
Age	Generally young children but adult variants	Median 27 yrs
Sex	No difference in childhood	F > M
Genetic influence	Yes	Some suggestive reports
Therapy		
Prognosis	Good with support	Generally fatal without specific Rx
Response to plasma Rx	Good	Good-excellent

REFERENCES

1. Moschcowitz, E.: An acute febrile pleiochromic anemia with hyaline thrombosis of the terminal arterioles and capillaries: an undescribed disease. Arch. Intern. Med. 36: 89, 1925.

2. Hosebye, K.O., Stickney, J.M. and Bennett, W.A.: Platelet thrombosis in leukemia. Ann. Intern. Med. 44: 975, 1956.

3. Ritama, V.: Granular capillary thrombi in acute familial leukemia. Ann. Med. Int. Fenn. 43: 305, 1954.

4. Komori, R.: Thrombotic microangiopathy in patients with malignant tumor. Acta Path. Jap. 12: 3: 379, 1962.

5. Jones, D.B. and Loring, W.E.: Glomerular thrombosis. Amer. J. Path. 27: 841, 1951.

6. Pagel, W.: Acronecrosis due to fibrin thrombi and endothelial cell thrombi. Amer. J. Med. Sci. 218: 425, 1949.

7. Singer, K.: Thrombotic thrombocytopenic purpura. Adv. Intern. Med. 6: 195, 1954.

8. Amorosi, E.L. and Ultman, J.E.: Thrombotic thrombocytopenic purpura: Report of 16 cases and review of the literature. Medicine (Baltimore) 139, 1966.

9. Gasser, C., Gautier, E., Siebenmann, R.E. and Dechslin, R.: Hamolytisch-uramische Syndrome: bilaterale Nierenrindennekrosen bei akuten erworbenen hamolytischen Anamen. Schweiz. Med. Wschr. 85: 905, 1955.

10. Gianantonio, C.A., Vitacco, M., Mendilaharzu, F. et al: The hemolytic uremic syndrome: renal status of 76 patients at long-term followup. J. Pediat. 72: 757, 1968.

11. Goldstein, M.H., Churg, J., Strauss, L. and Gribetz, D.: Hemolytic-uremic syndrome. Nephron 23: 263, 1979.

12. Kaplan, B.S., Thomson, P.D. and de Chaclarevian, J.P.: The hemolytic uremic syndrome. Pediatr. Clin. North. Am. 23: 761, 1976.

13. Dolislager, D. and Tune B.: The hemolytic-uremic syndrome-spectrum of severity and significance of prodrome. Am. J. Dis. Child. 132: 55, 1978.

14. O'Regan, S., Robitaille P., Mongeau, J.G. et al: The hemolytic uremic syndrome associated with ECHO 22 infection. Clin. Pediatr. 19: 125, 1980.

15. Raghupathy, P., Date, A., Shastry, J.C.M. et al: Haemolytic-uraemic syndrome complicating shigella dysentery in south Indian children. Br. Med. J. 1: 1518, 1978.

16. Kaplan, B.S. and Drummond, K.N.: The hemolytic-uremic syndrome is a syndrome. N. Engl. J. Med. 298: 964, 1978.

17. Harker, L.A. and Slichter, S.J.: Platelet and fibrinogen consumption in man. N. Engl. J. Med. 287: 999, 1972.

18. Jaffe, E.A., Nachman, R.L. and Merskey, C.: Thrombocytopenic purpura. A coagulation parameter in twelve patients. Blood 42: 499, 1973.

19. Kwaan, H.C., Gallo, C., Potter, E. et al: The nature of the vascular lesion in thrombotic thrombocytopenic purpura. Ann. Intern. Med. 68: 1169, 1968.

20. Kwaan, H.C.: The pathogenesis of thrombotic thrombocytopenic purpura. Semin. Thromb. Hemostas. 5: 184, 1979.

21. Ekert, H., Friedlander, I. and Hardisty, R.M.: The role of platelets in fibrinolysis. Studies on the plasminogen activator and antiplasmin activity of platelets. Br. J. Haematol. 18: 575, 1970.

22. Remuzzi, G., Misiani, R., Mecca, G. et al: Thrombocytopenic purpura - a deficiency of plasma factors regulating platelet action. N. Engl. J. Med. 299: 311, 1978.

23. Remuzzi G., Marchesi, D., Mecca, G. et al: Haemolytic-uraemic syndrome: deficiency of plasma factor(s) regulating prostacyclin activity. Lancet 2: 871, 1978.

24. Mant, M.J., Cauchi, M.N. and Medley, G.: Thrombotic thrombocytopenic purpura: a report of a case with possible immune etiology. Blood 40: 416, 1972.

25. Burns ER, Zucker-Franklin D.: Pathologic effects of plasma from patients with thrombotic thrombocytopenic purpura on platelets and cultured vascular endothelial cells. Blood 60: 1030, 1982.

26. Neame, P.B., Hirsh, J., Browman, G. et al: Thrombotic thrombocytopenic purpura: a syndrome of intravascular platelet consumption. Can. Med. Assoc. J. 114: 1108, 1976.

27. Harkness, D.R., Byrnes, J.J., Lian, E.C-Y. et al: Hazard of platelet transfusion in thrombotic thrombocytopenic purpura. JAMA 246: 1931, 1981.

28. Lian, E.C-Y., Harkness, D.R., Byrnes, J.J. et al: The presence of a platelet aggregating factor in the plasma of patients with thrombotic thrombocytopenic purpura. Clin. Res. 27: 780, 1979.

29. Lian, E.C-Y.: Effects of platelet inhibitors on platelet aggregation induced by plasma of patients with thrombotic thrombocytopenic purpura. Clin. Res. 27: 780, 1979.

30. Moake, J.L., Rudy, C.K., Troll, J.H. et al: Unusually large plasma factor. VIII. von Willebrand factor multimers in chronic relapsing thrombotic thrombocytopenic purpura. N. Engl. J. Med. 307: 1432, 1982.

31. Pareti, F.I., Capitanio, A., Mannucci, L., Ponticelli, C. and Mannucci, P.M.: Acquired dysfunction due to the circulation of "exhausted" platelets. Am. J. Med. 69: 235, 1980.

32. Kaplan, B.S. and Fong, J.S.C.: Reduced platelet aggregation in hemolytic uremic syndrome. Thromb. Haemost. 43: 154, 1980.

33. Mettler, N.E.: Isolation of a microtatobiote from patients with hemolytic uremic syndrome and thrombotic thrombocytopenic purpura and from mites in the United States. N. Engl. J. Med. 281: 1023, 1969.

34. Berberich, F.R., Cuene, S.A., Chard, R.L. et al: Thrombotic thrombocytopenic purpura. Three cases with platelet and fibrinogen survival studies. J. Pediatr. 84: 503, 1974.

35. Myers, T.J., Wakem, C.J., Ball, E.D. et al: Thrombotic thrombocytopenic purpura: Combined treatment with plasmapheresis and antiplatelet agents. Ann. Intern. Med. 92: (pt. 1) 149, 1980.

36. Reynolds, P.M., Jackson, J.M., Brine, J.A.S. et al: Thrombotic thrombocytopenic purpura - remission following splenectomy: report of a case and review of the literature. Am. J. Med. 61: 439, 1976.

37. Brown, R.C., Blecher, T.E., French, E.A. et al: Thrombotic thrombocytopenic purpura after influenza vaccination. Br. Med. J. 2: 303, 1973.

38. Frick, P.G. and Hitzig, W.H.: Simultaneous thrombotic thrombocytopenic purpura and agammaglobulinaemia. Lancet 2: 1401, 1960.

39. Glasgow, L.A. and Balduzzi, P.: Isolation of Coxsackie virus group A type 4 from a patient with hemolytic uremic syndrome. N. Engl. J. Med. 273: 754, 1965.

40. Austin, T.W. and Ray, C.G.: Coxsackie virus group B infections and the hemolytic-uremic syndrome. J. Infect. Dis. 127: 698, 1973.

41. Koster, F., Levin, J., Walker, L. et al: Hemolytic-uremic syndrome after shigellosis: relation to endotoxemia and circulating immune complexes. N. Engl. J. Med. 298: 927, 1978.

42. Karmali, M.A., Steele, B.T., Petric, M. and Lim, C.: Sporadic cases of haemolytic-uraemic syndrome associated with faecal cytotoxin and cytotoxin-producing escherichia coli in stools. Lancet 1: 619, 1983.

43. Boswell, D.C. and Sierra, G.: Probable 16-year course in a patient with thrombotic thrombocytopenic purpura. Illinois Med. J. 145: 29, 1974.

44. Upshaw, J.D., Jr.: Congenital deficiency of a factor in normal plasma that reverses microangiopathic hemolysis and thrombocytopenia. N. Engl. J. Med. 298: 1350, 1978.

45. May, H.V., Harbert, G.M. and Thornton, W.N.: Thrombotic thrombocytopenic purpura associated with pregnancy. Am. J. Obst. Gynecol. 126: 452, 1976.

46. Wunzel, J.W.: TTP lesions in placenta but not in fetus. N. Engl. J. Med. 301: 503, 1979.

47. Fuchs, W.E., George, J.N., Dotin, L.N. et al: Thrombotic thrombocytopenic purpura occurrence two years apart during late pregnancy in two sisters. JAMA 235: 2126, 1976.

48. Piver, M.S. et al: Thrombotic thrombocytopenic purpura during pregnancy. Am. J. Obst. Gynecol. 100: 302, 1968.

49. Caggiano, V., Chosney, B. and Way, L.W.: Thrombotic thrombocytopenic purpura, cholangiocarcinoma, and oral contraceptives. Lancet 2: 365, 1980.

50. Vesconi, S., Langer, M., Rossi, E. et al: Thrombotic thrombocytopenic purpura during oral contraceptive treatment. Thromb. Haemostas. (Stuttg.) 40: 563, 1979.

51. Robson, J.S., Martin, A.M., Ruckley, V.A. et al: Irreversible postpartum renal failure. Q. J. Med. 37: 423, 1968.

52. Brown, C.B., Clarkson, A.R., Robson, J.S. et al: Hemolytic uremic syndrome in women taking oral contraceptives. Lancet 1: 1479, 1973.

53. Wallace, D.C., Lovric, A., Clubb, J.S. et al: Thrombotic thrombocytopenic purpura in four siblings. Am. J. Med. 38: 724, 1975.

54. Paz, P.A., Elijovich, F. and Barcat, J.A.: Fatal simul-

taneous thrombocytopenic purpura in siblings. Br. Med. J. 4: 727, 1969.

55. Watson, C.G. and Cooper, W.M.: Thrombotic thrombocytopenic purpura. Concomitant occurrence in husband and wife. JAMA 215: 1821, 1971.

56. Hogewind, B.L., de la Riviere, G.B., van Eo, L.A. et al: Familial occurrence of the haemolytic uraemic syndrome. Acta Med. Scand. 207: 73, 1980.

57. Tune, B.M., Groshong, T., Plumer, L. et al: The hemolytic-uremic syndrome in siblings: A prospective survey. J. Pediatr. 85: 682, 1974.

58. Hagge, W.W., Holley, K.E., Burke, E.C. et al: Hemolytic-uremic syndrome in two siblings. N. Engl. J. Med. 277: 138, 1967.

59. Belobradkova, J.: The hemolytic uremic syndrome in sibs. Sb. Ved. Pr. Lek. Fak. Karlovy. Univ. (Suppl.) 20: 445, 1977.

60. Edelstein, A.O. and Tuck, S.: Familial haemolytic uraemic syndrome. Arch. Dis. Child. 53: 255, 1978.

61. Kaplan, B.S., Chesney, R.W. and Drummond, K.N.: Hemolytic uremic syndrome in families. N. Engl. J. Med. 292: 1090, 1975.

62. Shapiro, H.D., Doktor, D. and Churg, J.: Thrombotic thrombocytopenic purpura (Moschcowitz's disease): Report of a case with remission after splenectomy and steroid therapy. Ann. Intern. Med. 47: 582, 1957.

63. Rodriguez, J.R., Babb, D.F., Santiago, E.P. et al: Thrombotic thrombocytopenic purpura: Remission after splenectomy. N. Engl. J. Med. 257: 983, 1957.

64. Hill, J.M. and Loeb, E.: Massive hormonal therapy with splenectomy in acute thrombotic thrombocytopenic purpura: Report of three cases with one eight-year cure. JAMA 173: 778, 1960.

65. Bernard, R.P., Bauman, A.W. and Schwartz, S.I.: Splenectomy for thrombotic thrombocytopenic purpura. Ann. Surg. 169: 616, 1969.

66. Distenfield, A. and Oppenheim, E.: The treatment of acute thrombotic thrombocytopenic purpura with corticosteroids and splenectomy. Report of three cases. Ann. Intern. Med. 65: 245, 1966.

67. Goldenfarb, P.B. and Finch, S.C.: Thrombotic thrombocytopenic purpura: A ten year survey. JAMA 226: 644, 1973.

68. Reynolds, P.M., Jackson, J.M., Brine, J.A.S. et al: Thrombotic thrombocytopenic purpura - remission following splenectomy. Am. J. Med. 61: 439, 1976.

69. Sacks, P.V.: Splenectomy and steroid in thrombocytopenic purpura (letter). JAMA 228: 975, 1974.

70. Guttner, J.: Splenectomy, steroids, and dextran-70 in thrombotic thrombocytopenic purpura. JAMA 227: 397, 1974.

71. Kadri, A., Noinuddin, M. and de Leeuw, N.K.: Phagocytosis of blood cells by splenic macrophages in thrombotic thrombocytopenic purpura. Ann. Intern. Med. 82: 799, 1975.

72. Amorosi, E.L. and Karpatkin, S.: Antiplatelet treatment of thrombotic thrombocytopenic purpura (editorial). Ann. Intern. Med. 86: 102, 1977.

73. Rubenstein, M.A., Kegan, E.M., MacGilviray, M.H. et al: Unusual remission in a case of thrombotic thrombocytopenic purpura syndrome following fresh blood exchange transfusion. Ann. Intern. Med. 51: 1419, 1959.

74. Bukowski, R.M., Hewlett, J.S., Harris, J.W. et al: Exchange transfusions in the treatment of thrombotic thrombocytopenic purpura. Semin. Hematol. 13: 219, 1976.

75. Byrnes, J.J. and Khurana, M.: Treatment of thrombotic thrombocytopenic purpura with plasma. N. Engl. J. Med. 297: 1386, 1977.

76. Byrnes, J.J.: Plasma infusion in the treatment of thrombotic thombocytopenic purpura. Semin. Thromb. Hemostas. 7: 9, 1981.

77. Kaplan, B.S. and Thompson, P.D.: Heparin for the hemolytic-uremic syndrome. N. Engl. J. Med. 294: 846, 1976.

78. Monnens L., Kleynen F., Van Munster, P., Schretlen, F. and Bonnerman, A.: Coagulation studies and streptokinase therapy in the haemolytic uraemic syndrome. Helv. Paediatr. Acta 27: 45, 1972.

79. Stuart, J., Winterborn, M.H. and White, R.H.R.: Thrombolytic therapy in haemolytic uraemic syndrome. Br. Med. J. iii: 217, 1974.

80. Arenson, G.B. and August, C.S.: Preliminary report:

Treatment of the hemolytic uremic syndrome with aspirin and dipyridamole. J. Pediatr. 86: 957, 1975.

81. Thorsen, C.A., Rossi, E.C., Green, D. and Carone, F.A.: The treatment of the hemolytic-uremic syndrome with inhibitors of platelet function. Am. J. Med. 66: 711, 1979.

82. Remuzzi, G., Misiani, R., Marchesi, D. et al: Treatment of the hemolytic uremic syndrome with plasma. Clin. Nephrol. 12: 279, 1979.

83. Misiani, R., Apiani, A.C., Eedefonti, A. et al: Haemolytic uremic syndrome: therapeutic effect of plasma infusion. Br. Med. J. 285: 1304, 1982.

84. Lian, E.C-Y., Mui, P.T.K., Siddiqui, F.A. and Chiu, A.Y.Y.: Studies of thrombotic thrombocytopenic purpura (TTP): Purification and identity of TTP platelet aggregating factor inhibitor A. Blood 60 (Suppl 1): 189a, 1982.

CURRENT APPROACHES TO THE MANAGEMENT OF HEMOLYTIC UREMIC SYNDROME

Bernard S. Kaplan, M.B., B.Ch., F.C.P.(S.A.) and
Peter D. Thomson, M.B., B.Ch., F.C.P.(S.A.)

As exemplified by our own experience (1,2), there has been a considerable improvement in the results of treatment of patients with hemolytic uremic syndrome (HUS). In Johannesburg in 1970, we studied 67 patients retrospectively and found an overall mortality rate of 34% (1). Further analysis revealed that 71% of severely affected cases died; none of the cases judged to be mildly affected died (Table 1). However, early treatment of severely affected cases with peritoneal dialysis reduced the mortality rate to 29%; this compared with an 80% mortality for severely affected patients who were not treated with dialysis. We, and others (3,4,5),have come to the conclusion that early institution of peritoneal dialysis was the most important therapeutic measure that could favourably influence the outcome of severely affected cases (Table 2).

In 1976 (2), we reported the results of treatment of 44 consecutive cases who were managed as follows: careful control of hypertension; as few blood transfusions as possible; careful control of fluid and electrolyte balances, and acid-base status; and, where indicated, early and prolonged use of peritoneal dialysis. The overall mortality rate in these 44 patients was 4.5% (down from the previous rate of 31%) and the percentage mortality of the severely affected cases was 10% (compared with over 70% in the first series of cases) (1) (Table 3).

Table 1. Patient Fatality Rates According to Severity of the Disease (1)

Patients	Total	Alive	Dead	Mortality Rate (%)
Total No. of patients	67	46	21	34.3
Died on admission	3			
"Mild" patients	36	36	0	0
"Severe" patients	28	8	20	71.4

This is publication number 00000 of the McGill University-Montreal Children's Hospital Research Institute

Table 2. Results of Treatment in the Early, Late, and Nondialyzed Groups (1)

Dialysis	No. of Patients	Alive	Dead	Mortality Rate (%)
Early	7	5	2	28.5
Late	11	1	10	90.8
Not done	10	2	8	80

Table 3. Results of Treatment from August 1969 to November 1975 (2)

	Number	Alive	Dead	% Mortality	
"Mildly" affected	24	24	0	0	4.5
"Severely" affected (a)	19	18	1	10	
Progressive course	1	0	1		

(a) early peritoneal dialysis: usually 24 hours after onset of anuria

Our own experience has therefore shown that a considerable improvement in immediate survival can be achieved with the measures outlined above. These results have sometimes been equalled, but not improved upon, by introducing, until recently, other forms of treatment such as heparin (6-8), streptokinase (7,9,10), aspirin (10), dipyridamole (10,11), urokinase (12) and hemodialysis (13). Therefore, although it has become apparent that most mildly affected, and many severely affected patients can be saved with conservative care, a number of very important problems remain to be solved. From 5 to 15% of patients continue to die or to progress to end stage renal failure; these patients clearly require more than conventional treatment. Furthermore, although attempts have been made to determine which patients have a poor prognosis (14), these have been based largely on clinical impressions; reproducible biochemical indicators of prognosis are urgently required.

Recent observations on perturbations in the activity of certain prostaglandins (15), and their correction with fresh frozen plasma (FFP) and/or plasmapheresis (16) have opened up an exiting new era in the investigation and treatment of this syndrome. The purposes of this paper are to review these new findings and to attempt to place them within the broader context of the HUS. In addition, we shall present long-term follow-up data on patients from Johannesburg.

POOR PROGNOSTIC FEATURES

It is important to remember that many cases are mildly affected in that they do not have seizures, hypertension, or anuria. They are easily managed with one or two blood transfusions, restriction of fluid intake to equal replacement of fluid lost through skin, lungs, stool (insensible losses) and kidney, restriction or elimination of sodium, potassium and phosphorus, and correction of metabolic acidosis. Most recover within 7 to 10 days and their long-term prognosis is excellent. Our approach to their management is shown in Figure 1.

Severely affected patients are anuric, usually from the time of admission to hospital. They often have hypertension and may have seizures. Early use of peritoneal dialysis results in improvement in their fluid, electrolyte and acid-base status and enables adequate calories to be given orally or by nasogastric feeding, or in very ill patients, by intravenous infusion (Figure 2). Although most of these patients survive the acute illness, a percentage do not, and of those who do, some may have renal damage with elevated serum creatinine concentrations, active urinary sediments and hypertension (2,7.8).

There are some clinical clues that point to a poor prognosis (Figure 3). These include, by definition, patients with progressive or inexorable disease (2); a non-diarrheal prodrome (4); an older age of onset, especially in adults (15); familial involvement suggestive of an autosomal recessive (16) or dominant (17,18) mode of inheritance; HUS associated with pregnancy (19); intestinal gangrene; renal histopathological evidence of predominantly arteriolar changes, or acute

Management

Mild Cases

Do No Harm

As few transfusions as possible

FIGURE 1. Mildly affected cases may have hypertension or oliguria or seizures; do not have anuria.

Management

Severe Cases

Do No Harm

- As few blood transfusions as possible
- Meticulous control of BP, electrolytes, volume
- Early peritoneal dialysis
- Adequate nutrition

FIGURE 2. Severely affected cases are anuric for more than 24 hours.

diffuse cortical necrosis (20,21); HUS occurring sporadically (22); HUS with recurrent episodes (23); HUS complicating shigella (5); and possibly pneumococcal infections.

In our opinion, any new form of treatment should be tested in patients who are severely affected, or in those who have at least one poor prognostic feature.

PROSTACYCLIN (PGI_2) and HUS (Table 4)

Remuzzi and his colleagues (16) introduced a new era when they demonstrated that plasma from patients with HUS has a reduced ability to stimulate PGI_2 activity during the acute phase of the illness (15). For the sake of simplicity, these findings will be referred to in this paper as a reduction in plasma PGI_2 activity. They also found increased platelet thromboxane generation in a few patients (24). These observations led to the speculation that an imbalance between an anti-aggregating factor (PGI_2, derived from vascular endothelium) and a platelet derived aggregating agent, thromboxane, might result in intravascular platelet aggregation. This in turn could have an important role in initiating or promoting renal damage. Remuzzi <u>et al</u>

have suggested that reduced plasma PGI_2 activity might be the consequence of a reduction in a plasma stimulating factor of PGI_2 (15), but Levin et al (25) have shown that patients with a sporadic variety of HUS have an inhibitor of PGI_2 production in their plasma. This inhibitor was not found in plasma from patients with an epidemic variety of HUS (25). Therefore, Remuzzi et al and Levin et al may be defining two different subsets of HUS. In addition, patients with sporadic HUS had a poorer prognosis than those with epidemic HUS (22).

Plasma PGI_2 activity is transiently reduced in patients with the usual childhood form of HUS (26). This transient reduction is in contrast with a number of other interesting and potentially important findings: 1. Reduced plasma PGI_2 activity was demonstrated in a woman with recurrent episodes of HUS, while she was in remission (27). Two of her four children also had reduced PGI_2 activity. This lends credence to the suggestion that some patients have a genetic predisposition to develop HUS on an autosomal recessive basis (16). Equally interesting was the demonstration of reduced plasma PGI_2 activity in a 19-year-old man who progressed to end-stage renal failure; the plasma of his mother and her mother, but not of other family members, also failed to stimulate PGI_2 activity (28). These findings and those of another report in which reduced PGI_2 activity was found in a 2-year-old girl and her unaffected mother (29) are supportive of the concept that HUS can be inherited in some families by an autosomal dominant mode (17,18).

Poor Prognostic Features

- Inherited HUS especially dominant
- A gradually worsening course
- Older age of onset
- Pregnancy
- Predominant arteriolar injury; cortical necrosis
- Intestinal gangrene
- Pneumococcal infection
- Shigella infection
- Recurrences

FIGURE 3. A careful analysis of prognostic features has been done by Trompeter et al (Barratt TM, personal communication). They found that the probability of complete recovery of renal function was favoured by a younger age of onset, presentation in summer, and a diarrheal prodrome.

Table 4. Prostacyclin (PGI_2) activity in HUS*

	References
Transient reduction	Beattie *et al.* (26)
Permanent reduction	Remuzzi *et al* (46)
Reduction in family members	
-in offspring	Remuzzi *et al* (27)
-in a parent	Jorgensen & Pedersen (29)
-in a parent and grandparent	Wiles *et al* (28)
Mechanism	
Reduced plasma PGI_2 stimulating factor	Remuzzi *et al* (15)
Circulating inhibitor of PGI_2 production	Levin *et al* (25)
Reduced endothelial cell PGI_2 production	Speculation

*estimation of the ability of patient's plasma to liberate PGI_2 from exhausted rat aortic rings.

TREATMENT OF HUS WITH PLASMA AND/OR PLASMAPHERESIS

The value of fresh frozen plasma and/or plasmapheresis in the treatment of HUS has been demonstrated in a number of Case Reports (16) and in one uncontrolled series of patients (30). A convincing role for plasmapheresis (if a single Case Report can ever be convincing) was shown in a report by Denneberg *et al* (31). The response obtained was so dramatic that we have reproduced the Figure depicting the patient's course in this paper (Figure 4). In addition, Misiani *et al* (30) treated 17 patients (including 10 adults) with the regimen included in Table 5. Their results were outstanding, but regrettably uncontrolled. Fresh frozen plasma resulted in an increase in the platelet count, a reduction in hemolysis, and an improvement in renal function. Hypertension was not a problem despite infusion of up to 40 ml/kg in oliguric or anuric patients. This study has raised a number of important questions: Should fresh frozen plasma be given routinely to all cases? What are the indications for plasmapheresis? Should plasmapheresis be done only in conjunction with hemodialysis? Would a prospective, controlled trial be ethical? Is fresh frozen plasma (with/without plasmapheresis) *the* answer to the treatment of HUS?

FIGURE 4. An increasing urine volume appears to be related to the institution of frequent peritoneal dialysis (reproduced with permission).

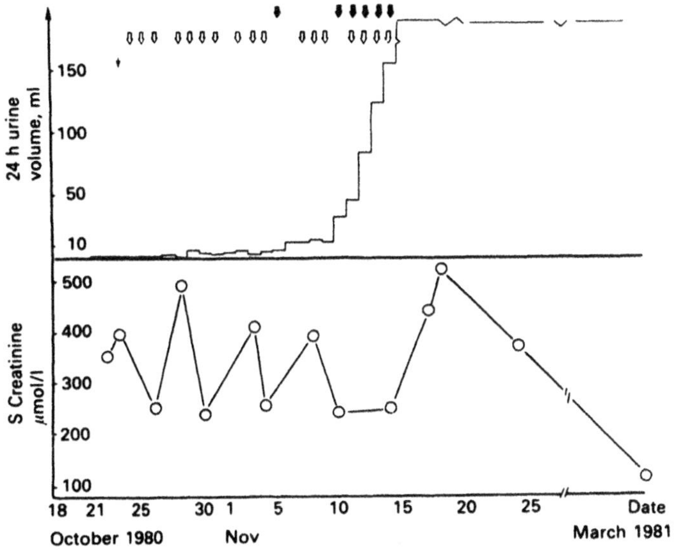

Plasmapheresis and hemodialysis treatment in an 8-month-old boy with severe HUS. ⬇, Plasmapheresis; ⇩, hemodialysis; ↓, peritoneal dialysis.

Unfortunately, only the last question can be answered, albeit only with partial certainty: because HUS is a syndrome, it is unlikely that all cases listed under this rubric will benefit from any single regimen. Indeed, there are a small number of reports in which fresh frozen plasma and/or plasmapheresis did not prevent progression to end-stage renal disease (32) or, in one of our patients and another reported case, death (33). It is possible that treatment failures occurred as a result of very serious complications such as gangrene of the colon, or late onset of treatment, or infusion of insufficient volumes of fresh frozen plasma, or infrequent infusions. On the other hand, it is also possible that reduced PGI_2 activity may be an epiphenomenon in some cases or that an entirely different pathogenetic mechanism may be operative in others.

Cogent evidence implicating PGI_2 and thromboxane in the pathogenesis of HUS is lacking. Demonstration of a reduction in the activity of one, the anti-aggregating agent, and an increase in the other, a platelet aggregating factor, does not prove complicity in causing renal damage. If PGI_2 is important in the pathogenesis of HUS and if fresh frozen plasma reconstitutes its activity and thus improves the outcome, how are we to reconcile the above with the observation of O'Regan *et al* (11) that patients treated with doses of aspirin known to inhibit PGI_2 production, do not fare worse than those not treated with ASA? One possibility is that the ASA also inhibits thromboxane production. However, if thromboxane is usually normal or increased in HUS, and may therefore stimulate platelet aggregation, how are we to reconcile this with studies that demonstrate reduced platelet reactivities and evidence of platelet exhaustion in the acute phase of HUS (34)?

PGI_2 is telling us something, perhaps a great deal, but not everything, about the pathogenesis of HUS.

A number of studies in HUS and in thrombotic thrombocytopenic purpura suggest that there may be other factors involved in the pathogenesis of these syndromes. These include the role of plasma anti-oxidants (35), plasma antithrombin-III (36), platelet agglutinating factor(s) and unusually large plasma factor VIII: von Willebrand factor multimers (37).

Before we accept the use of fresh frozen plasma as *the* answer to the treatment of HUS, we should pause for a moment and consider the fact that other regimens have also seemed to be *the* answer. Despite this caveat, we cannot help but feel that fresh frozen plasma has introduced hope for some patients with HUS who may otherwise have died. There is as yet insufficient information to enable us to comment on the use of infusions of PGI_2 in the treatment of HUS.

THE VALUE OF DIALYSIS IN HUS

Peritoneal dialysis was originally thought of as merely having a supportive role in the treatment of HUS by virtue of removing excess fluid, correcting electrolyte and acid-base balances and perhaps by allowing more calories to be given. It is possible, however, that peritoneal dialysis has a much more active role in preventing ongoing renal damage by removing large quantities of uric acid (38) and phosphate and by dialyzing other factors such as an inhibitor of fibrinolysis (39). Much evidence has been mounted in favour of the concept that phosphate has an important role in producing ongoing renal damage in patients and animals with kidney diseases (40,41). In addition, hyperphosphatemia *per se* can cause acute renal failure (42). Therefore, it is not an unreasonable speculation that dialysis may be valuable in preventing phosphate-induced renal damage from occurring in patients with HUS.

It has become the practice in some centers to insert a Tenckhoff catheter *ab initio* in patients with HUS requiring peritoneal dialysis. This allows for more protracted dialysis if required. Peritoneal dialysis is also being used more frequently in patients who are less severely affected, but there is no information on indications for, or the result of, this approach.

LONG-TERM FOLLOW-UP

Proesmans *et al* (8) have eloquently summarized the numerous shortcomings in the few papers which provide long-term follow-up data of patients who have had HUS. These include large numbers of cases lost to follow-up, lack of information on glomerular filtration rates, the absence of 24 hour urine protein measurements and in some papers, the paucity of actual values.

Table 5. Current Approaches to Management

1. Establish the diagnosis as quickly as possible.

2. Explain the serious nature of the illness to the parents but indicate that the outcome is usually good.

3. Measure blood pressure hourly, keep a careful record of fluid intake and output, and weigh twice daily.

4. Restrict fluid intake to 5% glucose in water and replace insensible water and renal losses only, unless dehydrated.

5. Do not give potassium or phosphate initially.

6. Half-correct metabolic acidosis with sodium bicarbonate.

7. Give packed cell transfusions if hemoglobin falls below 6 g/dl; do not raise hemoglobin above 8-9 g/dl.

8. Control hypertension carefully.

9. Decide each day whether or not to start peritoneal dialysis. We start peritoneal dialysis if the patient has been anuric for 24 hours, or if the metabolic complications cannot be controlled, or if there is fluid overload.

10. Fresh frozen plasma infusions can be given to all cases other than those who are mildly affected according to this schedule: 30-40 ml/kg of fresh frozen plasma; then 15-20 ml/kg daily until the platelet count has returned to normal and active hemolysis has abated (Misiani *et al*) (30).

11. Plasmapheresis may be indicated in patients who fail to respond to fresh frozen plasma infusions.

12. Encourage a good caloric intake while the child is being dialyzed.

In 1969, we planned to do a prospective study in which all of our patients would be followed up at regular intervals. We hoped to measure creatinine clearances, protein excretion, blood pressures and intended to do serial biopsies. Unfortunately, not all of these intentions were realized. However, we have been able to follow-up 64 of 72 patients (89%) initially treated by us. These 64 patients have been followed for a mean of 4½ years (8 months to 12 years) and the results of their progress are the basis of this report.

PATIENTS

From November 1969 to October 1981 (12 years), a total of 81 patients with HUS were seen at the Transvaal Memorial Hospital for Children (now transferred to the Johannesburg Hospital). Of these, 72 patients were treated *ab initio* by the authors (B.S. Kaplan from October 1969 to June 1970 and P.D. Thomson from July 1980 to October 1981). An

Table 6. Prodromal illnesses in 81 HUS patients in Johannesburg

Diarrhea ($\pm$ vomiting)	77%
Vomiting alone	6%
Upper respiratory tract infection	9%
Varicella	3%
DPT and polio shots*	3%

*within the previous month

additional 9 patients were treated and referred later to Transvaal Memorial Hospital by consulting pediatricians for treatment of complications.

The most frequent prodromal illness was that of diarrhea with or without vomiting (Table 6). Three percent of patients had recently been innoculated or had had varicella. An antecedent upper respiratory tract infection was noted in only 7 patients (Table 7). All of these 81 patients were white children; 36 were boys and 45 were girls; the mean age at onset was 14 months.

During the same period, only 3 definite cases were diagnosed in black children at Baragwanath Hospital; all three died. However, there were also 7 possible cases in black children, but no follow-up data are available.

Table 7. Patients with URTI Prodrome*

	Course
JF, M, 6 8/12	peripheral gangrene recovered; mild hypertension
A de V, F, 6 9/12	transient positive Coombs test transplantation
AJ, M, 5 11/12	progressive renal failure transplantation
JB, M, 1 6/12	recovered
CL, F, 1 5/12	recovered
LS, F, 7/12	recovered
EF, F, 8/12	recovered

*no differences were found between these patients and those with a diarrheal prodrome with respect to outcome if matched for age.

HUS occurred in three families; in each the onset in one child occurred within less than 2 months of the onset in the other sibling. In two families, the siblings were twins: the C twins were fraternal and the F twins were HLA identical. In the latter set, one was mildly, and the other, severely affected. None of the twins died. Both of the S siblings were severely affected, L was a 2½-month-old girl and R a 14-month-old boy; both are alive.

The major presenting features in the 81 patients are shown in Table 8. There were 36 mildly affected cases and 45 severely affected patients (1). Two patients with the progressive or inexorable form of HUS (1) are included in the severely affected group. None of the patients had a recurrence of HUS. Seizures and hypertension occurred significantly more often in the severely affected patients, i.e., those in whom anuria was documented for more than 24 hours.

TREATMENT

Our approach to the classification of severity (1) and treatment of these patients has previously been described in detail (1,2). The same protocol was used for the treatment of all of these patients. Mildly affected cases were treated with appropriate management of fluid, electrolytes, and blood transfusions were given if the hemoglobin fell below 6 g/dl. Elevated blood pressure was carefully controlled. Severely affected cases were managed in the same way except that peritoneal dialysis was started as soon as it was apparent that the child was anuric.

RESULTS

Seventy-two patients were treated by our unit initially, but only 64 patients have been followed for a mean of 4½ years (range 8 months to 12 years); 27 of these have been followed for more than 4 years (4 to 12 years).

The results of the 72 patients initially treated by us are shown in Table 9. The deaths of two patients out of 72 were related to HUS (2.8%). None of the mildly affected cases died; 4.4% of the severely affected patients died.

Table 8. Major Presenting Features

	No.	Seizures	Hypertension
No anuria ("mild")	36	11%*	46%°
Anuria > 24 hr ("severe")	45	57%*	98%°
Total	81	37%	75%

* $p < 0.01$, ° $p < 0.01$

Table 9. Immediate and Long-term Mortality

72 cases (a)	Death in 1st month	Death after 3 months	
		Renal	Non-renal
31 mild	0	0	1(b)
41 severe	1(c)	1(d)	0

(a) Treated ab initio by the authors

(b) Recovered completely from HUS; died from pneumonia several years later.

(c) 10 m girl. Died within 4 days of admission. Peritonitis, septicemia, meningitis.

(d) 6 y, 7 m girl, anuria, severe hypertension, peritoneal dialysis, marked arteriolar and minimal glomerular changes histologically; died 4 months after onset because parents refused hemodialysis and/or renal transplantation.

As noted above, 9 patients were referred, after initial treatment by consultant pediatricians, to our hospital. One died acutely, one developed end-stage renal disease, and the remainder survived.

Four out of our 64 patients proceeded to end-stage renal disease (ESRD) and are now on hemodialysis or have received allografts; one died 3 months after onset. Each of these was severely affected (Table 10). Therefore, the combined figures for mortality and loss of kidneys (ESRD) are 8.3% of 72 cases and 14.6% of severely affected patients.

Accurate serum creatinine determinations, blood pressure recordings and urinalysis were available in 64 patients: 5 were in end-stage renal failure (one died), 9 had hypertension (>2 S.D. above the mean systolic or diastolic pressure for age) and persistent proteinuria (≥ 3+ by Dipstick measurement)(Table 11).

PATIENTS WITH ESRD

As seen in Table 10, none of the patients who developed ESRD were mildly affected, 67% were girls (compared to 56% for the entire group) and 83% were older than 2 years at onset. In contrast, only 1 of 67 children under 2 years at onset proceeded to ESRD (1.5%). The mean age at onset of the entire group was 14 months and that of the 5 children with ESRD, 54 months.

Table 10. Patients With ESRD

Patient	Sex/Age (a)	Severe	Progressive	Treatment
AdeV	F/6 y, 9 m		+	Tx (b)
YdS	F/6 y, 5 m		+	Tx
JA	F/2 y, 6 m	+		Tx
RB	M/9 m	+		Tx
FdC	F/6 y, 7 m	+		Died(c)

(a) at onset

(b) transplant

(c) see footnote (d) Table 9

As noted above, 3 of the 9 patients were referred to Transvaal Memorial Hospital after being initially treated by consultant pediatricians: one of the 3 (aged 5 y 11 m) developed ESRD. One was left with severe hypertension, and the third, mildly affected, did well. Of the other 6, 2 were severely affected (one aged 7 years died acutely without dialysis treatment) and 4 were mildly affected.

Table 11. Follow-up of 64 Patients with Accurate Serum Creatinine and B.P. Determinations

	Severe	Mild	
End stage renal failure or increased creatinine for age	$5^{\Delta}/38$	0/26	$p < 0.05$
Hypertension (> 2 SD) above mean of systolic or diastolic)	9*/38	0/26	$p < 0.01$

$^{\Delta}$1 on dialysis; 3 transplanted
*All with significant proteinuria

RESULTS OF TRANSPLANTATION OF PATIENTS WITH HUS AT TRANSVAAL MEMORIAL HOSPITAL

Six patients with HUS have been transplanted at Transvaal Memorial Hospital (Table 12). This includes one child who presented in 1967; her blood pressure was poorly controlled and she had a residual mild hemiparesis. None of the transplanted patients has died and graft survival has been as good as that in non-HUS cases. Out of 16 related living donors, graft survival for HUS has been 4 out of 6, and for non-HUS cases, 9 out of 10 cases.

DISCUSSION

Before discussing these results, several caveats are in order: all the patients were treated by the same group of physicians, the treatment protocol was not changed during the 12 years, not all the patients could be followed up beyond the acute phase, these patients differ in certain important respects from those seen in other countries by virtue of age of onset (compared, for example, with Holland), and prodromal illness (compared with Shigellosis in India and Bangladesh) and the prevalence of atypical cases (compared with Montreal) (43). Two additional factors potentially detract from the value of this study: glomerular filtration rates were not done and there is no assessment of renal histology on follow-up.

Table 12. Results of Renal Transplantation

Patient	Age (Months) Onset	Age (Months) Tx	Follow-up Years	Results (a)	Donor (b)
AdV	81	93	5	Functioning graft	RLD
YdS	77	83	0.5	Functioning graft	RLD
JA (c)	30	60	2	Functioning graft	RLD
AL (d)	14	170	1	Graft failure	Cad
RB	9	129	3	Graft failure	RLD
AJ	71	83	5	Functioning graft	RLD

(a) No recurrences of HUS occurred post-transplant.

(b) RLD, related living donor; Cad, cadaver

(c) At onset of HUS had severe CNS involvement, was unresponsive to all stimuli and unable to swallow; recovered; temporary cortical blindness.

(d) Presented in 1967, was severely affected, did not receive peritoneal dialysis, had severe, poorly treated hypertension.

Habib et al have noted that although a reduction in the acute mortality rate has been achieved by improvements in the management of acute renal failure, this has been attended by an increase in the morbidity rate among the survivors (20). From 1950 to 1966, 35% of their cases recovered and residual renal symptoms were noted in 3%; however, from 1967 to 1979, 54% recovered and 23% had residual renal symptoms (20). In our series, only one child treated prior to 1970 developed end stage renal failure requiring transplant in contrast to 4 patients from 1971 to 1982. Furthermore, as stressed again by Habib et al (20), the prognosis appeared to be worse in older children than in infants. In our patients, an antecedent URTI did not seem to be associated with a poorer prognosis than the typical prodrome of diarrhea and vomiting. The results of transplant were not worse than those of non-HUS patients. Mildly affected patients have an excellent prognosis.

We have not studied prognosis in relation to renal histopathology. An excellent approach to this subject has been provided by Habib et al (20) who have defined three main patterns of histopathologic appearances: cortical necrosis, 3% complete recovery; predominant glomerular involvement (under 50% glomeruli affected), 19% complete recovery; (over 50% glomeruli affected) 2% recovery; predominant arteriolar involvement, zero% complete recovery.

The experience at The Montreal Children's Hospital has been very different from that in Johannesburg. Thirty patients have been seen from 1969 to 1983. Sixty percent were over 2 years of age at onset and 20% died. Of the 6 patients who died, 3 were siblings (16); one had had a recurrence followed by transplantation (44), and he then died 6 years later; one had severe shock; and one had interstitial gangrene and a progressive course. Of the 24 survivors, one has an elevated serum creatinine concentration, proteinuria and hematuria; and one has congestive heart failure. Two additional patients were atypical in other ways: one had a mixed picture of acute glomerulonephritis and HUS (45) and the other developed idiopathic thrombocytopenic purpura shortly after recovering from HUS (46).

REFERENCES

1. Kaplan, B.S., Katz, J., Lurie, A., et al.: An analysis of the results of therapy in 67 cases of the hemolytic-uremic syndrome. J Pediatr 78:420, 1981.
2. Kaplan, B.S., Thomson, P.D., and de Chadarevian, J-P.: The hemolytic-uremic syndrome. Pediatr Clin North Am 23:761, 1976.
3. Gianantonio, C.A., Vitacco, M., Mendilaharzu, F., et al.: The hemolytic-uremic syndrome. Nephron 11:174, 1973.
4. Tune, B.M., Leavitt, T.J., and Gribble, T.J.: The hemolytic-uremic syndrome in California: A review of 12 non-heparinized cases with long-term follow-up. J Pediatr 82:304, 1973.
5. Date, A., Raghupathy, P., Jadhav, M., et al.: Outcome of the haemolytic-uraemic syndrome complicating bacillary dysentery. Annals of Tropical Paediatrics 2:1, 1982.
6. Vitacco, M., Avalos, J.S., and Gianantonio, C.A.: Heparin therapy in the hemolytic-uremic syndrome. J Pediatr 83:271, 1973.
7. Monnens, L., van Collenburg, J., de Jog, M., et al.: Treatment of the hemolytic-uremic syndrome. Helv Paediatr Acta 33:321, 1978.

8. Proesmans, W., ki Muaka, B., Van Damme, B., et al.: The use of heparin in childhood hemolytic-uremic syndrome. In Remuzzi, G., Mecca, G., and de Gaetano, G. (eds.): Hemostasis,Prostaglandins and Renal Disease. New York, Raven Press, 1980.
9. Bergstein, J.M., Edson, J.R., and Michael, Jr., A.F.: Fibrinolytic treatment of the haemolytic-uraemic syndrome. Lancet 1:448, 1972.
10. Powell, H.R., and Ekert, H.: Streptokinase and anti-thrombotic therapy in the hemolytic-uremic syndrome. J Pediatr 84:345, 1974.
11. O'Regan, S., Chesney, R.W., Mongeau, J-G., et al.: Aspirin and dipyridamole therapy in the hemolytic-uremic syndrome. J Pediatr 97:473, 1980.
12. Jones, R.W.A., Morris, M.C., Maisey, M.N., et al.: Endarterial urokinase in childhood hemolytic uremic syndrome. Kidney Int 20: 723, 1981.
13. Ekberg, M., Holmberg, L., and Denneberg, T.: Hemolytic uremic syndrome: results of treatment with hemodialysis. Acta Paediatr Scand 66:693, 1977.
14. Fong, J.S.C., de Chadarevian, J-P., and Kaplan, B.S.: Hemolytic-uremic syndrome: current concepts and management. Pediatr Clin N Amer 29:835, 1982.
15. Remuzzi, G., Misiani, R., Marchesi, D., et al.: Haemolytic-uremic syndrome: Deficiency of plasma factor(s) regulating prostacyclin activity? Lancet 2:871, 1978.
16. Remuzzi, G., Misiani, R., Marchesi, D., et al.: Treatment of the hemolytic-uremic syndrome with plasma. Clin Nephrol 12:279, 1979.
17. Karlsberg, R.P., Lacher, J.W., and Bartecchi, C.E.: Adult hemolytic uremic syndrome. Arch Intern Med 137:1155, 1977.
18. Hogewind, B.L., de la Riviere, G.B., van Es, L.A., et al.: Familial occurrence of the haemolytic uraemic syndrome. Acta Med Scand 207: 73, 1980.
19. Segonds, A., Louradour, N., Suc, J.M., et al.: Postpartum hemolytic-uremic syndrome: A study of three cases with a review of the literature. Clin Nephrol 12:229, 1979.
20. Habib, R., Levy, M., Gagnadoux, M-F., et al.: Prognosis of the hemolytic uremic syndrome in children. In Hamburger, J., et al. (eds.): Proceedings of the Necker Hospital. Chicago, Year Book Medical Publishers, 1982.
21. Thoenes, W., and John, H-D.: Endotheliotropic (hemolytic) nephroangiopathy and its various manifestation forms (thrombotic microangiopathy, primary malignant nephrosclerosis, hemolytic-uremic syndrome). Klin Wochenschr 58:173, 1980.
22. Trompeter, R.S., Schwartz, R., Chantler, C., et al.: Haemolytic-uraemic syndrome: An analysis of prognostic features. Personal communication.
23. Kaplan, B.S.: Hemolytic uremic syndrome with recurrent episodes: An important subset. Clin Nephrol 8:495, 1977.
24. Remuzzi, G., Livio, M., Mecca, G., et al.: Prostacyclin and kidney disease: Focus on uremia and thrombotic microangiopathy. In Lewis, P.J., and O'Grady, J. (eds.): Clinical Pharmacology of Prostacyclin. New York, Raven Press, 1981.
25. Levin, M., Elkon, K.B., Buckle, A.M., et al.: An inhibitor of prostacyclin production in the plasma of some children with the hemolytic uremic syndrome and thrombotic thrombocytopenic purpura. Kidney Int 22:583, 1982.

26. Beattie, T.J., Murphy, A.V., and Arneil, G.C.: Studies on prostaglandin metabolism in hemolytic-uremic syndrome. Int J Pediatr Nephrol 2:130, 1981.
27. Remuzzi, G., Marchesi, D., Misiani, R., et al.: Familial deficiency of a plasma factor stimulating vascular prostacyclin activity. Thromb Res 16:517, 1979.
28. Wiles, P.G., Solomon, L.R., Lawler, W., et al.: Inherited plasma factor deficiency in haemolytic-uraemic syndrome. The Lancet i: 1105, 1981.
29. Jorgensen, K.A., and Pedersen, R.S.: Familial deficiency of prostacyclin production stimulating factor in the hemolytic uremic syndrome of childhood. Thromb Res 21:311, 1981.
30. Misiani, R., Appiani, A.C., Edefonti, A., et al.: Haemolytic uraemic syndrome: therapeutic effect of plasma infusion. Br Med J 285:1304, 1982.
31. Denneberg, T., Friedberg, M., Holmberg, L., et al.: Combined plasmapheresis and hemodialysis treatment for severe hemolytic-uremic syndrome following campylobacter colitis. Acta Paediatr Scand 71:243, 1982.
32. Beattie, T.J., Murphy, A.V., Willoughby, M.L.N., et al.: Plasmapheresis in the haemolytic-uraemic syndrome in children. Br Med J 282:1667, 1981.
33. Stuart, M.J., Spitzer, R.E., and Coppe, D.: Abnormal platelet and vascular prostaglandin synthesis in an infant with hemolytic uremic syndrome. Pediatr 71:120, 1983.
34. Fong, J.S.C., and Kaplan, B.S.: Impairment of platelet aggregation in hemolytic uremic syndrome: Evidence for platelet "exhaustion". Blood 60:564, 1982.
35. O'Regan, S., Chesney, R.W., Kaplan, B.S., et al.: Red cell membrane abnormalities in the hemolytic-uremic syndrome. Clin Nephrol 15: 14, 1980.
36. Brandt, P., Jespersen, J., and Gregersen, G.: Post-partum haemolytic-uraemic syndrome treated with antithrombin-III. Nephron 27:15, 1981.
37. Moake, J.L., Rudy, C.K., Troll, J.H., et al.: Unusually large plasma factor VIII: Von Willebrand factor multimers in chronic relapsing thrombotic thrombocytopenic purpura. N Engl J Med 307: 1432, 1982.
38. Kaplan, B.S., and Thomson, P.D.: Hyperuricemia in the hemolytic-uremic syndrome. Am J Dis Child 130:854, 1976.
39. Bergstein, J.M., Kuederli, U., and Bang, N.U. Plasma inhibitor of glomerular fibrinolysis in the hemolytic-uremic syndrome. Am J Med 73:322, 1982.
40. Ibels, L.S., Alfrey, A.C., Haut, L., et al.: Preservation of function in experimental renal disease by dietary restriction of phosphate. N Engl J Med 298:122, 1978.
41. Karlinsky, M.L., Haut, L., Buddington, B., et al.: Preservation of renal function in experimental glomerulonephritis. Kidney Int 17:293, 1980.
42. Kaplan, B.S., Hebert, D., and Morrell, R-E: Acute renal failure induced by hyperphosphatemia in acute lymphoblastic leukemia. Canad Med Assoc J 124:429, 1981.

43. de Chadarevian, J-P., and Kaplan, B.S.: The hemolytic uremic syndrome of childhood. In Rosenberg, H.S, and Bolande R.P. (eds.): Perspectives in Pediatric Pathology, Vol. 4. Chicago, Year Book Medical Publishers, 1978.
44. Barre, P., Kaplan, B.S., de Chadarevian, J-P., et al.: Hemolytic uremic syndrome with hypocomplementemia, serum C3NeF, and glomerular deposits of C3. Arch Pathol Lab Med 101:357, 1977.
45. de Chadarevian, J-P., Goodyer, P.R., and Kaplan, B.S.: Acute glomerulonephritis and hemolytic uremic syndrome. Canad Med Assoc J 123:391, 1980.
46. Kaplan, B.S.: Hemolytic-uremic syndrome followed by idiopathic thrombocytopenic purpura. Int J Pediatr Nephrol 2:97, 1981.

PANEL DISCUSSION: HEMOLYTIC UREMIC SYNDROME

Moderator: José Strauss, M.D.

QUESTION: In the first paper that you gave, you talked about the fact that platelet aggregation is already reduced in hemolytic uremic syndrome. So, then, what would be the use of giving prostacyclin which would reduce it even further? The second question is about the difference between the use of plasma infusion and plasmapheresis, where in the second case you are removing something and in the first case you are adding something. Do you think there is any difference?

RESPONSE: With respect to the infusion of prostacyclin, there are some who believe that it is of value not only because of its effect on platelets but also because it causes vasodilatation and increases renal blood flow. So, it's not clear to me that it is of any value if there is decreased platelet aggregation. On the other hand, our patient's platelets may not be acting normally because they already have been damaged by some process and perhaps there are some platelets that are still taking part in the process. I am just giving the other points of view. I don't subscribe to this view myself. So far, I am not impressed with the few case reports that I've seen of patients in whom prostacyclin has been infused. It does not seem to have done much. With respect to FFE and plasmapheresis, I've told you about what I think might be happening in FFE which is that I don't know what's happening. I don't think anybody really knows what's being added but certainly something good seems to be added including in thrombotic thrombocytopenic purpura where, incidentally, prostacyclin activity is reduced but there seem to be other factors operating as well. And with pheresis, is something being removed? Well, the only thing so far that is promising is the finding that there is an inhibitor of fibrinolysis which is removed by peritoneal dialysis in patients with HUS. If some similar inhibitor of something is being removed by plasmapheresis, I don't think anybody knows.

COMMENT: In TTP clearly the benefit is from the infusion and replacement of some deficient or inactive plasma factor. Plasmapheresis replaces the factor as long as you use fresh frozen plasma as the replacement fluid. In the hemolytic uremic patients that we have seen, particularly the adults, we have been forced to use plasmapheresis because of the oliguric state. We may (and we have on occasion) infuse plasma with volume control by dialysis but the oliguric state and the congestive failure generally necessitate plasmapheresis. Every once in a while a case report surfaces suggesting that in addition to replacing something some good may be obtained from the removal component also. But that is on much less firm grounds than clearly the replacement of a controlling factor, at least in TTP.

COMMENT: In the paper which you quoted, the one with the therapeutic trial with plasma infusion, there was one of those patients who did not respond to the infusion of plasma but did respond, apparently, to plasmapheresis. One gets the impression from some studies in aortic vascular rings, and in family members as well as in the few individual patients mostly with TTP but in some with hemolytic uremic syndrome also, that the absence of prostacyclin response is quite important. I understand your skepticism about this. When they infused plasma, they were able to replace the prostacyclin activity. It would appear that there are perhaps two things going on. One, as we were just told, we are removing something from the circulation (the striking results of Dr. Gianantonio with dialysis certainly suggests that, and the success with plasmapheresis also suggests the same sort of mechanism). Two, the administration of a factor in plasma that is apparently very beneficial as well. I certainly concur that there is an enormous need here for a controlled therapeutic trial because the disease, as you all have demonstrated, spontaneously can remit and exacerbate. This is the ideal situation for collaborative kinds of studies. There are differences in the endemic type and the sporadic type and very interesting - I suppose many of us, being pediatricians, have seen this article recently in the Journal of Pediatrics with the apple juice followed by a mini-epidemic of typical hemolytic uremic syndrome - a very interesting epidemiologic study. This happened in Toronto where there was something like 14 patients who came down, within a span of about ten days, with hemolytic uremic syndrome. All were traced to a fair in the outskirts of the city where they were served, or managed to get, some unfermented apple juice or cider. The one youngster who did not go to the fair managed to receive it from his father who had picked it up from a vendor at the same source. So, it is one of the clearest epidemiologic studies of this kind of hemolytic uremic syndrome and I hope that they have lots of plasma and blood stored on those patients.

COMMENT: They were overwhelmed by the clinical cases. They concentrated on the cider. They really looked very carefully at the cider. They were helped by the Center for Disease Control in Atlanta, Georgia. I don't know that they did that much on the patients. I wonder if I could make a comment about peritoneal dialysis. The patients who are doing well are also being dialyzed either peritoneally or by hemodialysis. Long ago we found very high uric acid levels in our patients. We thought that maybe removing the uric acid was making a big difference. One cannot prove this one way or another. We've reported two cases of acute cell lysis syndrome in leukemics, patients who went into acute renal failure but not as a result of hyperuricemia because they had relatively normal uric acid concentrations. What they had was profound hyperphosphatemia; after we treated their hyperphosphatemia they got better. There are lots of data now on the deleterious effects of hyperphosphatemia in the context of chronic renal failure. Also in nephritic rats, putting these rats on a phosphate depleted diet can decrease the amounts of proliferation in the glomeruli, decrease the amounts of calcium phosphate deposition in the kidney, and improve survival of the rats. So, here we gave things like uric acid, phosphates, the inhibiting factor, etc., and we don't know what they do. There just have to be so many different factors involved in whatever is causing the renal damage once the disease begins.

COMMENT: Regarding your comments about the hyperphosphatemia, there has been recent discussion that hyperphosphatemia may be one of the factors that leads to the acute renal failure seen in children with Burkett's lymphomas as opposed to uric acid per se. We have recently seen such an example. The other comment I would make in terms of peritoneal dialysis is that in our experience in dialyzing children with acute renal failure, most of whom have hemolytic uremic syndrome, it's very difficult to get the phosphorus levels to drop because of the ongoing hypercatabolism, cell turnover, etc. So that if the phosphate is the evil anion, it's hard to remove it with peritoneal dialysis.

COMMENT: I want to make a comment regarding the dialysis treatment. My feeling is that when we dialyze these infants what we do is nothing that may change the design that nature has about these kidneys. What we do is to keep them alive for a longer period of time. With the exception of a few infants who have bouts of disease, let's say, during the first weeks, these are progressive and uncommon in our experience. The other babies, when we dialyze them, we know that the damage already has been done. Let's suppose that we treat a baby with oligo-anuria of two or three days duration; he will be in anuria for a couple of weeks or three or four weeks. What we do with dialysis I don't think is to influence the pathogenetic mechanisms or the damage; we only keep the patient alive, that's all. This is my feeling. What we have seen is an improvement in the other aspects of the syndrome, the general compromise of the patient, a decrease in the blood levels of muscular enzymes; we have evidence of extensive skeletal muscle ischemic damage. I also think that we improve the CNS status. But I don't think with our schedule of treatment we are extracting something. Perhaps the only thing we do is to put the patient in a better general state, that's all. Because I would insist that in our kind of hemolytic uremics, by the time they get to the hospital, it has been settled what's going to happen with them; we feel that nothing we do from then on will change the prognosis. If we treat them badly, what we do is injure a patient; by not doing things or by doing too many things, we reduce the expectancy of recovery.

QUESTION: I want to ask a question from everybody here. How do you actually dialyze these children? What volumes of dialysate, how often do you do the exchanges? Do you dialyze continuously for the first few days? Do you add anything to the dialysate?

RESPONSE: I think we have had different experiences among the panel members. What we do is dialyze the patients (when we decide on dialysis) early: the severe cases on admission; the moderate cases, after a period of observation of a day or two at the most; the mild cases,we don't dialyze. We are using now Tenckhoff catheters in the patients in which we think the dialysis will be a prolonged procedure (over days) in order to avoid the need to re-introduce the other kind of catheters every two days. Initially, we use a small volume to fill the peritoneal cavity with a needle through the abdominal wall and then we put the catheter. We use volumes of about one-half the blood volume of the child - between a half and two-thirds - and we keep the fluid in the peritoneal cavity for about 45 minutes in order to attain what we feel is a good equilibration. In the case in which we are facing acute pulmonary edema, hypervolemia, and so on, the period is much shorter, let's say 15 minutes, 20 minutes for each exchange. And we do, as an average, six exchanges a day so that the baby can sleep and will not be bothered for twelve hours a day or 14-15 hours a day. And we want to do the procedure during the daylight hours because in our hospital we have more nursing problems at night than during the day and we want to check the baby very carefully. We weigh the baby after each exchange. We keep an external balance and an internal balance of fluid. So it will take, in the severe cases eight hours. One thing we did before, was 24 hours peritoneal "lavage". One of the consequences was that the baby was exhausted many times after this procedure because it is painful and it brings many changes in the patient - especially in the small baby, six months, eight months old. All is better the other way. So we do that and we are happy with the experience. We have no reason for doing the dialysis with some other schedule. We use standard fluids for peritoneal dialysis. In the small babies we don't use commercial fluids with lactate; we use bicarbonate. We prepare our fluids because we had lactic acidosis in some of the small infants.

MODERATOR: Regarding the use of Tenckhoff catheters, have you had a high rate of complication, specifically infections? We have tried the Tenckhoff catheters and we think that they work. Michael Freundlich in our group is particularly interested in that. We have had a couple of bad experiences in terms of infections, but the patients were obviously prone to severe infections anyhow. Have you had any problems of that type?

RESPONSE: Yes, we have had infections but we are not afraid of infections in the acute patient as we used to be before. The rigid catheters in which we used to have them are not well made in my country. They attract the omentum and once it is attached it is difficult to obtain a clear way for the input and output so we must change it; there is some bleeding in the cavity when you pull the catheter out, and sometimes then we have adhesions. We have lots of patients dialyzed with these kinds of catheters that had to be operated on months after the acute episode because of intestinal occlusion. Sometimes there were multiple adhesions. I think this is because of hemo-peritoneum, because of removal of the catheter. With the Tenckhoff we had better experience for a year and one-half or two years. We are happier with it. We have problems anyway but they are not so bad.

MODERATOR: Specifically, you have not seen more infections in the acute use of the Tenckhoff catheters ?

RESPONSE: No, I would say less.

QUESTION: By infections, are you talking about peritonitis or tunnel infections?

MODERATOR: Sepsis by Pseudomonas, localized infections. All types - obviously involving the peritoneal cavity and the area around the catheter with the little felt that surrounds the catheter. We had such a few patients treated that way that we said, well, you can't conclude anything. But in our hospital it is a joke now that each time we put a Tenckhoff for prolonged acute dialysis we are going to end up with Pseudomonas and so on. I just wanted for the record, your defense of this approach.

COMMENT: Our experience with the Tenckhoff catheter would suggest that as people use it more, learn to handle the catheter, and perhaps don't use to external cuff, that you generally have less problems with it. Most places that began to use the Tenckhoff catheter have gone through an experience of people not regarding the Tenckhoff catheter the same way that they think of a central hyperalimentation line and don't follow the necessary aseptic techniques to preserve the catheter. Consequently, they get a lot of infections. There are, of course, a number of people who use (but we don't) prophylactic antibiotic for a day or two after they put a Tenckhoff catheter in place for that reason. I think that unless you use it regularly and your intensive care unit is used to it, you are going to have a high incidence of infection.

MODERATOR: We are talking about a sophisticated group that is accustomed to handling catheters and with catheters implanted by surgeons. The statement is made by infectious disease people that by putting the Tenckhoff as opposed to the regular acute peritoneal dialysis catheter, we are inviting severe infections. We cannot see the rationale for that except for these two patients in whom we had this experience. We feel that the same type of care is applied and, again, the Tenckhoff is put by a surgeon under strict aseptic techniques.

QUESTION: Are there any data on prostacyclin activity in patients during the recovery phase and remission - particularly in those children who have other members of the family with low levels of prostacyclin?

RESPONSE: Yes to the first part, and no to the second. There are data from Belgium on prostacyclin activity in children with the usual epidemic form of HUS: low initially, and it gradually returns to normal. In fact, most of the patients return to normal by accepted criteria before the prostacyclin activity is returned to normal. With respect to siblings, there are not any data that I can think of.I just wanted to say that someone passed a note to me which says,"What kind of follow-up care would you recommend in a child recovered from severe HUS completely except for residual proteinuria? Do you expect late complications with neurologic, cardiac or renal function?" This is a very interesting question which I could try to answer except that I'm not sure what the person means by "residual proteinuria". How much proteinuria is there in the patient?

RESPONSE: She has about 3+ proteinuria.

QUESTION: Have you done a 24 hour collection?

RESPONSE: No, not after she recurred.

QUESTION: How old is the patient?

RESPONSE: She is four years old.

COMMENT: In general one can say, and this is not true for Dr. Gianantonio, but certainly from what I can gather in North America, that late development of chronic renal failure is the exception. It's very unusual. Dr. Habib has stated that perhaps a very small number of patients may develop chronic renal failure, perhaps ten years later. So, what I am saying is that this can occur in a small number of patients. If I have a patient who has hypertension or in whom the serum creatinine is not completely normal, or the urine sediment is active, or there is proteinuria, we would continue to see that patient every six months or every year, indefinitely. I don't think one can do anything about it but one would follow the patient, and if the patient goes into renal failure, of course, one would have to treat for that.

QUESTION: Do you follow these patients for 10-15 years?

RESPONSE: Well, I haven't had to follow anyone that long because I haven't had such a patient. But, if a patient continues to have abnormalities, yes, I would continue to follow that patient.

COMMENT-QUESTION: We routinely follow any child with HUS at least once a year so that we can look at his blood pressure, urine protein and sediment, and if necessary, anything else. We have two children who are now on chronic dialysis who allegedly had an episode of HUS a number of years ago, were presumably discharged fully recovered, and then came in with irreversible end-stage renal disease, perhaps related to severe hypertension. Their biopsies had the onion-skinning of malignant hypertension, etc. The question that I have is, if you have vascular disease of the kidney and some sort of local ischemia, does this set you up for the eventual development of hyperreninemia, and the whole sequence of events? If you don't follow the patient, you may miss it. Although I'm not sure in the children I am talking about, whether they actually recovered or not, but they certainly came to us with end-stage disease. It's a simple enough thing to do, not to let go of them, to see them periodically and monitor them. If the blood pressure is the culprit, then perhaps one has the possibility, if something happens, of treating it.

COMMENT: I would like to make a few comments not regarding the case you are discussing. First, if you are working with HUS patients and the mortality in the acute stage is very high, you are limiting the population of patients that may develop chronic renal sequellae, because the most severe cases are those who are most likely to go to chronic failure ten years later. Once you are saving them and keeping alive infants with mild and severe cases, you are increasing the population of patients with chronic renal failure.

The second is that our difficulty in the Children's Hospital was that our renal clinic was growing on the basis of the follow-up of hemolytic uremics. Once we had, let's say, the first seven hundred or one thousand patients that were alive and keeping contact with us, the problem was not only that it was difficult to manage but the families were kept in a continuous anxious state for years and years. We finally decided that if a child is normal by clinical criteria, with normal BUN, and urinalysis and normotensive for five years, we would tell the parents he is OK and there is no need to come back to the hospital. I think this is correct. We were receiving some girls who were coming with their boy friends to the hospital; they really were healthy in every respect but still were coming to see us as if they were sick.

The third is the last comment made by my colleague. I think this is very important - to follow-up hypertension in the patients who have it. Many times it is one of the most severe hypertensions you can find in pediatric patients. One of the few things we can do to help and avoid progression of vascular damage to the kidney, I deeply feel, is to follow hypertension and treat it energetically, with all the means we have. With this approach the progression of disease may be halted, not always forever, but at least it is slowed down in many cases.

MODERATOR: Let me ask the panel about the irregular progression of the disease. Recently we had a patient that we shared with some of the members of Dr. Gianantonio's group. The patient was looking really bad and we didn't expect to attain much improvement. We basically did not make any change in the treatment. The patient was ready to be dialyzed and apparently transplantation had been discussed already. This patient now is doing fairly well, has a slight elevation in the serum creatinine with a bit of a problem with hypertension but the patient is growing as a happy child, and the difference is almost magical. How often do you see that variability in the progression of the disease?

RESPONSE: It is not infrequent. These patients, this patient you mentioned, will end up in failure. That's the problem. Sometimes they get better but if they have high proteinuria, decreased glomerular filtration rate, and are hypertensive, in five years they will be in chronic renal failure. Let's suppose that we control the hypertension, that the glomerular filtration rate goes up, and that the patients feel better for a couple of years. But then they will come back again. We are now in a program of kidney transplantation. We have transplanted 29 children. All our adolescents, with one exception, that were transplanted in the adolescent years were hemolytic uremics. There are two groups of patients that recover. One has never had a normal glomerular filtration rate after the acute episode. They will decompensate and die in months or perhaps a year or two. The other one is the largest group, with patients who will grow and develop as normal children, with those exceptions that I mentioned where we check the patient, but they will go into failure many years after - let's say when they are 14, 15, 16, 19, 20 years old. That's the problem. It is a very slow process. Now that we are doing more biopsies, we find in most of them focal sclerosis, segmental sclerosis; it is a very slow process going on for many years.

QUESTION: In terms of biopsy, the question comes up, do you biopsy early in the course with low platelets and what do you do in terms of a hematologic work-up, making the decision to do a biopsy in the first few days of the disease?

RESPONSE: We don't do biopsies in the acute stage because we decided not to years ago when we lost several patients because of uncontrollable renal hemorrhage after the biopsy. Now we know, within our group, that there is no indication for an early renal biopsy because we are obligated to dialyze the patient until he dies or gets well. We have the longest period that a baby has been kept alive with dialysis while anuric: four months.

We may have a biopsy showing extensive vascular damage, perhaps cortical necrosis, but this is spotty in all our patients. It is not spread to the whole kidney; so, a needle biopsy may not give us the whole picture. This is my idea; some other people in my country are doing a biopsy for a prognosis in the acute stage. In the late stage we have been doing some biopsies because of investigational reasons but we don't like them either because this is a biopsy in a patient. After doing it,we don't know what to do with the patient. I would prefer not to do them unless there is something that somebody might suggest about the studies. We have recently completed our evaluation of immunofluorescence in these patients and this is definitely negative; we have no findings. The findings are the same as in the nephrotic syndrome - with segmental hyalinosis and sclerosis that's all. So we don't do biopsies for prognosis. We always follow the patient. One thing that's very useful in my experience is the ultrasound study, measuring the kidney size over the years. Very easily you can see that it correlates very well with glomerular filtration rate by square meter of body surface. This is a useful tool to determine whether or not the kidney is getting shrunken. In the acute stage we are using more and more gamma camera studies of perfusion of the kidney. We follow the the babies in this way when anuria is prolonged. The findings are very similar to acute rejection and very useful without traumatic studies.

MODERATOR: I know you want to make a comment. Would you please include in your comment your thoughts on the suggestion that has been made over the years that IgM in the glomeruli may have some information regarding the future of the disease and so on. I don't know exactly where we stand at this time but the question specifically pertains to IgM in the HUS patient.

COMMENT: With respect to kidney biopsies, we haven't biopsied a patient for a long time. That's not yet clear to me how a biopsy can be of any value. The Paris group and another group from Germany have constructed (especially in the latter case) very elaborate schematics telling how the biopsy can be of prognostic significance, talking about G1, G2, A1, A2, A3, etc., depending on whether they are talking about glomeruli or arterioles. I feel that the information they are offering overlaps so much that I don't really see that is it valuable to do a biopsy.

With respect to IgM, I didn't mention this but we found that serum IgG levels usually were low in the acute phase, and IgM levels were high in the plasma of patients on admission. With progression over the next week or so, the IgG levels rose and the IgM levels rose even more. I didn't really know what to make of this. I just sort of mentioned it in a paper once. Then other people were finding that IgM was present in the glomeruli of most cases. A group from Holland has also found IgM present in the skin vessels of patients with HUS. So, what does this all mean? Personally, I don't think that it means too much. It seems to me to be akin to the findings of elevated IgA in the plasma of patients with Berger's or Henoch Schöenlein, and IgA in the mesangium and in the skin of these patients. Perhaps it's telling us something but I haven't heard anything convincing about it.

MODERATOR: It's interesting that that initial presentation of low IgG and a high IgM that you described is similar to that of the patient with minimal change nephrotic syndrome.

QUESTION: Did I get right the concept that epidemic HUS can have as poor a prognosis as occasional cases of endemic HUS?

RESPONSE: No, I think what I was saying is that patients with epidemic HUS tend to have, as a group, a better prognosis than sporadic, according to a group from England. Still, there is no guarantee that they will survive just because they happen to get sick in an epidemic.

QUESTION: Has the institution of early peritoneal dialysis altered the long-term prognosis in your cases?

RESPONSE: Not at all, no.

QUESTION: In your last slide of your last talk, your second suggestion is to give fresh frozen plasma because it may be useful in very severe cases.

RESPONSE: Yes. I made that slide before the paper I referred to appeared in the British Medical Journal. At the moment it would be foolhardy to say that FFP should not be given because what people are writing about is that it seems to be of value. Certainly, what bothers me continuously when one talks about this, is that one first sees all the successful reports appearing in the literature. Are there cases of TTP or HUS where the results are not good? There are, but one has to try and understand why are the results poor? One of the things that I think about in my own experience is that perhaps we are not giving enough plasma. My colleague here could make that point more strongly than I could.

COMMENT: The amount of plasma that they gave is equivalent to the amount that we recommend: 30-40 ml/kg/body weight. So, it's close to total body plasma replacement. Certainly in TTP we have the advantage of a definite end point: either the patient survives or doesn't. In HUS it's more self-limited and obviously, as we discussed, controlled studies are necessary to demonstrate an improvement above the self-limiting nature of the disorder. One thing that was mentioned that I think bears some discussion, is platelet transfusions. It's our impression in TTP that they are hazardous, definitely contra-indicated, and in a number of reports in the literature, rapid neurologic deterioration after platelet transfusions have been documented. We have one particular experience we published in JAMA where a patient was thought to have ITP, a very mild TTP, and eventually was found to have an anemia and some GI blood loss, thought to require endoscopy,and platelet transfusions were ordered. Subsequently proteinuria, microscopic hematuria, and schistocytes became evident. The case fell into place as a TTP. However, the platelet transfusions weren't cancelled. They were given and the patient, who was completely neurologically intact before the platelet transfusions, a few hours after was comatose and shortly thereafter, dead. At post, the findings were classic TTP lesions throughout the body except the brain. Throughout the body there were all stages of thrombi with fibrin, platelets, microaneurisms, etc. However, in the brain there were just loose platelet aggregates, no fibrin, no endothelial proliferation, just as though the brain had been a platelet aggregometer and the platelets had been put in. On the basis of experience such as that, we feel that in TTP, platelet transfusions certainly add fuel to the fire and are contraindicated

QUESTION: Half of my point has already been mentioned. I mainly see adult patients and I sometimes find it difficult to differentiate between TTP and HUS, despite the comments. We probably tend to call most of these patients as having TTP, rather than hemolytic uremic syndrome. I just wonder, because it wasn't mentioned here, about coagulation. Really, you mentioned to us about the similarities but is there any striking difference between the children and adults to differentiate, and maybe you can comment about the coagulation.

RESPONSE: Only clinically, and as you can see from the presentations today, TTP in adults and the extrarenal manifestations talked about in children, it's very difficult to say hard and fast that one isn't at one end of the spectrum and the other at the other end. But, in the adults that I have seen with hemolytic uremic syndrome, the kidney is the focus of the action; the oliguria, the acute renal failure is the problem. There are generally not as severe or impressive CNS findings. The rest of the syndromes overlap. Maybe the studies I talked about with Von Willebrand's might provide a clue to a real difference. But, otherwise, it's just a slight difference in the syndromes. It's a very soft destinction.

Coagulation studies. Often in TTP and in the hemolytic uremic syndrome in adults, there is mild evidence of some DIC or fibrin turnover, fibrin split products are up, thrombin time is somewhat elevated, but the fibrinogen in TTP is generally within normal ranges.

QUESTION: I'm also an adult nephrologist. We have had a lady with biopsy proven hemolytic uremic syndrome who subsequently went on and received an A match living related kidney transplant and at about one year into the transplant started developing renal failure. On biopsy of the transplant she was found to have developed not hemolytic uremic syndrome but a transplant rejection. Have you seen anything like that in chilren? What has been the success rate of your transplants? Have you seen any recurrence of the hemolytic uremic syndrome in people who have been transplanted?

RESPONSE: As I mentioned before, our experience in transplant is limited, but we have not seen any recurrence of the hemolytic uremic syndrome. More than that - perhaps this is a chance occurrence - they are behaving as very good recipients. I've been talking about that with the group in Los Angeles. They have also a small group of patients transplanted because of the consequences of the hemolytic uremic syndrome and they also have behaved as good recipients. I don't know if my colleague could comment on that.

COMMENT: We transplanted a few children who have had no special problems. There are, however, scattered reports of the recurrence of HUS within a few weeks after transplant. The Minnesota group recorded that.

COMMENT: Quite a few reports, more than about half a dozen. The people in Toronto have been worried about this and they are trying to collect data on it. Certainly in Johannesburg, the experience is the same as yours - no recurrence of HUS. But there have been reports of it recurring. Its hard to differentiate between a recurrence of HUS and a rejection. That can be very difficult.

MODERATOR: We had a patient a few years ago who had systemic manifestations, active disease by biopsy, membrano-proliferative glomerulonephritis, and recurrent HUS. We treated empirically with immune suppression and transplanted the patient who did very well. We presented the patient here and a colleague from London was horrified at the treatment. We transplanted the patient when everything had quieted down,the sed rate and so on. The patient has done beautifully well for the past several years.

COMMENT: We reported a case of recurrent HUS who had C3 nephritic factor in his serum and C3 deposits in the kidney. His HUS recurred. He was transplanted and did well for about six years and then he died. But there have been a few reports now - not many, just a few - of this type of MPGN like picture, with C3 nephritic factor. Did your patient have C3 nephritic factor?

MODERATOR: We did not measure C3 nephritic factor, but the patient was hypocomplementemic.

COMMENT: Oh, he was. That's really interesting. That sounds again like another little sub-group of HUS, certainly different from what you think it is.

COMMENT: I want to stress what has been said. In our group we have seen a very few patients with recurrent hemolytic uremic syndrome, very few familial cases. What we do is to put them aside from the "usual" problems we face with the babies we treat monthly or weekly. In those other patients we have no experience about renal transplantation and recurrence; they may recur or not, I do not know. I have no experience, I have no data. But proportionally, this is a very insignificant bunch in the whole group of patients we are treating.

QUESTION: If I'm not mistaken, vincristine was used for TTP. I was wondering what the latest is on that, if it's been tried in HUS, if it's been abandoned in TTP, and what is the possible mechanism for its action.

RESPONSE: It certainly has been reported to be effective in TTP. I've not seen any reports that it is used in the hemolytic uremic syndrome. In Ohio a group reported five cases. The response there was less than dramatic and it took a while. It's our feeling that it certainly might be a second line form of therapy and that along with other immunosuppressive agents might help to terminate a case that is seeming to be chronic. There have been some cases where there has been an ongoing plasma requirement that's been terminated by cyclophosphamide and prednisone, prednisone alone, prednisone and azathioprine, and perhaps vincristine fits into that same pattern, too. I'm a bit skeptical about its usefulness. I've tried it in patients with TTP and have not had any luck.

QUESTION: We usually see an average of about three to four patients with hemolytic uremic syndrome each year. The average age is in the range of one to three or four years. We had a case that was younger than one year of age and the patient had persistent low platelets and hemolysis, and died. There was not a history of diarrhea or vomiting in that baby. Another patient we had was about a two year old boy in whom the hemolytic uremic syndrome occurred after an episode of chicken pox. The patient survived but ended up with chronic renal failure and hypertension.

What do we do for the patients? We may start them on peritoneal dialysis, but if the patient has good vascular access, we switch to hemodialysis. None of the speakers has commented about hemodialysis. I would like to see if there is any benefit for peritoneal dialysis as compared to hemodialysis.

RESPONSE: There is one study from England in Archives of Diseases of Childhood where this sort of comparison was made. No advantage was found with hemodialysis. Personally, I think that hemodialysis - and this again is just a speculation - may be indicated in a patient to whom one was giving large amounts of plasma, or perhaps a patient who has been plasmapheresed and who one would want to control better with hemodialysis. I can't really think of a reason to use it.

RESPONSE: The only times that we have used hemodialysis have been in children who have had bowel perforation. Otherwise, we have used peritoneal dialysis. In a number of children we used continuous peritoneal dialysis for a few days to manage all the problems in the hypercatabolic state.

RESPONSE: I have the same experience. We have used also hemodialysis in HUS babies who were wrongly operated upon, because the surgeon thought that his hemorrhage meant a surgical abdominal condition. We have another situation. In my hospital, peritoneal dialysis is much less expensive than extracorporeal dialysis. In our standard work, extracorporeal is practically limited to chronic patients and peritoneal to acute renal failure with a few exceptions. I would say that perhaps people who have large experience with extracorporeal dialysis, there is no reason why they shouldn't use it in these infants. I don't feel that there will be any basic difference in prognosis on the basis of which method is used.

MODERATOR: It has been said that peritoneal dialysis may remove larger particles, middle molecules. Do you have any thoughts on that?

RESPONSE: No.

COMMENT: I would like to reiterate something that was just said. Every couple of years we see a patient with HUS who is referred after he has had his "appendectomy", and that for people on the front lines looking at children, one ought to consider in the differential diagnosis of an acute abdomen, the hemolytic uremic syndrome and make sure that the smear is looked at reasonably carefully before the child goes to the operating room. In the few examples we've seen, when we went back and recovered the smear, there had been a microangiopathic smear although rather mild.

MODERATOR: We had such an experience with an older child. She was actually eight or nine and came comatose after an appendectomy with general anesthesia.

COMMENT: Related to this problem of experience versus lack of experience with the syndrome, I would say that one of the objections I have always made about the reports of mortality or prognosis in the acute stage relating epidemic versus endemic depends also on the experience of the people who see many of these infants over the whole year. If you have the bad luck of having an endemic problem of any kind - schizophrenia or anything - lead poisoning - in time you will be able to reduce mortality. If you have one case every two years, perhaps this child is going to have a poor prognosis. This I wanted to say because we are in some ways repetitive animals. The more we do one thing, the better we do it until we get bored; then, things go the other way. Really, the treatment of such diseases is very complex. Reye Syndrome is another example. We were seeing one every year and the child would die. Now we see more and we treat them better. I think that's important,too.

COMMENT: I don't agree completely because I have lived in two different situations - countries,and unless I lost my skills as I got older - which is possible - I find that we do have cases now which are different from those I had before. I used to believe as you do.

COMMENT: Since we got the discussion back to the technique, I wanted to comment that we have made good use of the Dean button in this kind of a situation where usually what happens is that the patient comes in acutely ill, we dialyze for a brief period of time, and there is recovery with no need for further dialysis. In some of the patients, of course, we do need to dialyze for prolonged periods of time and we will put a Tenckhoff catheter. But the Dean button has saved us from having to do the repetitive punctures in the child who looks as though there is some tendency towards improvement. I just wanted to mention that the creation of that little fistulous track, for any peritoneal dialysis that is going to be done repetitively, is very helpful. We never undertake acute peritoneal dialysis without making use of the Dean button just to save the child the puncture on a repeat acute dialysis.

MODERATOR: It has been a very exciting morning. Everybody must be exhausted. I would like to thank everyone for being here; particularly I want to thank Dr. Freundlich, Dr. Zilleruelo, and Dr. Retureta for their help with so many details this morning.

II

RENAL EMERGENCIES

PERINATAL ASPHYXIA: PATHOPHYSIOLOGY AND AN APPROACH TOWARDS THERAPY

RONALD N. GOLDBERG, M.D.

Perinatal asphyxia is an all too common phenomenon in the newborn nursery. Approximately 20% of all neonates weighing greater than 2500 grams receive Apgar scores under 7 at 1 minute and 2-3% receive Apgar scores under 7 at 5 minutes. In addition, if the Apgar score is below 3 at 1 minute or under 5 at 5 minutes and there are neurologic manifestations of asphyxia, approximately 20% of these infants die, 30% sustain marked and 15% minimal neurologic sequelae while only 35% are normal. In order to understand the full scope of this problem we must consider the amount of neurologic damage and loss of potential occurring secondary to asphyxia that cannot be measured. Windle noted that newborn monkeys who were subjected to sublethal asphyxia and who evidenced gross neurologic dysfunction which cleared within a few days or weeks had pathologic evidence of nerve cell loss and bilateral cerebral lesions at autopsy.(1) It is possible to extrapolate from these findings and postulate that even short asphyxial episodes, to which the human newborn is thought to be resistant, may blunt his potential and produce neurologic and developmental deficits that are difficult to detect clinically.(2)

PATHOPHYSIOLOGY OF CNS INVOLVEMENT

The brain is non-homogeneous in terms of anatomy, metabolism and circulation. This makes some areas more susceptible to asphyxia than others. The reasons for this are related to neuronal sensitivity, differences in metabolic rate, red cell aggregation, capillary compression secondary to edema, collateral circulation and regional differences in neurotransmitter content. These factors and their interaction will vary the pattern of cerebral damage secondary to an interruption of fetal respiration and circulation.(3)

Neuronal damage occurring after an asphyxia insult can be thought of as damage occurring during the insult and that developing after the event. This latter damage is related to the biochemical and physical sequelae of the initial asphyxial insult. This sequence and its timing are important in considering and evaluating therapy after the asphyxial episode.

Biochemical Changes During Asphyxia. During ischemia glycolytic activity is stimulated, resulting in rapid depletion of phosphocreatine, glucose, ATP and glycogen. After 30 minutes of anoxia most glycolytic intermediates are reduced to 30-50% of baseline values. This results in an elevation in lactate which is in part related to the increase in glycolytic activity. This rise in lactate and consequent decrease in brain pH plays a role in the pathogenesis of ischemic brain damage resulting in edema. Also because of the increase in glycolysis, the carrier mediated transport of glucose across the blood brain barrier may limit biochemical recovery after the asphyxial insult.

Protein synthesis remains intact during ischemia, but is disrupted when circulation is re-established. The increased cerebral excretion of ammonia and amino acids indicates increased proteolytic activity post-insult.

For the first 30 minutes after recirculation there is a 50-70% decrease in cerebral oxygen consumption. Within 1 hour the oxygen consumption has increased threefold. This hypermetabolism is believed to also aggravate any existing cerebral damage.

Ischemia results in release of neurotransmitters which according to Nemoto may lead to neuronal dysfunction, necrosis, and cerebral infarction.(3) During recirculation and re-oxygenation post-ischemia, catecholamine synthesis and release increases resulting in increased oxygen consumption, lipolysis, proteolysis, cell membrane permeability and glycolysis. It is postulated that the neonate's decreased sensitivity to asphyxia may in part be related to immaturity of central nervous system neurotransmitters with a resultant lower cerebral metabolic rate.

The pattern of pathologic changes occurring in the asphyxiated neonate varies depending on the severity and duration of the insult and the gestational age.

The increasing glycolytic and proteolytic activity results in an increase in osmolarity which varies depending on the metabolic rate of different areas of the brain. Areas with increased metabolic rate and high capillary density have a large pool of water from which to produce edema. The edema resulting from this and from the brain necrosis secondary to the initial insult may cause vascular compression. Edema also results in hemoconcentration and stasis which in the presence of acidosis may result in intravascular coagulation. These factors plus vasospasm and increased local tissue pressure result in what is known as the "no reflow phenomenon" once oxygenation and circulation are re-established. "No reflow" means that even with high cerebral perfusion pressures, areas of the brain will remain non-perfused after the ischemia because of the above mentioned pathophysiologic processes. The inadequate perfusion of cerebral tissue which results, plays a significant role in post-ischemic cerebral damage.

This "no reflow" phenomenon develops within 1 to 2 hours of the ischemic insult. It is felt that most of the brain damage occurs during the post-ischemic period and not as a result of the initial ischemic episode.

The belief that cerebral edema is an important feature in the pathophysiology of hypoxic-ischemic injury and that it causes subsequent tissue necrosis by compromising cerebral blood flow is based on studies of term newborn monkeys. In these studies asphyxia has been severe and prolonged.(4,5) In addition, intracranial and mean arterial blood pressures were not monitored. It is consequently not clear from these data whether cerebral edema is a major cause of decreased cerebral blood flow. It is possible that the brain swelling might occur as a consequence of brain necrosis rather than being the major cause of necrosis after the asphyxial episode.(6)

In the preterm infant the primary target of hypoxic-ischemic injury is the periventricular germinal matrix. Asphyxia with its attendant hypoxia and hypercarbia may result in damage to and disruption of the endothelial lining of the fragile capillaries of the germinal matrix, and a loss of cerebral vascular autoregulation with a resulting increase in cerebral blood flow. Cerebral terminal arterioles, which are maximally dilated secondary to hypercapnea and have lost the ability to autoregulate blood flow, expose the capillaries of the subependymal germinal matrix to fluctuations in blood pressure and volume. These variations in the presence of endothelial damage may cause vessel rupture and subependymal and intraventricular hemorrhage. Factors that have been associated with intraventricular hemorrhage in the preterm infant include infusions of hypertonic sodium bicarbonate or dextrose, rapid plasma expansion, and sudden elevation of arterial or central venous pressures in association with hypoxia.

Treatment of Asphyxiated infants

Fluid balance. It is commonly believed that asphyxiated infants are usually hypotensive and hypovolemic. In fact, hypertension is occasionally seen in the first hours after birth, and hypervolemia has been documented in these neonates.(7) Animal experimentation has demonstrated that during hypoxia there is placental vasoconstriction with redistribution of blood to the fetus. Blood volume studies in infants with perinatal asphyxia have revealed greater red blood cell and plasma volumes than controls even with early cord clamping.(8)

The kidney of the neonate is frequently involved in the hypoxic-ischemic injury produced by perinatal asphyxia.(10,11) Asphyxia directly causes renal ischemia by hypoxemia and indirectly by producing hypotension with decreased renal blood flow. Acute tubular necrosis involving all parts of the tubule can occur after asphyxia, and the presence of cellular casts should be considered as evidence of possible renal tubular injury.(12) Perinatal asphyxia has also been implicated in the etiology of renal medullary necrosis and more rarely in necrosis of the renal pyramids.(13)

The clinical presentation of post-asphyxial renal failure initially includes an oliguric phase which may be of short duration and is frequently overshadowed by the infant's other difficulties. Elevation in the blood urea nitrogen and serum creatinine may be found, but proteinuria is a variable finding. Hematuria, although more common in renal vein thrombosis, may also occur with post-asphyxial renal injury. The presence of casts in the urine correlates strongly with perinatal distress. Edema or dehydration may also be present, since the kidney may be unable to maintain a normal sodium balance. With post-asphyxial renal injury, a polyuric phase may follow the initial oliguria.

In addition, fluid management may be further complicated in that many asphyxiated infants will sustain subendocardial and papillary muscle damage.(9) This myocardial dysfunction may be worsened by hypocalcemia or hypoglycemia which frequently accompanies perinatal asphyxia.

Fluids may be retained if renal failure occurs as a consequence of hypoxemia and renal ischemia. Inappropriate ADH syndrome frequently accompanies perinatal asphyxia resulting in oliguria with fluid retention.(14) This resultant increase in total body fluids may worsen heart failure, possibly increase cerebral edema and may also increase lung water. It is essential therefore to avoid overhydration of infants who sustained perinatal asphyxia. Close monitoring of cardiovascular function, urinary output, serum and urine osmolarity and body weight are essential to maintain a normal fluid balance. Daily fluid intake must be initially restricted to 40-60 ml/kg body weight until adequate diuresis is established. In cases of heart failure, inotropic agents such as dopamine or dobutamine may be indicated. Low dose dopamine (2.5 µg/kg/min) has been shown to improve myocardial function and glomerular filtration rate in asphyxiated infants.(15,16)

In view of the aforementioned factors, it can be assumed that volume expansion without clear cut evidence of volume depletion may aggravate the cardiogenic shock present in some severely asphyxiated infants and should be avoided. Excessive volume expansion may also over-distend the fragile vessels of the subependymal germinal matrix in the preterm infant and result in intraventricular hemorrhage. In fact, we have noted that rapid volume expansion given in the absence of clear cut evidence of shock is associated with massive IVH in small preterm infants.(17)

In trying to assess which infants need volume expansion, it is important to remember that clinically subjective data, such as skin perfusion and color are helpful, but may accompany disparate clinical entities (i.e., ventilator malfunction, pneumothorax, pneumopericardium, cardiogenic shock, malpositioned endotracheal tube, hypoglycemia, hypothermia and IVH).

Prior to plasma infusion ,central venous pressure measurements may be helpful in differentiating cardiogenic and hypovolemic shock so that fluid overload is avoided.

Stabilization after resuscitation should include close monitoring of arterial blood gases, arterial blood pressure, glucose, calcium and fluids. Restoration and maintenance of arterial blood pressure within normal limits during the post-ischemic period may improve recovery of neurologic function.

Another aspect of supportive care which is frequently ignored is the effect of head position on intracranial pressure. Infants at risk for intracranial hypertension should be maintained with their head in the midline position and the head of their bed elevated 30° as this results in a lower intracranial pressure than other positions.(18)

Seizure Control. Seizure activity increases oxygen consumption and can cause central nervous system damage. It is therefore recommended that convulsions secondary to perinatal asphyxia be controlled rapidly with phenobarbital given as 10 mg/kg infusions. This dosage should be repeated if seizures are not controlled. Diphenylhydantoin (10 mg/kg) should be given intravenously if seizures persist and may be repeated if further seizure control is warranted. In order to achieve therapeutic levels of these drugs,15-20 mg/kg doses should be given initially as a loading dose. The maintenance dose of each drug is 3 mg/kg/day.

Severe perinatal asphyxia often leads to seizure activity. In the majority of patients the diagnosis is obvious. However, in the neonate paralyzed in order to improve ventilation, the motor manifestations of seizures are absent. Seizure activity that is not accompanied by muscular activity may result in the same sequelae as those with motor activity. We have noted that seizure activity in the paralyzed infant may be accompanied by clinically significant periodic fluctuations in blood pressure, heart rate, oxygen saturation and transcutaneous oxygen that may be demonstrated by continuous monitoring.(19)

As mentioned previously, most damage occurs within 1-2 hours of the ischemic episode and not as a result of the initial insult. What therapies may be beneficial in preventing the damage which occurs, for the most part, secondary to cerebral edema and the "no reflow" phenomenon, are unproven in the neonate. Problems arise in evaluating these therapies because of the difficulty in selecting eligible patients who are at an increased risk for developing cerebral palsy.

Brain Resuscitation. At present,data supporting the superiority of any particular mode of therapy aimed at the physiologic sequelae of perinatal asphyxia are lacking. As a consequence of this, our therapy is directed towards stabilization, fluid restriction and arterial blood pressure control. The following is a discussion of the possible therapies that are available to decrease intracranial hypertension and lower cerebral metabolism after an asphyxial episode has occurred.

Hyperventilation. Hyperventilation reduces intracranial pressure (ICP) by constricting cerebral vessels and decreasing cerebral blood flow. Both of these effects will decrease the volume of cerebral blood. Reduction of PCO_2 from 40 to 20 mmHg results in a 40-50% decrease in cerebral blood flow in adults. Others have shown in normal preterm infants that with inhalation of CO_2, cerebral blood flow (CBF) increases 8.6% per mmHg $PaCO_2$ change, suggesting that CO_2 is an important regulator of CBF. These changes, however, may not occur in the asphyxiated neonate whose cerebral vessel may have lost the ability to regulate blood flow.

Hypothermia. It is hypothesized that the homeostatic mechanisms that compensate for cold stress are inactivated during severe asphyxia. The infant could, therefore, decrease his metabolic demands when temperature is lowered. Survival after asphyxia has been shown to be longest at 15°C body temperature in guinea pigs, kittens, rabbits and puppies.(20)

Hypothermia to 32°C has been useful in the treatment of cerebral edema secondary to head trauma, anoxia and encephalitis in adults and pediatric patients. Uncontrolled studies in the human neonate suggest that hypothermia may have a cerebral sparing effect post asphyxial insult. At present this mode of therapy cannot be recommended until more extensive work is done to elucidate the metabolic sequelae of hypothermia in the neonate.

Steroids. Steroids have been used extensively in the adult and older pediatric age groups in the treatment of cerebral edema. They have been found to be most effective when administered prophylactically. Newborn rats subjected to prolonged asphyxia showed increased brain water which can be prevented by pretreatment with dexamethasone. Treatment after the insult can prevent or reduce brain edema, but only when used in large doses. The mechanism by which steroids produce their beneficial effects in cerebral edema is unclear. Steroids are thought to stabilize cell membranes and lysosomes and decrease protein leakage through the "blood brain barrier". At the present time, convincing data and experience with steroids in the neonate are lacking and the potential side effect of high dose steroids caution against its uncontrolled usage.

Osmotic Therapy. Lasix and mannitol have been shown to act synergistically to produce greater reduction in ICP for longer periods of time than either therapy alone. The use of mannitol is fraught with many potential problems. IVH has been related to infusions of hypertonic sodium bicarbonate and dextrose. In patients with widespread "blood-brain barrier" disruption, mannitol may penetrate into the brain, aggravating rather than ameliorating existing cerebral edema. For this reason we would strongly caution against its use in the asphyxiated preterm infant.

Barbiturate Therapy. Barbiturate therapy has been shown to ameliorate brain damage post-circulatory arrest in experimental animals by the following mechanisms: reduction of cerebral metabolism, suppression of catecholamine-induced brain hypermetabolism, prevention of cell membrane destruction by active free radicals, diminution of intra- and extra-cellular water, prevention of convulsions, and diminution of intracranial pressure.

Investigators have noted that morbidity in patients with intracranial hypertension due to different etiologies was directly related to the control of intracranial pressure, and that barbiturates were effective in controlling this intracranial hypertension. Elevated ICP has also been noted in neonates after perinatal asphyxia, but no data are available at present regarding the effect of barbiturate therapy on ICP or neurologic outcome after an asphyxial event. For this reason their routine use cannot be recommended.

Central nervous system damage secondary to perinatal asphyxia has been discussed as occurring in two stages. The first occurs in utero and the second results from a sequence of physiologic changes that are the sequelae of the initial insult. If our resuscitative efforts are to be successful in ameliorating the primary and secondary effects of asphyxia, then resuscitative efforts must be organized and carried out by a skilled team. In addition, asphyxiated neonates at risk for long-term neurologic sequelae must be identified early so that various modes of advanced brain resuscitation can be evaluated in a controlled manner.

REFERENCES

1. Windle WF: Brain damage by asphyxia at birth. Sci Am, 221:76, 1969.
2. Bancalari E, Goldberg RN: Perinatal asphyxia and meconium aspiration. The diagnosis and management of respiratory disorders in the newborn. Ed by L Stern, Addison-Wesley Publishing Co. (in press)
3. Nemoto EM: Pathogenesis of cerebral ischemia. Crit Care Med, 6:203, 1978.
4. Myers RE, Beard R, Adamsons K: Brain swelling in the newborn versus monkey following prolonged partial asphyxia. Neurology, 19:1012, 1969.
5. Selzer ME, Myers RG, Holstein SB: Prolonged partial asphyxia: Effects on fetal brain water and electrolytes. Neurology, 22:732, 1972.

6. Volpe JJ: Neurology of the newborn. Philadelphia: W.B. Saunders, 1981, p 163.
7. Yao AC, Lind J: Blood volume in the asphyxiated term neonate. Biol Neonate, 21:199, 1972.
8. Oh W, Omori K, Emmanouilides G, et al: Placenta to lamb fetus transfusion in utero during acute hypoxia. Am J Obstet Gynecol, 122:316, 1975.
9. Setzer E, Ermocilla R, Tonkin I, et al: Papillary muscle necrosis in a neonatal autopsy population: Incidence and associated clinical manifestations. J Pediatr, 96:289, 1980.
10. Dauber IM, Krauss AN, Symchych PS, et al: Renal failure following perinatal anoxia. J Pediatr, 88:851, 1976.
11. Daniel SS, Husain MK, Milliez J, et al: Renal response to fetal lamb occlusion of umbilical cord. Am J Obstet Gynecol, 131:514, 1978.
12. Tan K, Hull D: The excretion of cells in urine following perinatal asphyxia. Pediat Res, 3:228, 1969.
13. Anand SK, Northway JD, Smith JA: Neonatal renal papillary and cortical necrosis. Am J Dis Chil, 131:773, 1977.
14. Feldman W, Drummond KN, Klein M: Hyponatremia following asphyxia neonatorum. Acta Paediat Scand, 59:52, 1970.
15. DiSessa TG, Leitner M, Ching CT, et al: The cardiovascular effects of dopamine in the severely asphyxiated neonate. J Pediatr, 99:772, 1981.
16. Leitner MJ, Mc Neal R, Knapp RA, et al: Glomerular filtration rate in the severely asphyxiated neonate treated with dopamine. Pediatr Res, 14:622, 1980.
17. Goldberg RN, Chung D, Goldman SL, et al: The association of volume expansion and intraventricular hemorrhage. J Pediatr, 96:1060, 1980.
18. Goldberg RN, Joshi A, Moscoso P, et al: The effect of head position on intracranial pressure in the neonate. Crit Care Med (in press).
19. Goldberg RN, Feller R, Goldman SL: Detection of seizure activity in the paralyzed neonate. Pediatrics, 69:583, 1982.
20. Westin B, Nyberg R, Miller JA, et al: Hypothermia and transfusion with oxygenated blood in the treatment of asphyxia neonatorum. Acta Paediatr Scand, Suppl 139:7, 1962.

SEIZURES IN RENAL DISEASES

Richard G. Curless, M.D.

Seizures occurring as a complication of chronic renal failure represent part of the generalized encephalopathy which occurs in about 15% of children with prolonged renal dysfunction (1,2). Clinical epileptiform activity often follows myoclonus and is almost always generalized in nature. Focal seizures suggest structural brain disease such as that produced by a major intra - cerebral hemorrhage. In 1977 Foley described a progressive encephalopathy in 5 of 35 infants and children with chronic renal failure; their age range was 9 months to 5 years . The symptoms occurred from 4 to 5 years following the initial diagnosis of renal disease. The onset of symptoms could not be related to dialysis, hypertension, or the duration of renal failure. All of the patients had evidence of slowing on EEG in addition to polyspike activity which became worse on repeated records. Only 2 of the 5 children responded well to anticonvulsants. Finally, the 2 patients in Foley's series which were transplanted did not demonstrate improvement in terms of the neurological signs and symptoms of encephalopathy.

Encephalopathy in chronic renal failure may be related to a number of features including 1) uremia, 2) calcium dysmetabolism, 3) hypertension, 4) dialysis, or 5) heavy metal intoxication, in particular aluminum. The question of whether or not uremia is important in the development of cerebral symptomatology remains uncertain since the BUN may be as low as 25 or as high as 400 at the time of neurological symptomatology. Calcium metabolism problems may occasionally contribute in a dramatic fashion. While an elevated parathyroid hormone in conjunction with a normal or low calcium is common in chronic renal failure, an occasional patient has high serum calcium along with a high PTH at the time of encephalopathic symptomatology. In these unusual cases a parathyroidectomy may produce a significant benefit in cerebral function (2,3).

Hypertensive encephalopathy may be manifested by 1) headache and altered consciousness, 2) nausea and vomiting with associated visual disturbances, 3) generalized seizures or 4) focal neurological signs and symptoms including focal seizures. In a recent review emphasizing clinical pathological correlation, Chester et al. identified 20 cases with post mortem results (4). In addition to the symptoms and signs just mentioned, they pointed out that all of these adults had opthalmological changes generally associated with hypertension and all had significant uremia. Symptoms 1 and 2 were the most common and the visual disturbances were described as principally blurred vision. Seizures and vocal findings were considerably less common than categories 1 or 2. The neuropathological findings in all cases included fibrinoid necrosis of the arterioles, thrombosis of arterioles and capillaries, micro-infarcts, and petechial hemorrhages. No significant edema was noted.

Another author reported on 9 children with significant hypertension secondary to renal disease associated with neurological signs or symptoms. The most pronounced features in these children were altered mental status and bilateral upper motor neuron signs. The optic fundi were normal in 6, with papilledema present in 2 and flame hemorrhages present in 1. Two of these 9 children had abnormal CT scans with a hemorrhage in 1 and a large area of decreased attenuation in another. Of significance is the fact that all 9 children recovered without neurological residual (5).

The disequilibrium syndrome or dialysis encephalopathy has no single proven etiology. The areas receiving consideration over the past several years include dopamine depletion, slow virus infection, asparagine deficiency, potassium dilution or depletion, rapid change in acid base balance, urea lag, or heavy metal accumulation. It is of interest that in one study serial EEGs appeared to predict the development of encephalopathy in several patients by the appearance of diffuse slowing with spike and wave abnormalities several days prior to neurological symptomatology (6).

There are a number of reports which weave together a body of evidence in support of aluminum as being an important consideration. The features which make aluminum toxicity an important cause include: the syndrome is most common in areas with a high aluminum in the city water, there are several reported cases which improved after decreasing the aluminum intake, in more than one case a blood aluminum level of well over the normal range of 40 was discovered during the encephalopathic symptomatology, and the neuropathological picture fails to demonstrate any structural cause suggesting a metabolic or toxic etiology (6). It should also be pointed out that animal work initially performed some 40 years ago clearly indicates that if aluminum is directly applied to the cerebral cortex an epileptiform model is produced (7).

Other studies have shed doubt on the aluminum theory. There are a number of published cases with a normal blood aluminum during neurological symptomatology (2). In one child the post mortem evaluation of brain aluminum levels failed to reveal any significant elevation. Similarly, in the series by Foley, mentioned earlier, aluminum phosphate binding gel was used in all 35 children while only 5 developed encephalopathy, unfortunately no aluminum levels were obtained (1)

The kinetic patterns of anticonvulsants in the presence of renal failure have been inadequately evaluated. Only phenytoin has been studied to a significant degree. This drug is 90% protein bound, but in uremia or following dialysis there may be a 30% unbound fraction . Therefore, therapeutic levels of 5 to 10 micrograms per ml are acceptable rather than the usual 10 to 20. As a general rule these values can be obtained without adjusting the phenytoin dosages. Uremia and/or dialysis also reduces the adult T-½ from the usual +24 hours to approximately 8 hours. No good studies of T-½ are available in children. This necessitates a minimum of Q8h dosing. It has also been shown that total phenytoin does not dialyze to a significant degree so that no dosage change is necessary during dialysis (8).

Valproic acid may have a pattern similar to phenytoin since it is also 90% protein bound. However, there are no good studies of kinetics in patients with renal disease. Unfortunately, there is also very little information on the other commonly used drugs including phenobarbital, primidone (Mysoline), carbamazepine (Tegretol), ethosuximide (Zarontin), or clonazepam (Clonopin). Relatively little Clonopin or Zarontin is excreted in the kidneys suggesting the likelihood of minimal effect in chronic renal failure. However, no in-depth studies are available for any of these modes of therapy.

In summary, approximately 15% of children with chronic renal failure will develop an encephalopathy which may include seizures. How frequently dialysis or aluminum provide a major contribution is unclear; however hypertension and uremia may not be major contributors.

REFERENCES

1. Foley, C.M. et al. The Encephalopathy of Chronic Renal Failure in Childhood. Ann. Neurol (Abst.) #2, 254, 1977.
2. Geary, P.F. et al. Encephalopathy in Children with Chronic Renal Failure. J. Ped. 97: 41, 1980.
3. Tyler, H.R. Neurologic Disorders in Renal Failure. Am. J. Med. 44: 734, 1968.
4. Chester, E.M. et al. Hypertensive Encephalopathy: A Clinicopathologic Study of 20 Cases. Neurology 28: 928, 1978.
5. Benjamin, D. Hypertensive Encephalopathy in Children. Abs 80; Child Neurol. Soc. 1980; Pub. in program only.
6. Dunen, G. et al. Role of Aluminum in Dialysis Dementia. Ann. Int. Med. 88: 502, 1978.
7. Kopeloff, L.M. et al. Recurrent Convulsive Seizures in Animals Produced by Immunologic and Chemical Means. Am. J. Psych. 98: 881, 1942.
8. Asconape, J.J. and Penry, J.K. Use of Antiepileptic Drugs in the Presence of Liver and Kidney Diseases: A Review. Epilepsia 23 (Suppl. 1): 565, 1982.

ABDOMINAL MASS IN THE NEWBORN

Jorge L. Lockhart, M.D. and Robert K. Rhamy, M.D.

Among all abdominal masses in newborns, more than half are of non-surgical nature, and of those which are surgical, more than half originate in the urinary tract.

Accurate diagnosis is essential, and in some children, we have the diagnosis of a mass and the nature of this mass made in the intra-uterine period through ultrasonography. If this is the case, intervention can be done during the intra-uterine period or we can proceed with immediate evaluation and treatment in the newborn.

Physical examination of the newborn will detect the nature of the mass in many instances. In the newborn, the kidneys are normally in a relatively low position and are readily palpable. Dehydration or emaciation may result in less resistance of subcutaneous tissue, allowing the kidneys to be more easily felt. In the newborn the kidney retains its fetal lobulations and these can be palpated, especially when there is any renal enlargement. Obviously, the ectopic kidney can easily be palpated as a mass, usually located in the region of the pelvis.

After palpation of the abdomen, transillumination of the mass should be attempted. Urinary obstructive lesions and cystic lesions of the kidneys can readily be evaluated by transillumination. To transilluminate the abdomen, the child is placed in the lateral decubitus position. The end of a fiberoptic probe is placed in the upper quadrant of the side of the abdomen which is in a superior position. Pressure with the probe will displace the loops of bowel and the observer views the costovertebral angle from the posterior side. Presence of a hydronephrotic kidney, cystic renal structures or solid tumors can be readily discerned by this procedure. The accuracy is very good by this method, but infantile polycystic disease of the kidneys (Potter's Type I) is not easily identified by transillumination in children less than one year of age. Transillumination may also demonstrate hydroureter on occasion, but with less accuracy. The bladder in the neonate is readily transilluminated in almost all children. Abnormal enlargement can easily be demonstrated. The bladder descends in the pelvis normally and becomes much more difficult to transilluminate after age one year.

Ultrasonography provides a valuable tool with no radiation exposure and also has the advantage of being non-invasive. The technique essentially is as done in the adult with the child usually being placed in the prone position. In young infants, sedation may be necessary for adequate examination. In neonates, a 5 NHz transducer is best, while in children a little older, a 3.5 NHz transducer is used. This provides a higher frequency for the probe than the standard 2.25 NHz used in teenagers and adults. Localization of the kidneys with transverse scans is done with several longitudinal cuts at 0.5 centimeters intervals. The right kidney may be separated from the liver by doing the examination in the supine position,

Major Abdominal Masses in the Neonate

URINARY	GASTROINTESTINAL	GENITAL	LIVER AND BILE DUCTS	MISCELLANEOUS
Midline	Meconium	Hydrocolpos	Subcapsular hematoma	Adrenal hematoma
Bladder	Imperforate anus			
Urachal cyst	Meconium plug syndrome	Ovarian cyst		Neuroblastoma
Urachal diverticulum			Choledochal cyst	
		Meconium ileus		Sacrococcygeal teratoma
Bilateral flank	Duplication of bowel	Primary hamartoma	Hemangio-endothelioma	
Hydronephrosis				Hepatoma
-with posterior urethral valves	Mesenteric cyst			
			Cystic disease	Splenic hematoma
-with ureteroceles	Pyloric stenosis			
Hydroureters				Splenic cyst
Polycystic disease	Intussusception			
Unilateral flank				
Multicystic kidney				
Hydronephrosis				
Mesoblastic nephroma				
Engorged kidney (renal vein thrombosis)				
Wilms' Tumor				

while the left kidney may be separated from the spleen by doing the examination in the right lateral decubitus position. Adequate examination differentiates solid from cystic lesions, if the masses are cystic; ultrasonography also establishes if it is a solitary or multiple cystic disease and its contour. Among the solid masses, it determines if the lesion is renal or extra-renal. In neonates with non-visualization of the collecting system on excretory urography, ultrasonography will establish the presence or absence of the kidney and in some instances, the nature or the etiology of the non visualization.

The conventional standard of radiographic evaluation of the abdomen, the KUB,may reveal much information concerning the location and the diagnosis of the mass. The KUB should be inspected for detail of soft tissue and bony structures. The position of the bowel gas with any displacement of the bowel gas will facilitate determining the location and the extent of the mass. The nature, the type and the position of any calcifications are helpful in discerning the type of mass.
mass

The initial evaluation of renal function is determined by radionuclear studies. This is a much more accurate way of determining the amount of renal function, the distribution of function between the two kidneys, and the degree of vascular flow and the gross appearance of the urinary tract. We prefer this method of evaluation over the injection of iodinated contrast materials, since the iodine compounds are poorly concentrated and excreted in infants and sometimes the gas patterns impair an adequate evaluation and visualization of the urinary tract. The radionuclear isotopes give much less radiation, they by-pass the intra-abdominal gas and permit a better determination of renal function. Against the radionuclear scan and the renogram would be the fact that the urinary tract anatomy is less well delineated. Isotopic cystography is a valuable form of investigation to detect or to rule out vesicoureteral reflux. Because of the accuracy of other tests, cystourethroscopy with retrograde filling of the catheters with contrast media is, at the present time, because of these newer diagnostic modalities,rarely indicated. Computerized tomography is being investigated for its use in the diagnosis of abdominal masses in the neonate and can provide useful information in some isolated cases. The newer CT scanning equipment with its decreased time for each cut and the increased delineation,with the ability to make cuts closer to one another, have increased its accuracy, but usually still requires some sedation in order to facilitate its performance. Against CT scanning is the fact that there is a scarcity of fatty tissue between the organs of the newborn, making delineation between these areas more difficult.

Percutaneous puncture of a cystic mass associated with the injection of contrast media can provide both a diagnostic and a therapeutic solution to difficult clinical situations. This is of particular value in obstructive hydronephrosis when the point of obstruction cannot be clearly established by other examinations and at the same time, percutaneous puncture will provide adequate decompression of the collecting system, prior to considering an open surgical procedure. Other useful tests are renal arteriography, particularly when partial nephrectomy or surgery in solitary kidneys is being considered; inferior venacavography in the presence of tumor in order to determine whether or not there has been tumor extension and/or invasion into the inferior vena cava.Both of these procedures, particularly renal arteriography, are being used with much less frequency at the present time. If a neuroblastoma is found to be present, biopsies of the bone marrow and/or any skeletal lesions are essential. The most common abdominal mass in the neonate is the multicystic kidney and throughout the first month of life, up to six months of life, hydronephrosis predominates. In bilateral cystic lesions, we should consider hydronephrosis, multicystic kidneys and polycystic disease. Among the solid masses, the mesoblastic nephroma predominates, although the surgeon should ascertain the presence of a neuroblastoma because of its ominous prognosis. Abdominal masses in children are rarely surgical emergencies. In a case of cystic lesions, satisfactory drainage with decompression of the urinary tract and improvement of renal function can initially be achieved and surgery delayed until after the neonatal period. The most common clinical emergency due to cystic masses is in boys with urethral valves and in the girls with bilateral ureteroceles. In both situations, initial treatment should be correction of the electrolyte imbalance and elimination of the sepsis simultaneous with the provision of drainage of the urinary system. Particular emphasis should be done for the case with a multicystic kidney. Surgery should be done when the lesion is infected, when it produces elevation of the blood pressure, or other problems, such as gastrointestinal symptoms, related to a large space-occupying lesion in the abdomen. Those are the only situations in which early surgery should be considered. Since the multicystic kidney is a functionless mass of dysplastic tissue and chances of malignancy do exist, later surgery should be considered. However, a non-symptomatic, multicystic kidney is not an emergency and we believe should be delayed until after the infancy period.

REFERENCES

Pediatric Transillumination. Steven M. Dorn and Lawrence R. Kubus. Yearbook Publishers Inc. New York, 1983.

Ultrasound in Urology. Martin I. Resnick and Roger C. Sanders. Williams and Wilkins Co. Baltimore, 1979.

Pediatric Urology. S. Innes Williams. Appleton-Century-Crofts. London, 1968.

Visible and Palpable Lesions in Children. C. Everett Koop. Grune and Stratton, New York, 1976.

Palpable Abdominal Masses in Infants and Children: A report based on a review of 653 cases. Meyer E. Melicow and Aurelio C. Uson. J. Urol. 81:705, 1959.

Near-Drowning and The Kidney

Bernard M. Holzman, M.D.

The problem of immersion incidents and the consequences produced by them, commonly called drowning and near-drowning, have been discussed at great length in the literature since the first monograph on the subject, written by Dr. Jerome Modell, was published in 1971 (1). Although numerous articles had previously appeared, the work by Modell provided the first comprehensive review of the problem. It is this body of information which has formed the foundation for, and has established many of the principles upon which current treatment is based.

The Magnitude of the Problem

Drownings are responsible for 10% of the accidental deaths which occur in the United States annually. Nationally each year more than 7000 people die as a result of immersion incidents in bodies of water. Children are the most common victims with 40% of all drownings occurring in children under 4 years of age, and a further 15 to 20% occurring in the 5-20 year age group. Three of 4 victims are males. Almost half of all pool drownings occur in home pools, 10% in motel or hotel pools, 10% in pools of multiple dwellings and 20% at public facilities.

In Florida, amongst children under 14 years of age, drowning is the third leading cause of death from any means, coming just after neonatal deaths and automobile accidents (2). In Miami, despite it's coastal location, only 10% of the total immersion incidents in children occur in salt water. In this area, because of its unique lifestyle centered around the water, the common sites of immersion incidents primarily occur in and around the home with over 70% occuring in bodies of water within the confines of the private residence including home pools, bathtubs, buckets of water and toilets. Even more distressing is that over half of the victims of near drowning are children under the age of three years (Table 1). Clearly, the problem is in large measure one of inadequate

Table 1. Near Drowning - Body of Water

1970-1980 UM/JM

CHILDREN		99 (73.3%)
0 - 36 mos.	56 (56.6%)	
36 mos. - 10 yrs.	26 (26.3%)	
10 - 16 yrs.	17 (17.1%)	
ADULTS (> 16 years)		26 (26.7%)
TOTAL		125 (100%)

supervision. Equally distressing, and somewhat more pertinent to the discussion at hand,is that 20% of all children who are removed from bodies of water following an immersion incident ultimately die or are severely damaged neurologically (2,3).

Terminology

The first step in understanding this subject is to be familiar with the terms which are conventionally used (Table 2), as they were first

Table 2. Conventional Terms

Drowning
Near drowning
Drowning with apiration
Drowning without aspiration
Near drowning with aspiration
Near drowning without aspiration
Delayed death subsequent to near drowning
Secondary drowning

proposed by Dr. Modell (1). Drowning implies death by suffocation as a result of immersion in a liquid media. Near-drowning implies a period of viability following removal from the liquid media, and if death then ultimately occurs it is called a delayed death subsequent to near-drowning. In addition to this distinction between drowning and near-drowning, consideration is also given to whether there has been aspiration of the fluid media into the lungs. Secondary drowning is used by some (4), although not Dr. Modell, to describe a deterioration of pulmonary function that follows deficient gas exchange due to loss or inactivation of surfactant.

There is a growing feeling amongst some (5), however, that this myriad of terms should be discarded and the event simply described as an immersion incident, specifying the pathophysiologic problem which results, whether it is an aspiration pneumonia, hypoxic encephalopathy, or water intoxication.

Pathophysiology

Much of the current thinking about the pathophysiology which results from an immersion incident stems from a series of animal experiments done by Dr. Modell and his colleagues which are concisely summarized in his monograph (1). These experiments described many of the changes which occurred when different fluid media were instilled into the intubated trachea of anesthetized animals.

Within three minutes of fresh water being instilled into the trachea of an intubated dog, the blood volume of the animal increased, and the magnitude of the increase in the blood volume was directly proportional to the volume of fluid instilled into the trachea (6). Not only did the blood volume increase, but the free plasma hemoglobin concentration rose as well. Clearly, there appears to be some absorption of the hypotonic fresh water from the alveolus, transversing the alveolar-capillary membrane and entering the intravascular space (Figure 1), thus expanding the blood volume and leading to lysis of red cells and release of hemoglobin into the plasma.

Figure 1.

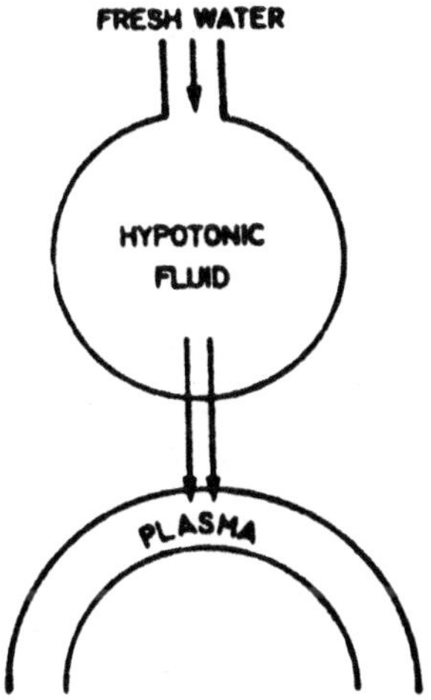

If this is the case when fresh-water is instilled into the intubated trachea, then one might expect instillation of salt water to produce consequences which are opposite (Figure 2). When the whole blood density is measured, and compared following the instillation of fresh or salt water, one sees an increase in the blood density following instillation of salt water, and a decrease after fresh water is instilled (7). As with fresh water, there is a shift of free water, although this time the water flows from the plasma space into the more hypertonic alveolar space. In the case of salt water instillation, there is a shift of various ions and electrolytes from the hypertonic alveolar fluid into the plasma (8). The end result then, is that the plasma electrolyte concentration increases following instillation of salt water into the intubated trachea of the anesthetized animal, and falls following instillation of fresh water (6,9).

Figure 2.

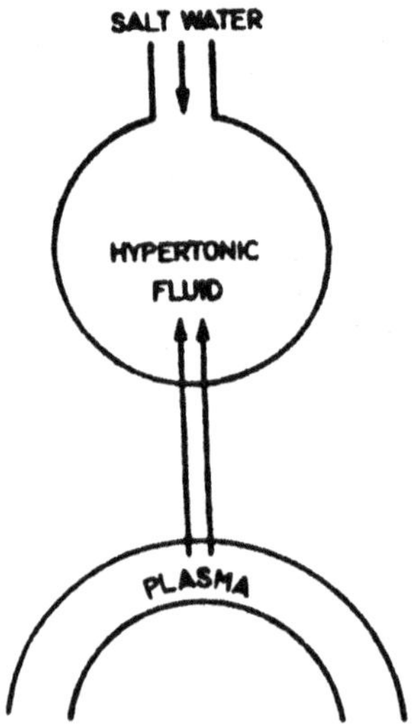

The Human Experience

The next step in the scientific method is to apply data derived in the laboratory animal to humans. If we again examine electrolyte concentrations, but this time look at humans who have died as a direct result of the immersion incident, that is, drowning victims, we can see that the electrolyte concentrations differ depending on the fluid media in which the person drowned, and parallel in a nearly identical manner the information which was derived from dogs. Those individuals who have drowned in fresh water had lower than normal electrolyte concentrations, and those who met their demise in salt water had higher concentrations of electrolytes in their serum (10). In going further, however, keep in mind these are individuals who had died as an immediate consequence of their immersion in a fluid medium.

Examining the electrolyte concentrations of survivors of immersion incidents, near-drowning victims, we fail to find any significant difference between serum electrolyte concentrations regardless of the tonicity of the fluid media in which the incident occurred (3).

This discrepancy between the animal and human drowning data, and the data in near-drowning victims can be explained by several factors. First, the animal data were delivered by instilling upwards of 22 ml of fluid per kilogram of body weight into the endotracheal tube (6). This volume is an extremely large volume, one which is twice normal human tidal volume and approaches total lung capacity. It is unlikely that this volume could be aspirated in the clinical situation. Secondly, by the time the near drowning victim arrives to the emergency room, there has been sufficient time for equilibration to have occurred,and the electrolyte concentrations are at or close to normal values. And in the case of children, we feel there is a third, and most important reason which accounts for this lack of difference between the consequence of salt water immersions and those in fresh water. We feel that children develop acute laryngospasm as they are submerged, and thus, rather than aspirating fluid,suffocate by virtue of an obstructed airway. Others have shown that reflex airway closure occurs from aspiration of fluid (11), and Modell estimates that even in the case of adults, some 10-15% of patients undergo laryngospasm and fail to aspirate fluid (1). Furthermore,it appears that even those adult drowning victims who die, and have obvious changes associated with apiration of fluid into the lungs, initially close their glottis as they begin to suffocate, and it is only as a preterminal event that the glottis relaxes and the natural elasticity of their adult chest wall draws fluid into the airway and fills the lungs. And, in fact, it is only those individuals who have died while in the fluid medium who do demonstrate changes in serum electrolyte concentrations (10). Children have significant differences in chest wall elasticity which does not favor this inflow of fluid in the flacid state. Additionally, their more vigorous glottic closure mechanism may also contribute to the infrequency of fluid aspiration in cases of childhood immersion incidents. Indeed, there is highly suggestive indirect evidence in the literature to support this contention (2,3). Fandell and Bancalari (2) in a review of 34 pediatric patients who were victims of immersion incidents,demonstrated that less than half had any radiographic evidence of aspiration of fluid, and less than one-quarter had any clinical signs or symptoms consistent with aspiration of fluid or pulmonary edema.

Certainly it is not uncommon to see patients who present in the emergency room after fresh water immersion incidents, and have clear chest radiographs when they arrive, only to develop signs of increasing lung water 6 to 12 hours later. If, in fact, a significant volume of fresh water is aspirated, and finds its way first into the alveoli and then into the vascular space, one would expect initial radiographs to have more evidence of increased lung water. Once the fluid has been absorbed into the vascular space, radiographs taken 6 to 12 hours after the incident should be clear. This, in fact, does not occur. It is the subsequent films which invariably have more evidence of increased pulmonary water. In fact, if we examine the electrolyte concentrations of children at presentation to the emergency room,we find there is no significant difference between fresh water and salt water immersion incidents (3). Neither is significantly abnormal, implying that no significant aspiration of fluid occurs.

We feel that rather than being primarily a lung process, near-drowning in children is primarily an entity in which the morbidity and mortality results almost solely from hypoxia. And in most cases the hypoxia is the result of laryngospasm. When the trachea of dogs is acutely obstructed the PaO_2 falls very rapidly while the $PaCO_2$ rises more slowly (1). It is this rapid fall in the PaO_2 which results in severe neurologic injury, and which, in part, is the cause of the renal injury which occurs. In fact, in reviewing the literature it is evident that it is the extent of the neurologic injury which is the determinant of the ultimate outcome (2,12). In the child the outcome clearly does not relate to the lungs. Fandel and Bancalari (2) found that the morbidity and mortality following immersion incidents related directly to the neurologic status at the time of presentation. Those patients who were comatose on admission, following resuscitation,had poor ultimate outcomes. Jim Orlowski (13) has developed a prognostic scoring system (Table 3) which is

Table 3. Prognositc Scoring System in Drowning

Age less than 3 years.

Estimated maximum submersion time greater than 5 minutes.

No attempt at mouth-to-mouth at the scene.

Patient in coma with fixed and dilated pupils on admission.

Arterial pH < 7.10

One point for each.

Score less than or equal to 2 = 90% chance of recovery.

Score greater than 2 = 5% chance of recovery.

---

from Orlowski, Critical Care Medicine 6:94, 1978.

intended to be applied to patients at the time they arrive to the emergency room. With careful examination of these factors, however, it is evident that each specifically relates to the degree of hypoxia to which the patient has been exposed. As can be seen, the second and last items relate to the length of time the patient was hypoxic. The age is important, not because of a greater sensitivity of the young brain to hypoxia, but rather because the immersion incidents of young children occur in an environment where there are no other individuals around. These young children wander away from supervision and are not removed from the water until someone notices that they are missing and begins to look for them. They inevitably remain in the water for far longer periods of time than do older children whose immersion incidents occur in the presence of possible rescuers and therefore are removed from the water far more expeditiously. It is obvious that the number of these prognostic factors which directly apply to a patient relates directly to the risk of death.

Renal Effects of Immersion Incidents

The renal consequence of immersion incidents relates to two general factors: those as a consequence of the incident itself and those which are consequences of our therapy (Table 4).

By far, the most important cause of renal injury following immersion incidents is tissue hypoxia. This hypoxia, in children, seems to be primarily caused by larygospasm, as discussed, and in contradistinction to the case with adults where the hypoxia seems related to aspiration of the

Table 4. Renal Consequences of Immersion Incidents in Children

I. Tissue hypoxia at time of incident
   a. asphyxia secondary to laryngospasm/alveolar filling
   b. hypoxia/ischemia secondary to cardiac arrest
   c. ischemia secondary to diving reflex

II. Consequence of therapy
   a. mannitol
   b. bicarbonate
   c. therapeutic dehydration
   d. PEEP (?)

III. Theoretic factors
   a. hemoglobinuria
   b. myoglobinuria

---

fluid media. In a review of pediatric immersion victims seen at the University of Miami (Table 5) hypoxia severe enough to cause central nervous system injury occurred in 30% of all victims, yet there was evidence of aspiration of the fluid media in only 12% of the patients.

Table 5. Near Drowning

Primary System Affected on Admission

1970-1980 UM/JM	Children	
Asymptomatic	30	(30.3%)
CNS only	27	(27.3%)
CNS and pulmonary	3	(3.0%)
Pulmonary only-clinical disease	9	(9.1%)
- x-ray only	30	(30.3%)
TOTAL	99	(100%)

Clearly, the hypoxia occurs without fluid aspiration as a consequence of laryngospasm. In many patients the hypoxia is further complicated by ischemia resulting from cardiac arrest. Even in those patients in whom cardiac arrest does not occur, there may be hypoxic injury to the kidneys, as well as other organ systems such as the bowel. It seems likely, at least in part, that the mechanism of this injury is that the immersion incident elicits a diving reflex (14) which augments the tissue hypoxia resulting from laryngospasm. The diving reflex, which is highly developed in deep diving aquatic mammals such as seals and dolphins, redistributes cardiac output preferentially away from the bowel, kidney and skin and toward the heart and brain (15). Numerous studies have shown that vagal bradycardia in man can be produced by the immersion of the face in cold water, and in fact, this has been used therapeutically to terminate supraventricular tachycardia in children (16-19). Goodwin (14) demonstrated evidence of acute tubular necrosis in patients following immersion incidents which were not associated with any evidence of hypoxic injury to the brain. By using a radioisotopic technique in volunteers, he demonstrated that when the face was immersed in cold water there was ischemia to the kidney, while their cognitive function remained normal, implying a reflex decrease in renal perfusion with preservation of blood flow to the brain.

Other causes of renal injury are listed in table 4. Hemoglobinuria resulting from hemolysis induced as hypotonic fresh water is absorbed from the alveolus has been demonstrated experimentally in animals (20,21) and an increase in free plasma hemoglobin has been documented in man (22). However, we feel this problem, at least in children, is more theoretic than real in that we have been unable to document any cases of hemoglobinuria in the 135 cases of immersion incidents which we have reviewed to date.

Complications of overly vigorous therapy have become increasingly more common as measures designed to control increased intracranial pressure have come into our therapeutic armamentarium. Osmotic diuresis with mannitol, and therapeutic dehydration have led to acute tubular necrosis and renal failure, most likely by means of significant decreases in glomerular filtration rate and damage to tubular cells.

Conclusion

One final note is appropriate in closing. There recently has been a suggestion that with the development of prognostic scoring systems which can be applied soon after resuscitation, one can project the recoverability of patients, and then can allocate scarce resources to those patients who have the potential to recover. While the scarcity of resources is, no doubt, eventually going to mandate some sort of triage for patients, such criteria must be very selectively and carefully applied to pediatric patients who are victims of immersion incidents. A case in point is illustrated by a case report (table 6). This child was 10 months old when she fell off a houseboat into the Miami River. By best estimates she was in the water in excess of 10 minutes and the initial arterial blood gas and physical findings supported this estimate. When she arrived

---

Table 6.

KN: 10 month old female - near drowning/Miami River
Estimated submersion time - 10 minutes
CPR by Fire Rescue - 10 minutes
CPR in Emergency Room - 45 minutes
Initial laboratory values
ABG (FiO_2=0.7) pH 6.68, $PaCO_2$ 72, HCO_3 8, BE - 27
Serum: Na=134, K=3.9, Cl=95, CO_2=15, BUN=12
Examination: Areflexic, apneic, flacid , no response to pain, pupils fixed and dilated.
Mechanical ventilation 6 days
Hospitalized 34 days

---

in the emergency room she was in complete cardiopulmonary arrest, with fixed and dilated pupils and severely acidotic. Following resuscitation she was begun on a program of brain resuscitation which included mechanical hyperventilation, envolemic dehydration and osmotic diuresis, and control of intracranial pressure with high dose barbiturate infusion and hypothermia (table 7). At the time of her discharge from the hospital she had reasonably normal brain stem function, but very poor motor control and minimal responsiveness to the environment. She was begun on a program of early stimulation and she has remained in this program for three years. She is now a precocious three and a half year old child whose only neurologic deficit is a slightly broad-based gait and a mild degree of hyperactivity. Even though cases like this are certainly not the majority, they do occur with sufficient regularity to warrant complete efforts on any child who is resuscitated in the emergency room following an immersion incident.

Table 7. Standard Therapy of ACI Patients

Head Position

Controlled Intubation (Sedation/Paralysis)

Antacid Therapy

Fluid Restriction

Mechanical Hyperventilation ($PaCO_2$ = 25 - 27 torr)

Steroids - Decadron

Paralysis and Sedation

Mannitol (Serum Osmolarity = 310 - 320 mOsm/L

Normothermia

Barbiturate Coma - Pentobarbital - Loading
dose 3-4 mg/kg over 5-10 minutes followed
by constant infusion 1-4 mg/kg/hr.
Serum Pentobarbital level 2.5-5.5 mg/dl

Hypothermia - surface cooling to 34° C (94° F)

References

1. Modell, J.H.: The pathophysiology and treatment of drowning and near-drowning. Charles C. Thomas, Springfield, Ill., 1971.

2. Fandel, I., Bancalari, E.: Near-drowning in children: clincal aspects. Pediatrics 58:573-579, 1976.

3. Peterson, B.: Morbidity of childhood near-drowning. Pediatrics 59:364-370, 1977.

4. Jacobsen, J.B., Neilson, H., Ringsted, C., Anderson, P.K.L.: Drowning and near-drowning. Crit. Car. Med. 8:529-530, 1980.

5. Pearn, J.H.: Secondary drowning in children. Brit. Med. J. 281: 1103-1105, 1980.

6. Modell, J.H., Moya, F.: Effects of volume of aspirated fluid during chlorinated fresh water drowning. Anesthesiology 27:662-672, 1966.

7. Swann, H.G., Brucer, M., Moore, C., Venzien, B.C.: Fresh water and sea water drowning: a study of the terminal cardiac and biochemical events. Texas Rep. Biol. Med. 5:423-437, 1947.

8. Redding, J.S., Cozine, R.A., Voigt, G.C., Safar, R.: Resuscitation from

drowning. J.A.M.A. 178:1136, 1961.

9. Modell, J.H., Moya, F., Newby, E.J., Ruis, B.C., Showers, A.V.: The effects of fluid volume in sea water drowning. Ann. Intern. Med. 67: 68-80, 1967.

10. Modell, J.H., Davis, J.H.: Electrolyte changes in human drowning victims. Anesthesiology 30:414-420, 1969.

11. Colebatch, H.J.H., Halmagyi, D.F.J.: Reflex airway reaction to fluid aspiration. J. Appl. Physiol. 17:787-794, 1962.

12. Conn, A.W., Montes, J.E., Barker, G.A., Edmonds, J.F.: Cerebral salvage in near-drowning following neurologic classification by triage. Can. Anaesth. Soc. J. 27:201-210, 1980.

13. Orlowski, J.P.: Prognostic factors in pediatric cases of drowning and near-drowning. J.A.C.E.P. 8:176-179, 1979.

14. Goodwin, N.M.: The importance of the diving reflex in man in relation to near-drowning and resuscitation. Crit. Care Med. 8:226, 1980.

15. Yoncey, L.R., Falkow, B.: The integration of the cardiovascular response to diving. Am. Heart J. 79:1-4, 1970.

16. Mathew, P.K.: Diving reflex: another method of treating supraventricular tachycardia. Arch. Inter. Med. 141:22-23, 1981.

17. Besset, G.S. III, Gaum, W., Kaplan, S.: The ice bag: a new technique for interruption of supraventricular tachycardia. J. Ped. 97:593-595, 1980.

18. Whitman, V., Friedman, Z., Bermann, W. Jr., Maisels, M.J.: Supraventricular tachycardia in newborn infants: an approach to therapy. J. Ped. 91:304-305, 1977.

19. Whitman, V., Zakeosian, G.M.: The diving reflex in termination of supraventricular tachycardia in childhood. J. Ped. 89:1032-1033, 1976.

20. Farthmann, E.H., Davidson, A.I.G.: Fresh water drowning at lowered body temperature: an experimental study. Amer. J. Surg. 109:410-415, 1965.

21. Spitz, W.U., Blanke, R.V.: Mechanisms of death in fresh water drowning. I: an experimental approach to the problem. Arch. Path. (Chicago) 71:661-668, 1961.

22. Modell, J.H., Davis, J.H., Giammona, S.T., Moya, F., Mann, J.B.: Blood gas and electrolyte changes in human near-drowning victims. J.A.M.A. 203:337-343, 1968.

INTOXICATIONS IN CHILDREN: A NEPHROLOGICAL APPROACH

Gaston Zilleruelo, M.D., Michael Freundlich, M.D. and José Strauss, M.D.

INTRODUCTION

Intoxications are serious world-wide problems affecting all social levels and posing questions as to prevention and treatment. These intoxications may involve drugs or poisons, and only in the United States affect two million children each year (mostly under five years of age) of which 400 die (1).

Despite several preventive and educative efforts, the prevalence of poisoning remains exceedingly high. Industry developments have increased the availability and risk of exposure to different chemicals and poisons. In addition, there has been an increased incidence of narcotic and sedative intoxications as suicidal attempts with the use of drug mixtures. In children, 75% of all poisonings occur from ingestion of "in-sight" compounds and only 25% from those hidden or "out-of-sight" (2). Accidental poisoning has a cumulative frequency of near 80% under 5 years of age and the suicidal attempts have a peak incidence in the age group of 13-30 years (3). The mortality rate remains high, ranging from 5 to 38% in hospitalized patients in stage 4 coma (4). In addition, important morbidity and sequelae are observed in a number of these patients.

In this review we will concentrate on some aspects of the management of intoxications in children from the nephrological point of view. The readers interested in more complete details should consult published thorough reviews on several clinical and diagnostic aspects of different types of intoxications (1,5).

GOALS OF TREATMENT

Intoxication always constitutes a medical emergency; thus, prompt diagnosis is essential for a good outcome. For instance, with salicylate poisoning, a mortality rate of 2% was reported in patients in whom the diagnosis was made upon admission to the hospital, while mortality was 25% when the diagnosis was delayed, regardless of the coma stage (6). Frequently, the diagnosis of accidental poisoning in a child arises from a good clinical history. In suicidal attempts, many times it is only the toxicology screen which will give the necessary information on the drugs involved. Treatment must be efficient in order to prevent additional morbidity and sequelae. Management should include three main aspects: 1) supportive therapy; 2) poison inactivation; 3) poison removal.

1) Supportive therapy: This represents the keystone of the management of intoxicated children. First of all, we must assure a permeable airway and adequate oxygenation of the patient, even if mechanical ventilation is required , and a close hemodynamic monitoring with vital signs assessment, correction of fluid and electrolyte imbalance, adequate caloric intake, and treatment of complications such as shock, convulsions, cerebral edema, respiratory depression, renal or liver failure.

2) Inactivation: There are certain substances called "antidotes" which will combine with the poison impeding its absorption to the body, making it harmless. The best example of an antidote is activated charcoal, a porous substance which adsorbs the drug or toxin, thus impeding its gastrointestinal absorption (7).

There are other substances with a protective action against specific toxics. These substances are useful when the intoxicant is known; an example is acetylcysteine, used in intoxications with acetaminophen in order to protect the liver (8), penicillamine for certain heavy metal intoxications (5), or deferoxamine for iron poisoning (9).

Other substances, which are called "antagonists" have the opposite pharmacologic action to the intoxicant. For instance, atropine is used to counteract the effect of organic phosphate compounds present in insecticides (5). Specific antibodies directed against the whole molecule or part of the intoxicant have become the most efficient way of treating certain intoxications. An example is the use of Fab-fragments of digoxin-specific antibodies to decrease active digoxin when present in toxic levels (10).

3) Removal: The most simple and rapid approach is the induction of vomiting by pharyngeal stimulation or by ingestion of ipecac syrup. The use of ipecac syrup has been controversial but there are many situations in which it is helpful if used early. Induction of vomiting and gastric lavage are contraindicated in intoxications with petroleum derivatives, caustics, or if the patient is in coma. The use of large amounts of oral activated charcoal is helpful in the management of intoxications not only by affecting absorption of the drug, but by producing an increased gastrointestinal clearance or removal; this seems to apply to phenobarbital, acetaminophen and aspirin (11).

Enhanced excretion by the use of forced diuresis is commonly recommended for drugs normally handled by the kidneys. A sustained diuresis of 2-3 times normal should be achieved in order to decrease tubular reabsorption and increase glomerular excretion rate of these drugs. In addition to intravenous fluids, the use of osmotic substances (mannitol) or loop diuretics (furosemide) may be considered. Ionized diuresis is based on the principle that renal excretion is favored when a drug is maintained in its ionized state. Forced alkaline diuresis may be helpful in enhancing removal of drugs with a low pK; in this category are salicylates, phenobarbital and uric acid (12,13). Best clearances of salicylates are obtained with urine pH > 7.5 (12). Forced alkaline diuresis can be attained with a large volume of any type of fluids (an essential component of any treatment of intoxication provided there is no cardio-pulmonary failure), plus bicarbonate or THAM, and diuretics like acetazolamide (Diamox^R) (14,15). However, forced alkaline diuresis is frequently misused and abused; it has been reported to produce severe alkalemia, hypokalemia and even pulmonary edema (16). With sodium bicarbonate or THAM, one of the problems is depression of the respiratory center, while Diamox induces a metabolic acidosis.

Other techniques for the removal of drugs include exchange transfusion which has been used mainly to treat endogenous intoxications due to hyperbilirubinemia, hyperammonemia and Reye Syndrome; also, it has been used to treat exogenous intoxications with inorganic phosphates, salicylates, phenobarbital, digitalis and antimicrobials (5). Dialysis (either hemo or peritoneal) and hemoperfusion, also have been used for toxic or drug removal. They will be reviewed separately in the next section of this chapter.

USE OF DIALYSIS AND HEMOPERFUSION IN THE MANAGEMENT OF INTOXICATIONS

There are some basic criteria for the selection of hemodialysis in the management of intoxications. The dialysis membrane must be permeable to the drug in question and there must be a drug distribution in plasma water with a known time/dose/cytotoxic relationship. The latter is the relationship of blood/drug concentration, body's exposure time to the drug and drug's toxicity (17). Severity of clinical manifestations and potential mortality depend on the level attained after a certain period of time following ingestion of the drug (17). This concept applies only to acute one time ingestions.

For salicylate intoxication, the use of peritoneal dialysis has been proposed as a significant addition to decrease plasma salicylate levels and to correct associated metabolic disturbances (metabolic acidosis, electrolyte abnormalities) (12). The addition of protein to the dialysate (usually 5% albumin) has been reported to enhance excretion of different drugs which are highly protein bound (18). The list of substances that have been reported to be efficiently removed by peritoneal dialysis is presented in Table 1.

Removal of toxic substances and drugs can also be accomplished by the use of hemodialysis (19). Advantages of this technique over peritoneal dialysis include greater speed of drug removal and efficiency since there is a much higher clearance. However, disadvantages are related to personnel required and the fact that it is a complex procedure which requires a vascular access. The latter can be attained through an arterio-venus shunt or through the use of femoral or subclavian catheters. The currently known dialysable drugs and poisons are listed in Table 1.

Hemoperfusion has been used over the past several years either experimentally or therapeutically for the management of different poison and drug intoxications (20,21). It consists of the direct passage of blood through various adsorbent materials such as charcoal or polystyrene resin (Fig. 1) and is used to remove toxic compounds from the circulation. Substantial advances have taken place in the design and composition of hemoperfusion cartridges which have enhanced the biocompatibility of these adsorbents and prevented charcoal embolization.

Since there is a large priming volume required for the cartridge and lines (the combined minimum volume is approximately 400-500 ml) and since the extracorporeal circuit volume should not exceed 10% of the child's estimated circulating blood volume, whole blood is frequently needed to prime the system. Recently, we treated a two month old infant with hemoperfusion and hemodialysis because of chloramphenicol intoxication (22). This baby developed the "Gray-baby syndrome" with

Table 1. Dialyzability of drugs by peritoneal dialysis (PD) and hemodialysis (HD).

DRUG	PD	HD	DRUG	PD	HD
ANTIMICROBIALS					
Amikacin	Yes	Yes	Nafcillin	No	No
Aminosalicylic Acid	?	Yes	Neomycin	?	Yes
Amoxicillin	?	Yes	Nitrofurantoin	?	Yes
Amphotericin B	No	No	Oxacillin	No	No
Ampicillin	No	Yes	Penicillin G	No	Yes
Aziocillin	?	Yes	Pentamidine	No	?
Carbenicillin	Slight	Yes	Pyrimethamine	No	?
Cefamandole	No	No			
Cefazolin	No	Yes	Quinine	No	Yes
Cephalexin	Yes	Yes	Rifampin	No	No
Cephalothin	Yes	Yes	Streptomycin	Yes	Yes
Cephapirin	?	Yes	Sulfamethoxazole		
Cephradine	Yes	Yes	trimethoprim	Yes	Yes
Chloramphenicol	No	Yes	Sulfisoxazole	Yes	Yes
Chloroquine	No	No	Tetracycline	No	No
Clindamycin	No	No	Ticarcillin	Yes	Yes
Cloxacillin	No	No	Tobramycin	Yes	Yes
Colistimethate	Yes	No	Vancomycin	No	No
Dicloxacillin	No	No			
Doxycycline	No	No	ANALGESICS		
Erythromycin	Yes	No	Acetaminophen	No	Yes
Ethambutol	Yes	Yes	Acetylsalicylic		
5-Fluorocytocine	Yes	Yes	Acid	Yes	Yes
Gentamicin	Yes	Yes	Methadone	No	No
Isoniazid	Yes	Yes	Methaqualone	?	Yes
Kanamycin	Yes	Yes	Propoxyphene	No	No
Lincomycin	No	No			
Methanamine mandelate	No	?	ANTIARRHYTHMICS		
Methicillin	No	No	Lidocaine	No	No
Metronidazole	?	Yes	Procainamide	Yes	Yes
Minocycline	No	No	Propranolol	No	No
			Quinidine	Yes	Yes

Table 1. (Cont.)

DRUG	PD	HD
ANTICOAGULANTS		
Heparin	No	No
ANTIHYPERTENSIVES		
Clonidine	?	No
Diazoxide	Yes	Yes
Guanethidine	No	?
Hydralazine	No	No
Methyldopa	Yes	Yes
Nitroprusside	Yes	Yes
Reserpine	No	No
CORTICOSTEROIDS		
Cortisone	No	No
Methylprednisolone	?	No
CARDIAC GLYCOSIDES		
Digitoxin	No	No
Digoxin	No	No
DIURETICS		
Aminophylline	Yes	Slight
Furosemide	No	No
IMMUNOSUPPRESSIVES		
Azathioprine	?	Yes
Cyclophosphamide	?	Yes
5-Fluorouracil	?	Yes

DRUG	PD	HD
NEUROLOGIC AGENTS		
Diphenylhydantoin	Yes	No
Gallamine	Yes	Yes
SEDATIVES, HYPNOTICS, TRANQUILIZERS		
Amitriptyline	No	No
Chlordiazepoxide	No	No
Chlorpromazine	No	No
Diazepam	No	No
Ethchlorvynol	No	Yes
Flurazepam	No	?
Glutethimide	No	No
Imipramine	No	No
Lithium carbonate	Yes	Yes
Meprobamate	Yes	Yes
Nortriptyline	No	No
Pentobarbital	No	No
Phenobarbital	Yes	Yes
Secobarbital	No	No
MISCELLANEOUS		
Cimetidine	Slight	Slight
Folic Acid	Yes	Yes
Vitamins (water soluble)	Yes	Yes

?=Insufficient data available
Yes=Alteration in drug dosage recommended

Chart compiled by Cleo J. Richard R.N., M.S.N. Reproduced from Dialysis and Transplantation 10(6):474, June 1981, with permission.

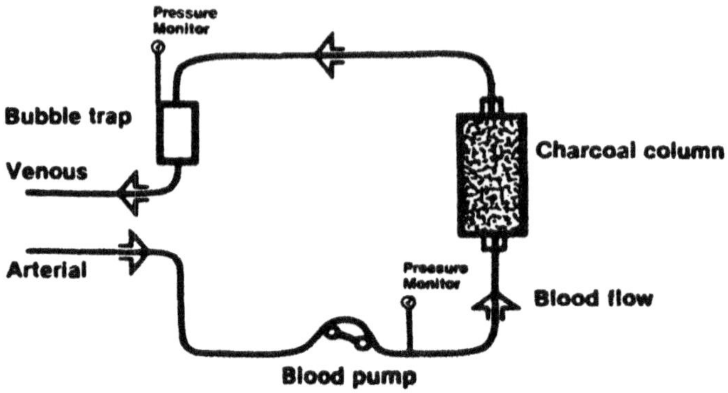

FIGURE 1. Hemoperfusion circuit. From p. 1043 of Papadopoulou ZL and Novello AC: The use of hemoperfusion in children. Past, present and future. Pediatr. Clin. N. Amer. 29:1039, 1982, with permission.

profound hypotension, hypothermia and coma, and required this procedure as an heroic measure. After two unsuccessful exchange transfusions, there was a definite decrease in the serum chloramphenicol levels from a mean of 150 to less than 50 mcg/ml at the end of four hours of hemoperfusion.

To calculate drug clearance, the arterial minus venous concentrations of the drug are divided by the arterial concentration and multiplied by the blood flow rate to the cartridge. Using this formula, the calculated maximal clearance by hemoperfusion was compared to other techniques for removal of different toxins (Table 2), and hemoperfusion was found to be the most efficient method (23). While several recent reviews (19,20) support the benefit of dialysis or hemoperfusion in the management of endogenous or exogenous intoxications, some continue to question its clinical value (24). Others have suggested that conservative supportive treatment alone is to be preferred in all poisoned patients regardless of the compound involved or the degree of intoxication (25). The decision as to whether a patient should undergo dialysis or hemoperfusion is not an easy one; therefore, we do not suggest that every patient suffering from an overdose of a dialyzable drug should necessarily undergo dialysis. There are certain guidelines, generally agreed upon, which should be considered for these more aggressive forms of treatment (Table 3).

A list of the most common substances removed by charcoal or resin hemoperfusion is given in Table 4. Hemoperfusion has also been used in cases with hepatic coma and Reye Syndrome, thyrotoxicosis with removal of T3 and T4, chemotherapy overdose with removal of the offending agents, and antibody removal as treatment of immune disorders (21).

Still, there are limitations in the use of hemoperfusion. We have mentioned already the technical limitations in small children in whom large priming volumes (>10% of total blood volume) are used. In addition, most drugs have a distribution space which includes intracellular water; in those cases, the drug is not readily available for removal through the blood and even a high plasma clearance will result in the removal of only small amounts of the drug. Therefore, caution should be placed

Table 2. Calculated Maximal Clearances by Hemoperfusion and Other Elimination Techniques.

	Resin Hemoperfusion	Charcoal Hemo-Perfusion	Hemo-Dialysis	Peritoneal dialysis	Forced diuresis
Barbiturates:					
Short acting, e.g., quinalbarbitone	220 mL/min	120	65	9.7	5
Medium acting, e.g.,					
amylobarbitone,	300	120	95	10.2	-
secobarbitone	333	-	-	-	-
Long acting, e.g., phenobarbitone	300	120	110	6.3	17
Glutethimide	280	125	90	10	10
Tricyclics:					
Amytriptyline	240	-	-	-	-
Nortriptylene	280	-	-	-	-

From Trafford A, Horn C, Sharpstone P et al. Hemoperfusion in acute drug toxicity. Clin. Toxicology 17: 551, 1980, with permission.

Table 3. Guidelines for Dialysis and/or Hemoperfusion

Need for prolonged, assisted ventilation
Persistent hypotension or need for vasoactive drug therapy
Persistent coma or progressive clinical deterioration unresponsive to medical therapy
Associated hepatic or renal disease impairing the excretion or metabolism of the intoxicant
Associated cardiac or pulmonary disease aggravated by the prolonged coma or hypotension
Ingestion and probable absorption of a potentially lethal amount of drug (after gastric lavage)
Plasma concentration reported as lethal of an intoxicant known to be cleared effectively from the blood with dialysis or hemoperfusion

in the interpretation of results of high plasma clearance of some drugs as an explanation for a rapid clinical recovery after hemoperfusion. Like hemodialysis, hemoperfusion is an expensive method requiring skilled personnel and access to the circulation through arterial and venous lines with an increased risk of potentially lethal infections. This complex procedure may also interfere with the general supportive measures for the patient by distracting the personnel in charge of the patient. Hemoperfusion has known complications such as hypotension, hypocalcemia, hypoglycemia, hypothermia, thrombocytopenia, and charcoal embolization (21). The latter risk has decreased with new devices, because of encapsulation of the charcoal particles within the cellulose. In addition, the use of hemodialysis in series with charcoal hemoperfusion has prevented the development of electrolyte imbalances and hypothermia because temperature can be corrected as the blood goes through the dialyzer. The sequential use of hemoperfusion and dialysis has been recommended whenever intoxication with an unknown drug has taken place (26).

In summary, conservative medical management is sufficient in the vast majority of intoxicated children. Specific indications for dialysis or hemoperfusion should be followed, based on the clinical status and type of drug or toxin involved. These procedures should always be performed in adequate facilities and by skilled personnel; their limitations and potential complications should be recognized. It is clear that there is a need for more controlled studies in order to assess their true efficacy under different circumstances. It is possible that in the near future, the improvement of dialysis membranes, and particularly hemoperfusion devices, will allow more efficient drug removal and extend their applications to many exogenous and endogenous intoxications. Still, overall prognosis will depend on early identification of the intoxication and prompt and adequate management in a medical center experienced with this type of emergency.

Table 4. Compounds Removed by Charcoal or Resin Hemoperfusion*

Analgesics
- Acetyl salicylic acid
- Methylsalicylate
- Acetaminophen (paracetamol)

Alcohols
- Ethyl alcohol (ethanol)

Antiasthmatics
- Theophylline

Antimicrobials
- Chloramphenicol
- Gentamycin
- Isoniazid

Anticancer Agents
- Adriamycin
- Methotrexate

Anticonvulsants
- Carbamazepine
- Phenytoin

Antidepressants
- Amitriptyline
- Clomipramine
- Desipramine

Barbiturates
- Amobarbital
- Butabarbital
- Medinal (Russian)
- Pentobarbital
- Phenobarbital
- Quinalbital
- Secobarbital

Nonbarbiturate Hypnotics, Sedatives, and Tranquilizers
- Ethchlorvynol
- Glutethimide
- Methyprylon
- Methaqualone

- Diazepam
- Chloral hydrate
- Carbromal
- Chlorpromazine
- Promazine
- Promethazine

- Meprobamate

Cardiovascular Agents
- Digoxin
- Procainamide
- N-Acetylprocainamide

Plant/Animal Toxins, Herbicides/Insecticides
- Amanita phalloides
- Amanitin
- Phalloidin

- Chlorinated insecticides
- Polychlorinated biphenyls
- Methyl parathion
- Demeton-S-methyl sulfoxide
- Dimethoate
- Nitrostigmine
- Paraquat, diquat

Solvents/Gases
- Carbon tetrachloride
- Ethylene oxide

Endogenous Toxins
- Amino acids
- Uric acid
- Creatinine

- Cholic acid
- Polyamino acids
- Polypeptides

- Uremic toxins

Table 4. Compounds Removed by Charcoal or Resin Hemoperfusion* (Cont.)

Endogenous Toxins (Cont.)
- Indicans
- Phenolic compounds
- Organic acids
- Middle molecules

- Thyroxine
- Triiodothyronine
- Immune proteins

Metals/Inorganics
- Mercury

Miscellaneous
- Cimetidine
- Epinephrine
- Norepinephrine
- Phenylbutazone
- L-Dopamine
- Methoxamine
- Serotonin
- Nucleotides
- Cholic acid
- Vitamin B_{12}
- Folic Acid
- Bromosulphthalein
- Inulin
- Sucrose dilaurate

Adapted from Winchester JF, Gelfand MC, Knepshield JH et al.: Dialysis and hemoperfusion of poisons and drugs - update. Trans. Am. Soc. Artif. Intern. Organs 23:762, 1977, by Papadoulou ZL and Novello AC: The use of hemoperfusion in children. Past, present and future. Pediatr. Clin. N. Amer. 29:1046, 1982, with permission.

REFERENCES

1. Deeths TM and Breeden JT: Poisoning in children. A statistical study of 1,057 cases. J. Pediatr. 79:299, 1971.
2. Arena JM: Poisoning, Toxicology, Symptoms, Treatments. Springfield, Illinois Charles Thomas,1974, pp 3-4.
3. Carmi J, Frati M, Martin ML: Acute poisoning in Barcelona, Spain. Clin. Toxicology 17:421, 1980.
4. Arieff AI and Friedman EA: Coma following non-narcotic drug overdosage. Management of 208 adult patients. Am. J. Med. Sci. 266:405, 1973.
5. Arena JM: The treatment of poisoning. Ciba Clinical Symposia 30:3, 1978.
6. Anderson RJ, Potts DE, Gabow PA et al: Unrecognized adult salicylate intoxication. Ann. Intern. Med. 85:745, 1976.
7. Greensher J, Mofenson HC, Picchioni AL and Fallon P: Activated charcoal updated. JACEP 8:261, 1979.
8. Rumack BH, Peterson RC, Koch GG and Amara IA: Acetaminophen overdose: 662 cases with evaluation of oral acetylcysteine treatment. Arch. Intern. Med. 141:380, 1981.
9. Robotham JL, Lietman PS: Acute iron poisoning: a review. Am. J. Dis. Child. 136:875, 1980.
10. Murphy DJ, Brenner WF, Haber E et al: Massive digoxin poisoning treated with Fab-fragments of digoxin specific antibodies. Pediatrics 70:472, 1982.
11. Levy G: Gastrointestinal clearance of drugs with activated charcoal. New Engl. J. Med. 37:676, 1982.
12. Winters RW: Salicylate intoxication. In Winters RW (ed). The Body Fluid in Pediatrics. Boston: Little Brown and Co., 1973, pp 483.
13. Lessen NA: Treatment of severe acute barbiturate poisoning by forced diuresis and alkalinization of the urine. Lancet 2:338, 1960.
14. Cirksena WJ, Bastian RC, Malloy JP and Barry KG: Use of mannitol in exogenous and endogenous intoxication. New Engl. J. Med. 270:161, 1964.
15. Fernstein RC, Finberg L, Fleishman E: The use of acetazolamide in the therapy of salicylate poisoning. Pediatrics 25:215, 1960.
16. Mathew H: Acute poisoning: some myths and misconceptions. Brit. Med. J. 1:519, 1971.
17. Done AK: Salicylate intoxication. Significance of measurements of salicylate in blood in cases of acute ingestion. Pediatrics 26:800, 1960.
18. Etteldorf JN, Dobbins RL, Summit WT et al: Intermittent peritoneal dialysis using 5% albumin in the treatment of salicylate intoxication in children. J. Pediatr. 58:226, 1961.
19. Knepshield JH, Schreiner GE, Lowenthal DT and Gelfand MC: Dialysis of poisons and drugs. Annual review. Trans. Am. Soc. Artif. Intern. Organs 19:590, 1973.
20. Winchester JF, Gelfand MC, Knepshield JH et al. Dialysis and hemoperfusion of poisons and drugs. Update. Trans. Am. Soc. Artif. Intern Organs 23:762, 1977.
21. Papadopoulou ZL and Novello AC: The use of hemoperfusion in children. Past, present and future. Pediatr. Clin. N. Amer. 29: 1039, 1982.
22. Freundlich M, Cynamon H, Tamer A et al: Management of chloramphenicol intoxication by charcoal hemoperfusion. J. Pediatr. 103:485,1983.
23. Trafford A, Horn C, Sharpstone P et al: Hemoperfusion in acute

drug toxicity. Clin. Toxicology 17:547, 1980.
24. Merril JP: Treatment of drug intoxication by hemoperfusion. New Engl. J. Med. 284:911, 1971.
25. Mathew H: Early treatment of the unconcious patient suffering from drug overdose.Med. J. Aust. 1:752, 1969.
26. Jose PA, Qinchester JF and Gelfand MC: Hemoperfusion of poisons and drugs in children. Contr. Nephrol. 27:61, 1981.

TREATMENT OF SEVERE HYPERTENSION IN CHILDREN WITH RENAL DISEASE

Alan B. Gruskin, H. Jorge Baluarte, Martin S. Polinsky, Bruce A. Kaiser, Sharon A. Perlman, and Bruce Z. Morgenstern.

Severe hypertension and hypertensive emergencies in children most often occur in association with secondary forms of high blood pressure and may develop in children with previously unrecognized disease or as a sudden change in children with known hypertension. The term hypertensive crisis or hypertensive emergency is used to denote a clinical situation in which the blood pressure has been elevated for some period of time and ought to be lowered over minutes, or hours depending on the patient's clinical status. The clinical presentation of hypertensive emergencies varies. Life threatening hypertensive symptoms, such as acute heart failure, pulmonary edema or neurologic changes require immediate lowering of the blood pressure. (Table I)

TABLE I - Clinical Presentation of Hypertensive Emergencies

Cardiac Failure	Epistaxis - uncontrolled
Central Nervous System Dysfunction	Toxemia [Pregnancy]
Increased intracranial pressure	
Encephalopathy	Visual signs and symptoms
Ischemic attack	Hemorrhage
Stroke	Papilledema
Subarachnoid hemorrhage	Blindness
Drug withdrawal	Renal Failure
Clonidine	

Appropriate management of disorders associated with high blood pressure requires recognition of the problem, knowledge of its natural history, appreciation of the pathophysiology involved, and understanding of the pharmacodynamic and toxic effects of therapy. Five aspects of severe hypertension in children will be considered: 1) clinical features 2) guidelines for acute antihypertensive therapy; 3) the physiology of blood pressure regulation 4) approaches to treating severe hypertension associated with specific renal disorders and 5) an overview of the pharmacologic agents used in treating severe hypertension in children with genitourinary disorders.

CLINICAL ASPECTS OF SEVERE HYPERTENSION

Effects of High Blood Pressure

The major clinical syndromes related to severe hypertension involve the central nervous system, heart and kidney. Severe hypertension may present as hypertensive encephalopathy (Table II), stroke, or subarachnoid hemorrhage; cardiac effects include myocardial ischemia presenting as angina and congestive heart failure; renal damage ranges from alterations in GFR to rapidly progressive renal failure.

Table II - Clinical Features of Hypertensive Encephalopathy

1. Alteration in consciousness
2. Blurred vision - cortical, retinal
3. Cranial nerve palsies
4. Focal neurologic signs
5. Headache
6. Hypertension - sudden onset or abrupt increase
7. Papilledema
8. Vomiting
9. Seizures

Hypertensive encephalopathy results when autoregulation of cerebral blood flow fails and blood flow to the brain increases. (1) Symptoms and signs include severe headache, irritability, dizziness, lassitude, altered mental capacity, seizures and coma. Sensory and motor deficits and transient ischemic episodes often precede more prominent symptomatology.

Two major theories regarding the pathogenesis of hypertensive encephalopathy exist: arteriolar spasm and decompensation of cerebral autoregulation. Both processes involve changes in cerebral blood vessels. Spasm of cerebral arterioles, followed by edema and infarction has been noted in conjunction with the development of hypertension.[2] Autoregulation is a normal homeostatic process whereby cerebral vascular resistance increases with increasing blood pressure, thereby maintaining a constant rate of blood flow, until the autoregulatory range is exceeded.[3] Autoregulation of cerebral blood flow normally occurs in adult animals within a blood pressure range of 70-200 mm Hg.[4] Failure of cerebral autoregulation is followed by the transcapillary movement of plasma, with cerebral edema and infarction occurring when cerebral perfusion pressure reaches a critical level. Cerebral blood flow and pressure are also influenced by changes in acid base status: alkalosis or hypercapnia may cause vasodilation, whereas acidosis or hypocapnia may lead to vasoconstriction.[5]

Strokes occur predominantly in patients with sustained hypertension. Although more common in adults, both hemorrhagic and thrombotic strokes occasionally occur in hypertensive children. The nature of the resultant neurologic deficit depends upon the site involved. A child suspected of having had a hypertensive stroke should have a CAT scan with a contrast agent as part of the evaluation. Our limited experience with hypertensive strokes in children suggests that children have a marked ability to recover neurologic function.

Subarachnoid hemorrhage occurs infrequently in children with high blood pressure. It has been observed in hypertensive children undergoing maintenance hemodialysis and receiving heparin.

Amaurosis can occur in children with acute post infectious nephritis and is associated with acute elevation of blood pressure.[6]

Chronic hypertension increases myocardial work and can lead to concentric left ventricular hypertrophy and eventually to cardiac decompensation. Whereas acute cardiac decompensation usually does not develop as a result of sudden elevations of blood pressure in older children, acute volume overload and pulmonary edema in association with the increased left ventricular preload does occur in patients with acute severe hypertension. Neonates and infants with severe high blood pressure, (especially those with coarctation of the aorta or renal vascular lesions), present with congestive heart failure more frequently than do older children.[7,8]

The most common cause of severe or malignant hypertension in children is intrinsic kidney disease; conversely, the kidney may also suffer the effects of sustained severe hypertension. Malignant hypertension may be defined as a syndrome associated with vascular lesions localized to the kidney [9] and retina.[10] Prior to the availability of antihypertensive treatment, progression to renal failure occurred in most patients over a period of a few months to one year.[11] Some have attempted to classify patients with lesser degrees of high blood pressure as having premalignant or accelerated hypertension, which is defined in adults as diastolic pressure in excess of 110 mm Hg accompanied by vascular lesions of the retina without papilledema.[12] Because most children with sustained moderate or severe high blood pressure are admitted to the hospital for diagnosis and therapy, it is clinically less important to distinguish between accelerated and malignant hypertension in pediatrics.

CRITERIA FOR DIAGNOSING HYPERTENSION IN CHILDREN

During the past decade, normal blood pressure ranges for children have been developed.[13] Blood pressure increases gradually throughout childhood, and the causes for these changes appear to be multifactorial. An approximation of the age-related ninety-fifth percentile value for blood pressure in children can be obtained by using the following formula: systolic blood pressure equals 100 plus (age in years times 3); diastolic blood pressure equals 70 plus (age in years times 1.5). For example, a 10 year old child would be expected to have a blood pressure below 130/85 [(100 + (10x3)]over [(70 + (10x1.5)]. We utilize this formula to approximate the upper limit of normal, for children above the age of one year with a maximum of 140/90 mm Hg.

Age-related data defining the relationship between blood pressure and clinical symptomatology are not available. As a working guideline for pediatric populations, we have adapted the criteria reported in adults for mild, moderate, severe and acute hypertensive emergencies.(14) The values which we utilize are summarized in Table III and are based upon the concept that it is the percent increase in diastolic blood pressure above the age-related upper limits (95%) that constitutes the major risk for hypertensive complications.

	Adults		Children
Severity	Diastolic BP	Percent elevation above normal limit	Percent elevation above age related upper limits (diastolic)
mild	95-105 mm Hg	5 - 16%	5 - 16%
moderate	105-120 mm Hg	16 - 33%	16 - 33%
severe	120-140 mm Hg	33 - 55%	33 - 55%
potential acute problem	>140 mm Hg	> 55%	> 55%

TABLE III - Severity of Diastolic Hypertension: Criteria for classifying the degree of hypertension as mild, moderate and severe in adults in either mm Hg or as a percent increase above normal. The definitions of mild, moderate and severe hypertension for children are based on the percent increase above age related upper limits for diastolic blood pressure (taken to be 70 mm Hg plus 1.5 times age in years until a value of 90 mm Hg is reached).

The upper limit of normal for diastolic blood pressure is taken to be 90 mm Hg in adults. Values between 90 and 95 mm Hg are considered borderline. A diastolic blood pressure of 105 mm Hg in an adult would be 16% above the upper limit (105 ÷ 90), and the patient would be considered to have a moderately elevated blood pressure. Mild, moderate, and severe hypertension correspond to blood pressure elevations in the range of 5-15%, 16-33%, and 33-55% above upper limit respectively. Blood pressure values exceeding 55% of the age related upper limit of diastolic blood pressure are an indication for acute therapy. For example, a 5 year old child's diastolic blood pressure should not exceed 77-78 mm Hg, i.e. (70 + (5.0 yr x 1.5). If the diastolic blood pressure were increased by more than 55%, to a level exceeding 121 mm Hg (1.55 x 78 mm Hg), acute antihypertensive therapy ought to be instituted.

Although the above criteria are based on measured diastolic pressures, it is our clinical impression that significant problems including target organ changes and hypertensive encephalopathy can also occur in children with less obvious hypertension. We have observed, for example, cortical blindness and a generalized seizure in a 6 year old child with post streptococcal glomerulonephritis, mild renal insufficiency and an admission blood pressure of 110/80 mm Hg. Full recovery occurred and the blood pressure at discharge was 75/50 mm Hg. We believe that this child may have had "relative" hypertension, with a fifty percent elevation in both systolic and diastolic blood pressure. Thus, when evaluating a hypertensive child, thought should be given to the concepts of both absolute and relative hypertension. The availability of blood pressure measurements taken as part of routine health care maintenance may prove helpful in understanding clinical features of diseases known to give rise to high blood pressure.

BLOOD PRESSURE REGULATION AND ANTIHYPERTENSIVE TREATMENT

Hypertension results from the complex interplay of the multiple factors known to influence the physiologic transformation (volume times vasoconstriction) of the basic formula for blood pressure (blood pressure = blood flow x resistance).[15,16] The physiologic factors influencing the two limbs of the blood pressure formula are summarized in Table IV. Therapy for hypertension may be specifically directed toward modulation of a discrete factor known to influence BP regulation, or therapy may be more nonspecitic in nature, with effects on more than a single factor involved.

TABLE IV - Factors Influencing Volume and Vasoconstrictor Limbs of the Blood Pressure Formula

Volume

Degree of mineralocorticoid activity

Non hormonal regulation of sodium by the kidney

Small vessel compliance

Cardiac output

Vasoconstriction

Sympathetic nervous system activity

Circulating catecholamines

Kinin system activity

Renin-Angiotensin activity

The sites of action of antihypertensive agents classified by their mode of action is summarized in Figure 1. The mainstay of treatment of hypertensive emergencies is an intravenous vasodilator often combined with the simultaneous use of potent diuretics.[17-27] Long term control of severe hypertension involves the judicious use of combinations of oral antihypertensive agents having different modes and sites of action.

Figure 1: The nature and site of the pharmacologic action(s) of antihypertensive agents (contained within boxes) in relation to the physiologic components involved in blood pressure regulation.

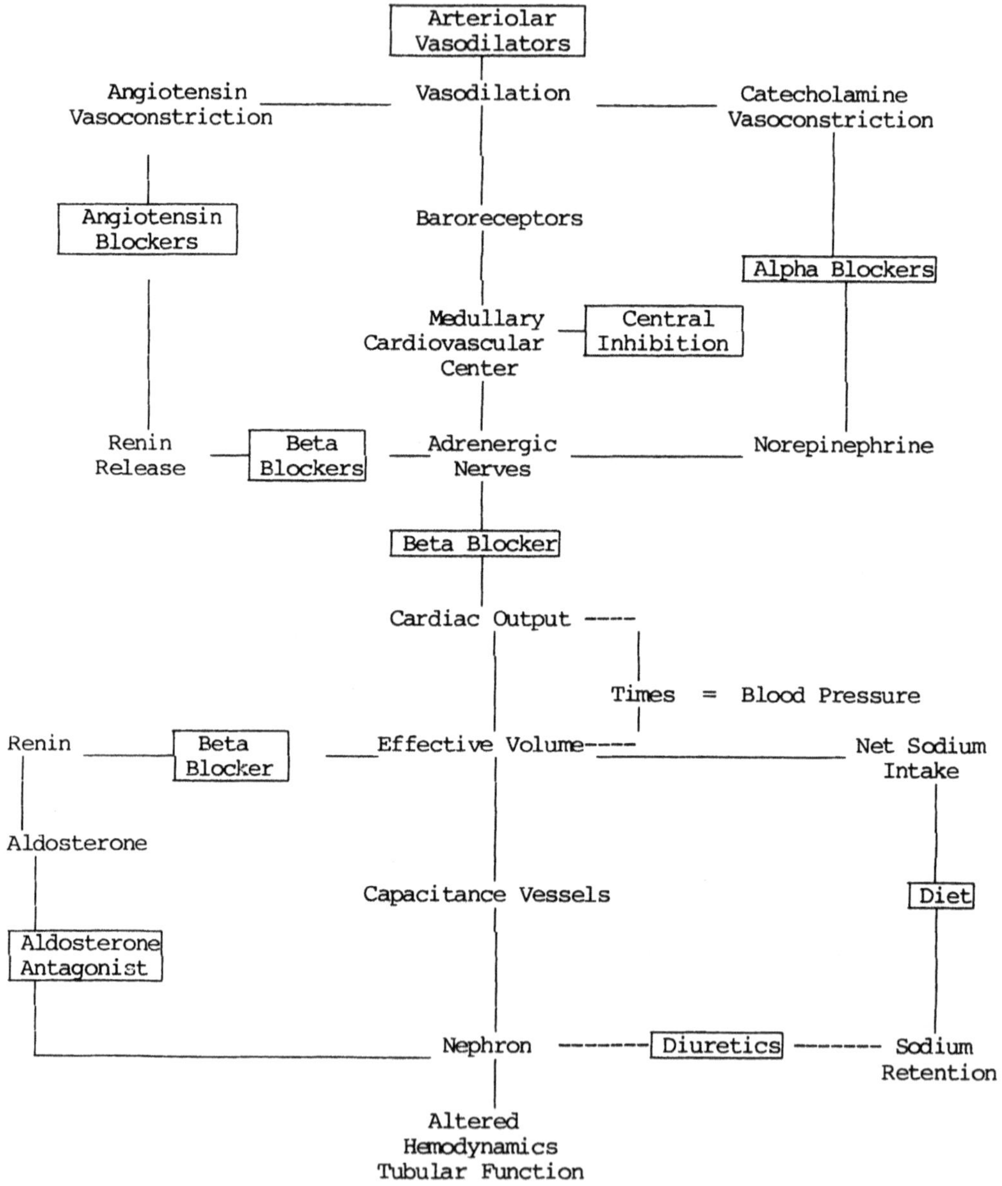

SPECIFIC APPROACHES TO TREATING SEVERE HYPERTENSION

Two clinical routes are available for treating severe hypertension. The first is based on the principle that therapy directed against any factor known to raise blood pressure will be successful. Because this approach fails to consider the pathophysiology involved, not only may the acute reduction of blood pressure be unsuccessful, but a smooth transition to more sustained control may be precluded. The steps in the non-specific approach to treating hypertensive emergencies usually involve the use of progressively more potent intravenous vasodilators starting with hydralazine and progressing to diazoxide and then nitroprusside. Salt and water restriction together with the administration of a potent diuretic are often begun simultaneously.

The alternative therapeutic approach is based on an understanding of the pathophysiology of the hypertensive process involved; it attempts to alter the hypertensive process by employing a combination of pharmacologic and physiologic interventions. This approach is more precise, allows for a smoother transition to chronic therapy, enables therapeutic failures to be viewed in a physiologic fashion and may diminish or prevent the development of side effects.

ANTIHYPERTENSIVE THERAPY FOR RENAL DISORDERS

Severe hypertension or hypertensive crises can occur in a wide variety of renal diseases (Table V). It is the nature of the renal disease which determines the specifics of treating the associated hypertension. The somewhat different yet overlapping therapeutic approaches used to treat children with acute post infectious nephritis, rapidly progressive renal failure, end stage renal disease and structural lesions will be individually considered.

Table: V Childhood Renal Disorders Associated with Hypertensive Crisis

Vascular Disorders

- Hemolytic Uremic Syndrome
- Renal Artery Lesions
- Renal Venous Thrombosis
- Renal Cortical Necrosis
- Medullary Necrosis

Sickle Cell Nephropathy

Glomerulonephritis

Post Infectious Nephritis

Henoch Schönlein Purpura

Membranoproliferative Glomerulonephritis

Focal Segmental Glomerulosclerosis

Rapidly Progressive "Crescentic" Nephritis

Chronic Glomerulonephritis

Collagen Vascular Disorders

Acquired Structural Disorders

Pyelonephritis

Reflux Nephropathy

Trauma

Congenital Anomalies

Polycystic Kidneys - Infantile and Adult Forms

Tuberous Sclerosis

Medullary Cystic Disease

Renal Cortical Microcysts (Multiple Syndromes)

Hydronephrosis

Therapeutic Approach to the Child with Acute Poststreptococcal Glomerulonephritis (PSGN)

The hypertensive process in patients with PSGN and mildly to moderately reduced renal function is primarily due to acute salt and water retention because of the continued intake of food and beverage despite a rapidly falling GFR. The renin-angiotensin system apparently responds appropriately in such patients since plasma renin activity (PRA) in children with PSGN is usually appropriately suppressed.[28] The response, however, may occasionally be inappropriate with relative hyperreninemia.

Hypertension in PSGN may range from mild to severe and lead to hypertensive encephalopathy, pulmonary edema and cardiac failure. Treatment should be based on the nature and severity of the clinical findings. The development or progression to severe hypertension may be prevented by appropriately restricting salt and water intake. Fluid management should be planned to ensure that negative salt and water balance occurs; indeed, in severely hypertensive children with PSGN, we have on occasion withheld all fluids for 12-24 hours except for fluids required to administer drugs. Rotating tourniquets may help lower blood pressure transiently in children with pulmonary edema and heart failure. While other therapies are being started, diuretics may satisfactorily lower blood pressure in children with PSGN because of the marked volume overload. Patients with moderately elevated blood pressure often respond to intravenous furosemide with a diuresis and a lowering of blood pressure (Table VI).[29] The initial dose of furosemide is 2 mg/kg given intravenously. If a significant diuresis does not occur in the ensuing 1-2 hours, a second intravenous dose of 4 mg/kg is given; the maximum dose used is 8 mg/kg.

If fluid control does not adequately lower blood pressure, then vasodilators are used. Our first choice of vasodilators to treat moderate and severe hypertension in children with PSGN is intravenous hydralazine starting at a dose of 0.15 mg/kg (Table VI). If an adequate response does not occur, a repeat dose of 0.30 mg/kg and then 0.45 mg/kg up to a maximum of 20 mg is given at 30 minute intervals. Should hydralazine fail to satisfactorily lower blood pressure, or if the patient has neurologic signs or symptoms, diazoxide is given, starting with a dose of 2.5 mg/kg repeated at 30 minute intervals and increasing stepwise to a maximum of 10 mg/kg or 300 mg.

Should such therapy fail, the next drug of choice would be nitroprusside. Although nitroprusside has been successfully used to treat the hypertension of PSGN,[30] we have not found it necessary to use nitroprusside to treat hypertensive complications of PSGN. Our practice of severely restricting salt and water, often in combination with the use of diuretics and vasodilators, may account for this.

Although reserpine[31] and methyldopa have been used effectively to lower blood pressure in children with PSGN, their sedative properties may mask developing signs of encephalopathy. The availability of other effective agents has led to diminished use of these agents as initial treatment for the acute hypertension associated with PSGN.

Antihypertensive Therapy for Rapidly Progressive Renal Failure

Although therapy for severe hypertension in children with rapidly progressive renal failure is similar to that discussed in the above section, some differences in approach do exist. The more symptomatic the patient and the higher the blood pressure the more urgent the need to rapidly lower blood pressure. The patholophysiology of the hypertensive process in such patients often reflects a combination of factors including increases in angiotensin II, aldosterone, and salt and water retention; changes in cardiac output; and perhaps, alterations in vasodepressor renal hormones. Therapy depends upon affecting these processes either singly or in combination.

We initiate therapy with intravenous vasodilators for severe hypertension in children with rapidly progressive renal failure based on the premise that vasoconstrictive forces are the ones leading to the severe elevation in BP. Therapy is begun with standard doses of intravenous hydralazine increased stepwise at intervals of 45-60 minutes until either adequate control of blood pressure is achieved or a maximum dose is reached. If the patient is more than mildly symptomatic or fails to rapidly respond to hydralazine, we next use diazoxide given in bolus doses and increase the doses at intervals of 30 minutes until a maximum dose is used, or a response obtained. Diazoxide can also be given as a continuous infusion or administered at regular time intervals. If diazoxide fails or if the child is thought to have had a cerebral vascular accident, a nitroprusside drip would be started at its minimally effective dose (0.5 mcg/kg/min) and increased. Because the cyanide moiety of nitroprusside increases in plasma as GFR falls, it is important to monitor thiocyanate levels as well as serum creatinine if nitroprusside is used either in high doses or over a prolonged period of time.

The use of antagonists of the renin angiotensin system as initial agents in treating such patients has only recently begun. Continuous infusions of intravenous saralasin have been reported to be effective in a few patients in acutely lowering and maintaining the lowered blood pressure for a number of days. Captopril, which is currently used primarily after therapy with multiple oral agents has failed, or after stabilization with intravenous vasodilators, has been used as initial therapy in severely hypertensive and/or symptomatic patients. The precise role of the currently available antagonists of the renin angiotensin system in treating acute severe hypertension should be delineated in the next few years. Minoxidil which is a peripheral vasodilator has been used in a similar manner.

The failure in most children of the blood pressure to acutely fall to acceptable levels with vasodilators alone, is often due to the concomitant expansion of extracellular fluid. Also it is possible that volume overload is the primary factor leading to severe hypertension in such patients. In severely hypertensive patients attempts to induce a diuresis in such patients should be begun simultaneously with the administration of vasodilators for two reasons: 1) most potent vasodilators cause sodium retention and 2) extracellular fluid accumulation occurs in most patients with a rapidly falling GFR. To insure that ECF contraction occurs, fluid intake should be either severely limited or even withheld during the acute phase of management. The aseptic insertion of a bladder catheter and use of a closed drainage system for 12-24 hours to monitor urine output can be helpful in monitoring the response to diuretics in previously undiagnosed critically ill children who are unable to void spontaneously.

Attempt to increase sodium and water output during the acute phase of therapy begins with the use of intravenous furosemide. The dose of furosemide is increased at intervals of 30-60 minutes if a bladder catheter is in place or at 90-120 minutes if no catheter has been inserted. If no diuresis has occurred despite doses of 7-8 mg/kg and the child is adequately or excessively hydrated, subsequent management should be planned on the assumption that advanced renal failure, i.e. GFR less than 20% of normal, has developed.

Two additional therapeutic maneuvers have been used to induce a diuresis and/or to convert low output to high output renal failure. Intravenous albumin 0.5 to 1 gm/kg given over a few hours and followed by intravenous furosemide may be helpful in patients with RPGN and the nephrotic syndrome. Mannitol 0.5 gm/kg given as an intravenous infusion over 45-90 minutes, followed by intravenous furosemide 30-45 minutes after the infusion has been started, may also be helpful. Because both albumin and Mannitol increase intravascular volume, and because most children with rapidly progressive renal failure already have an expanded extracellular volume, the use of these agents should be undertaken only after an extremely careful evaluation of the child's cardiopulmonary status. When these agents are used, the ongoing monitoring of vital signs, urine output, and repetitive physical examinations are mandatory. Such therapy should be discontinued if blood pressure rises significantly, a gallop rhythm or rales develop, or if urine output fails to increase. Repeat trials are contraindicated.

A successful diuresis, by acutely lowering extracellular volume, may help dramatically lower blood pressure, reverse cardiac failure and/or pulmonary edema, and increase GFR either by improving cardiovascular hemodynamics or lowering renal vascular resistance. In an occasional child, phlebotomy or the use of rotating tourniquets may be life saving, while other therapies are being instituted.

Acute peritoneal dialysis, or hemodialysis, or ultrafiltration alone is indicated to rapidly lower extracellular volume when more conservative maneuvers have failed. We prefer to use hypertonic peritoneal dialysis rather than hemodialysis to remove excess sodium and water in the newly diagnosed child for a number of reasons: an acute peritoneal dialysis can usually be started in a pediatric setting more quickly than hemodialysis; sodium and water removal can be extended as long as necessary to achieve the desired effect; and since peritoneal dialysis is "slower" than hemodialysis, the cardiovascular responses occur more slowly, and ongoing monitoring and therapeutic intervention is somewhat easier.

We insert a Tenckhoff catheter if it is felt that the need for dialysis will extend for more than 48 hours. One rapid in and out exchange is performed to ensure catheter function; and then, exchanges with 4.25% dextrose are begun at a volume of 30-50 ml/kg as tolerated, not to exceed 2000 ml. A total cycle length of 30-45 minutes is used. In children with compromised respiratory function, dialysis should be begun with smaller volumes and increased with each succeeding exchange until the desired volume is achieved. Blood sugars should be monitored frequently and treated with insulin if they exceed 300-500 mg/dl, or ultrafiltration may become impaired. End points and time frames for therapy should be predefined and redefined as therapy progresses.

Therapeutic Approach to Severe Hypertension Associated with Advanced Chronic Renal Insufficiency and End Stage Renal Disease (ESRD)

Severe hypertension occurs in the child with ESRD as part of the primary disease process itself and/or because of the patient's inability to alter life style and dietary intake in order to limit expansion of the extracellular volume (ECF). Because of the dynamic interplay of these factors, hypertensive crises frequently occur in such children despite ongoing antihypertensive therapy. Treatment of hypertensive children with advanced renal failure, including those undergoing maintenance dialysis, is based on altering one or both limbs of the blood pressure formula, BP = volume times vasoconstriction.[32-34] Treatment of the volume component is based primarily on the use of dietary restrictions, and occasionally on high doses of loop diuretics and dialysis to remove excess volume. The vasoconstriction limb is altered by the use of vasodilators, renin antagonists, and agents which influence nervous system regulation of resistance vessels. Four aspects of blood pressure control in children with ESRD need consideration. 1) reduction of ECF; 2) use of oral antihypertensive agents; 3) bilateral nephrectomy and 4) treatment of acute hypertensive episodes.

In our experience, an expanded ECF is the major issue needing immediate attention in the majority of severely hypertensive children with advanced renal insufficiency. Severely restricted sodium diets and high dose diuretics may be tried in children not yet on dialysis, but generally this approach is not very successful. We have been more successful when we have utilized a palatable diet containing a reduced sodium content combined with loop diuretics, primarily oral furosemide, in a daily dose of 4-8 mg/kg/day divided in two to four doses. Although furosemide is not likely to be very effective when the glomerular filtration rate is less than 15 ml/min/1.73m^2, it may have a beneficial effect even when the GFR is very low. Because the rate of excretion of sodium varies with both the severity and etiology of the renal failure, periodic measurements of the daily urinary sodium excretion can be helpful in prescribing the amount of sodium which ought to be ingested. In children with an obligate sodium loss, too severe a dietary restriction of sodium may result in volume contraction, the response to which may be one of excessive renin release and worsening hypertension. Fluid intake during the predialysis stage of uremia is limited to insensible water loss plus urinary water excretion. The water content of food must be taken into account. The training of patients and parents to alter fluid intake and/or doses of diuretics, based on weights obtained once or twice a day, can be very helpful.

Oral antihypertensive agents are used to chronically control hypertension when the diastolic and/or systolic blood pressure consistently exceeds the 95 percentile for age. Once children begin dialysis, we try to encourage children to limit weight gain between dialyses to 3-5% of dry weight. Weight gains (water retention) of this amount can be safely reduced by hemodialysis without causing unpleasant side effects. Children on CAPD can usually tolerate larger amounts of fluid without developing severe hypertension and can be managed by training families to alter the glucose content of the dialysate according to twice daily weights and measured drainage volumes. Excessive weight gains in the child on maintenance dialysis predisposes to developing congestive heart failure and hypertension. We have found the help of the nursing staff, especially one oriented toward primary care, a pediatric nutritionist, play therapist, and pediatric social worker to be essential in accomplishing the goal of good fluid compliance.

Three approaches can be used to treat children with excessive interdialytic weight gain and high blood pressure. First, we try to help the child cope with his attitudes toward life style and chronic dialysis by providing ongoing psychosocial and nutritional counselling to the child and family. Second, despite the ability of current dialyzers to remove large amounts of water during a given dialysis session, we try to restrict the amount of ultrafiltration per dialysis session to a quantity no greater than 5% of body weight regardless of the patient's weight gain, provided that he is not symptomatic. Our experience has been that the maneuver of setting limits on rates of ultrafiltration combined with positive reinforcement about fluid control, etc., may help function as a deterrent to children gaining excessive weight. Third, we have, when absolutely necessary, increased the frequency of dialysis to daily dialysis for 4-6 days.

Most children undergoing maintenance dialysis require antihypertensive agents at one time or another to satisfactorily control their blood pressure. It is often possible to modify drug therapy after maintenance dialysis has begun because of the effect of volume contraction, especially in those on CAPD.

Although the indications and doses of the drugs are widely used and discussed in the pediatric nephrology literature, many of these medications have not been approved for use in hypertensive children by the Food and Drug Administration. The starting and maximal doses of oral antihypertensive agents used to treat severe hypertension in our patient population are summarized in Table VII. Insofar as possible, we prefer to increase the dose of a given agent until the desired effect is achieved, or side effects require the lowering of the dose rather than using small doses of many drugs. When more than one agent is needed, the newly added agent should have a different mechanism of action. Lower doses of two agents may be used to avoid undesirable side effects. In such situations it is an individual's decision as to whether agents with similar and/or dissimilar modes of actions should be used. When treating severe hypertension in children with a low GFR, it should be remembered that the metabolic half life of some antihypertensives may be prolonged, and too rapid a lowering a blood pressure may further reduce and/or transiently lower GFR. There are no prospective controlled trials of antihypertensive agents in children with ESRD.

Because many antihypertensive agents interfere with the normal homeostatic reflexes involved in the cardiovascular reactions elicited by acute volume depletion, i.e. increased cardiac output and vasoconstriction, the dose of antihypertensive agent (s) given prior to dialysis may need to be reduced and/or omitted. The usual dose of antihypertensives, however, should be given when the predialysis blood pressure is extremely high or the child is symptomatic. When antihypertensives which are readily removed by dialysis (diazoxide, nitroprusside, methyldopa, and captopril) are used, these agents may need to be given during and/or immediately after dialysis.

There are some children whose blood pressure cannot be reduced to normal levels despite the use of maximal doses of antihypertensive agents and adequate ultrafiltration. Bilateral nephrectomy should be considered in such patients.[35-37] Measurements of peripheral PRA should be obtained prior to beginning antihypertensive therapy and whenever problems with blood pressure control develop. Knowledge of the PRA may be helpful when selecting antihypertensive agents and in deciding upon bilateral nephrectomy.

The removal of kidneys eliminates the contribution of the renin angiotensin system to the elevation of the blood pressure. Blood pressure usually falls to normal levels within a few days to a few weeks after nephrectomy. The failure of the blood pressure to return to normal after a bilateral nephrectomy suggests that the dry weight of the child may be lower than it was assumed to be, or that the baroreceptor reflexes have been reset at a higher level. We have on rare occasion recommended bilateral nephrectomy in a non-compliant child based on the premise that the blood pressure after nephrectomy will be lower for a given degree of volume expansion.

Bilateral nephrectomy may also be indicated in children with moderately elevated blood pressure levels because of the known relationship of chronic hypertension and cardiovascular disease. The presence of additional cardiovascular risk factors, such as hyperlipidemia, family history, and the documentation of hypertensive end organ damage, help influence the decision to recommend bilateral nephrectomy.

Episodes of marked elevations in blood pressure are not uncommon in children undergoing chronic dialysis. The usual cause is a sudden expansion in extracellular volume although a change in renal renin release may lead to similar hypertensive emergencies. When such a situation develops, steps to reduce extracellular volume need to be instituted while intravenous vasodilators are administered in a manner similar to that described in the section on rapidly progressive renal failure. Food and fluid intake should be lowered transiently to the amount necessary to administer drugs. If, as is often the case, excessive weight gain has occurred, an emergency acute dialysis should be arranged if life threatening medical complications have developed. During such a dialysis the child may be "bled" into the dialyzer. Ultrafiltration, possibly followed by regular dialysis, may be used to achieve extra removal of fluid. In patients on maintenance peritoneal dialysis, hypertonic exchanges are begun and utilized until adequate fluid removal is achieved, provided hyperglycemia does not intervene. In a few children with pulmonary edema, anemia, heart failure and advanced renal failure not yet started on dialysis, we have successfully utilized partial exchange transfusions and/or phlebotomy in conjunction with a carefully monitored transfusion of packed red blood cells to lower blood pressure and to treat concomitant anemia.

In some children with kidneys in place and who are on maintenance hemodialysis, excessive fluid removal, by acutely stimulating renin release, may result in an acute hypertensive crisis toward the end of a dialysis treatment. Should intravenous hydralazine fail to lower blood pressure, an infusion of saline and/or mannitol may lower blood pressure by acutely expanding intravascular volume.

Generalized seizures occur in a number of children with ESRD in conjunction with acute elevations in blood pressure. The therapeutic measures which we institute in such patients follows: be sure that the child's airway is patent and that he is adequately oxygenated; and give either intravenous diazepam (Valium) in the amount of 0.1-0.3 mg/kg or intramuscular phenobarbital 10 mg/kg up to a total dose of 250 mg. Steps should be undertaken to simultaneously lower blood pressure. If full recovery from a seizure associated with an acute hypertensive episode occurs within 24-48 hours, we generally do not undertake further studies to evaluate the central nervous system. Children with focal seizures, abnormal fundoscopic findings and/or repetitive seizures should undergo a complete neurologic evaluation. If it is felt that a cerebral vascular accident has occurred, nitroprusside, rather than bolus hydralazine or diazoxide therapy, may be a better agent to initially use to treat severe hypertension because it permits more precise control of the blood pressure to occur.

Anatomic Defects of the Genitourinary System Associated with Severe Hypertension in Children

The ideal form of management in these children is surgical correction of the defect. Specific guidelines for lowering blood pressure in such children are not available, and blood pressure control is often difficult to achieve. Most lesions are associated with excessive renin release and/or sodium retention. During the initial work-up and while awaiting definitive procedures, our approach to blood pressure control is based on the pathophysiology involved. As regards pharmacologic intervention the details of antihypertensive management are similar to those discussed in other sections, (Table VI, VII). A combination of intravenously administered vasodilators, starting with hydralazine followed by diazoxide if necessary, in conjunction with a loop diuretic would be used to treat hypertensive crises in such patients. Oral therapy would initially consist of antirenin agents such as Inderal followed, if required, by the addition of Apresoline and Aldomet. Diuretics might be used initially if the hypertension were felt to be due primarily to sodium and water retention; they are also used to deal with compensatory responses of other agents leading to expansion of the ECF. Captopril or minoxidil would be used if the above failed to maintain the blood pressure within acceptable limits.

A large number of primary anatomic disorders giving rise to severe hypertension in children occur infrequently and will not be discussed. Four types of anatomic lesions: renal vascular lesions, intrarenal mass lesions, obstructive uropathy and transplantation will be discussed because they occur more commonly.

In the past few years, percutaneous transluminal angioplasty (PTA) has been widely used in the treatment of renovascular hypertension.[38] Technical success has been reported in 87% and 67% of adults with fibromuscular hyperplasia and atherosclerotic disease respectively.[39] Blood pressure control over time was significantly better in the group with fibromuscular disease. Relatively few reports of the use of this technique in children are available. Most are individual case reports in which long-term success was reported. We are aware of at least two failures of PTA, involving unilateral and bilateral lesions. PTA, because of its limited risk and the potential to avoid major surgery, is worth trying in children with renal vascular lesions, but its precise role remains to be defined. Selection of children for PTA should be based on the demonstration of ipsilateral excessive renin release and contralateral renin suppression.[40] Stenotic lesions near the origin of the renal artery often respond poorly to PTA. Surgical repair continues to be the major form of correction of stenotic lesions.

Intrarenal lesions associated with severe hypertension include Wilms and juxtaglomerular cell tumors, cystic disorders, and trauma. Selective renal embolization has been successfully used to infarct kidneys with large tumor masses prior to surgical removal. Its use in small children has been associated with embolization of the contralateral kidney. Surgery may be curative.

The treatment of severe hypertension associated with various forms of polycystic kidney disease is often difficult and usually requires multiple antihypertensive agents, including agents such as minoxidil or captopril. Drainage of cysts or unilateral nephrectomy has not been effective in lowering blood pressure. Infants with progressive cystic disorders have survived to a size large enough to undergo transplantation because of our increasing ability to manage their hypertension.

Children with obstructive uropathy occasionally present with severe hypertension or develop severe hypertension during the initial few days after surgical correction. Severe hypertension would be treated parenterally as outlined above; and a beta blocker, because of its antirenin effect, would be our initial choice for chronic oral maintenance control until surgery is performed. Therapy should be discontinued over a few days after recovery from surgery with elevations in blood pressure used as a guideline for reinstituting or readjusting therapy.

Reflux nephropathy, especially when complicated by infection, may lead to unilateral or bilateral scarred kidneys associated with severe hypertension.(41) Treatment of acute hypertensive crises is similar to that considered in the section on RPGN. Antirenin agents may be helpful in chronically controlling hypertension. Nephrectomy in unilateral disease may be curative. Hypertension may be prevented in some patients by early detection of reflux and its surgical corrections. The correction of reflux usually does not improve hypertension once it is present.(41)

Post transplant hypertension may result from one or more of the following: ATN, rejection, vascular lesions, obstructive uropathy and the use of corticosteroids. Patients with glomerular lesions experience more transplant hypertension than those with obstructive uropathy. Post transplant patients tend to have their highest blood pressure during the night. When large doses of corticosteroids are being used, the blood pressure may be particularly refractory to antihypertensive agents. Therapy depends on the nature of the lesion; and in the absence of surgically identifiable lesions, therapy is similar to that already discussed. The hypertension associated with renal artery stenosis has been successfully managed by percutaneous transluminal angioplasty, surgical repair, and/or antihypertensive agents. Vasodilators, intravenous diuretics and renin inhibiting agents have been used in varying combinations to treat severe hypertension. Since the most common factors included in the hypertension process post transplant are volume overload and hyperreninemia, the combination of beta blockers and diuretics is often successful.

Table VI - Parenteral Antihypertensive Agents Available For Treatment of Hypertensive Emergencies in Children

Agent- Generic, Trade, and how supplied	How given	Dose	Interval
Alpha-methyldopa (Aldomet) (250 mg/5ml)	IV drip	5-10 mg/kg given in 5% D/W over 30-60 min. Max = 500 mg	q 6-8h
Diazoxide (Hyperstat) (300 mg/20ml)	IV push rapid IV infusion	2.5-10 mg/kg may repeat in 30 min if no response 7.5 mg/kg at a rate of 7.5 mg/min/70kg	prn 10% loading dose q6h or as continuous infusion
Hydralazine (Apresoline) (20 mg/ml)	IV push	0.1-0.5 mg/kg/dose maximum dose 20 mg	q 3-6h
Nitroprusside (Nipride) (50 mg vials)	IV infusion by pump	0.5-10 ug/kg/min diluted in 5% D/W	continuous infusion
Saralasin Acetate (Sarenin) (18 mg/30 ml)	IV infusion by pump	0.05-15 ug/kg/min min	continuous infusion
Furosemide (Lasix) (10 mg/ml)	IV infusion	1-7 mg/kg at a rate < 0.06 mg/kg/min	q 1-12 prn

Overview of Pharmacologic Agents Used to Treat Severe Hypertension in Children (Tables VI, VII)

Hydralazine (Apresoline)^R

Hydralazine(42) lowers blood pressure by decreasing vascular resistance. It directly relaxes smooth muscle and can lower vascular resistance up to 75%.(43) Its effect is less than theoretically expected because of

Table VI - Parenteral Antihypertensive Agents Available For
(Cont'd) Treatment of Hypertensive Emergencies in Children

Onset of action	Duration of action	Major Acute Problems	Agent- Generic, Trade, and how supplied
2-6 hrs	10-16 hrs	Sedation, delayed onset, paradoxical pressure response, diarrhea, orthostatic hypotension	Alpha-methyldopa (Aldomet) (250 mg/5ml
1-3 min minutes	1/2 - 24 hr 5-6 hrs	Hyperglycemia, hyperuricemia, acute hypotension, nausea, vomiting, flushing, arrhythmia, sodium retention	Diazoxide (Hyperstat) (300 mg/20ml)
5-30 min	4-6 hrs	Tachycardia, headaches, flushing, nasal congestion, palpitations, vomiting, diarrhea, acute hypotension, myocardial ischemia	Hydralazine (Apresoline) (20 mg/ml)
Immediate	Only effective during infusion	Thiocyanate intoxication (maintain thiocyanate levels below 10mg/dl); chest pain, abdominal pain, headaches, rigidity, GI upset, seizures	Nitroprusside (Nipride) (50 mg vials)
Immediate	Only effective during infusion	Pressor responses, rebound hypertension, marked lowering of blood pressure, headaches	Saralasin Acetate (Sarenin) (18 mg/30 ml)
5 min	2-3 hrs	Hearing loss, dehydration, interstitial nephritis, hyperglycemia, contraction alkalosis	Furosemide (Lasix) (10 mg/ml)

baroreceptor induced sympathetic discharge which increases heart rate, stroke volume and cardiac output. Vasodilators also cause sodium and water retention by altering the kidneys' perception of "effective" vascular volume. Hydralazine neither increases venous capacitance nor significantly alters renal blood flow. These responses limit the antihypertensive effect of hydralazine when it is used acutely or repetitively as a single agent, and the addition of other antihypertensive medications may be required.

Table VII - Oral Agents Commonly Used for Treatment of Severe Hypertension in Children

Agent - Generic, Trade and Tablet size	Dose(mg/kg/day) Initial	Max	Do not exceed per day	Dose Interval	Onset hours
Alphamethyldopa (Aldomet) 125,250 mg	10	60	2 gm	8-12 h	3-5
Captopril (Capoten) 25, 50, 100 mg	0.9	8	8 mg/kg	8-12 h	.25-1.5
Chlorothiazide (Diuril) 250,500 mg 50 mg/ml	10	20	2 gm	12-24 h	2
Clonidine (Catapres) 0.1, 0.2 mg	(0.05) Individual dose	(1.2)	2.4 mg	12 h	0.5 1.0
Guanethidine (Ismelin) 10, 25 mg	0.2	0.5	?	24 h	48-72
Hydralazine (Apresoline) 10,25,50,100mg	1.0	4	200 mg	6 h	1-2
Minoxidil (Loniten) 1,2.5,5,10 mg	0.1	0.5	40 mg	12-24 h	1.5-3
Furosemide (Lasix) 20,40,80 mg and 10 mg/ml	0.5	8	8 mg/kg	6-24 h	1
Hydrochlorothiazide (Hydrodiuril) 25,50 mg	1	4	200 mg	12-24 h	2

Table VII - Oral Agents Commonly Used to Treat Severe Hypertension in Children

Duration hours	Maximum response days	Frequency of Changing dose, days	Major Problems	Agent - Generic, Trade and Tablet size
8 - 12	7	3-6	postural hypotension sedation, liver enzymes positive Coombs	Alphamethyldopa (Aldomet) 125,250 mg
8 - 12	10-14	2-14	Neutropenia, proteinuria, membranous, nephropathy, hypertension, hyperkalemia, dysequesia	Captopril (Capoten) 25, 50, 100 mg
6-12	14	1-3	hypokalemia, hyperuricemia volume contraction hyperglycemmia	Chlorothiazide (Diuril) 250, 500 mg 50 mg/ml
8	5-7	1-4	rebound hypertension, sedation, dry mouth, coma, constipation, dizziness	Clonidine (Catapres) 0.1, 0.2 mg
1-3 wks	14	12-14	postural hypotension, headaches, impotence bradycardia, diarrhea	Guanethidine (Ismelin) 10, 25 mg
4-6	3-4	1-3	Tachycardia, lupus like syndrome, headaches-nausea	Hydralazine (Apresoline) 10,25,50,100mg
12-72	2-4	1	Tachycardia, fluid retension hypertrichosis	Minoxidil (Loniten) 1,2.5,5,10 mg
4-8	14	1-3	hypokalemia, alkalosis, ototoxicity, interstitial nephritis, leukopenia, pancreatitis	Furosemide (Lasix) 20,40,80 mg and 10 mg/ml
6-12	14	1-3	same as chlorothiazide	Hydrochlorothiazide (Hydrodiuril) 25, 50 mg

Table VII (Cont'd from p. 166)

Prazosin (Minipres) 1, 2, 5 mg	0.014	0.45	20-40 mg	6-12 h	1/2
Propranolol (Inderal) 10,40,80 mg	1	6	10 mg/kg	8-12 h	2-72
Spironolactone (Aldactone) 25 mg	2	4	200 mg	6-12 h	2-12

Hydralazine can be used in conjunction with diazoxide, methyldopa, propranolol, reserpine, or diuretics. If hydralazine is used on a chronic basis, the simultaneous use of oral beta blockers and diuretics will improve blood pressure control by inhibiting reflex tachycardia, and sodium retention.

Major side effects include headaches, nausea, vomiting, diarrhea, myocardial ischemia and the cardiovascular effects mentioned above. Certain patients, less able to metabolize hydralazine due to a reduced activity of hepatic-acetyl-transferase,[(42)] require a lower dose for therapeutic effect; in addition, toxicity is more common in slow acetylators. Major side effects which can occur with the chronic use of hydralazine include a lupus like syndrome,[(44)] drug fever, skin rashes and peripheral neuropathy.

Alpha Methyldopa (Aldomet)[R]

Methyldopa is capable of acutely lowering the blood pressure in children with severe hypertension. Its use in such circumstances, however, is limited by three factors: 1) too rapid an infusion may enable the drug to function as false neurotransmitter and paradoxically elevate blood pressure; 2) blood pressure falls gradually over a few hours when methyldopa is infused over 30-60 minutes (to avoid the paradoxical elevation in blood pressure), and such a rate of lowering may be unacceptably slow and 3) somnolence is a common side effect and may mask developing CNS symptomatology. Methyldopa lowers blood pressure by a combination of actions including a direct relaxation of arteriolar smooth muscle,[(45)] a central nervous system effect,[(46)] and an antirenin effect.[(47)]

Table VII (Cont'd from p. 167)

6-24	3-4	2	syncope, tachycardia, hypotension, sedation, headaches, weakness	Prazosin (Minipres) 1, 2, 5 mg
48	3-5	2-6	bradycardia, bronchospasm, hypotension, hypoglycemia	Propranolol (Inderal) 10,40,80 mg
24-48	2-3	3-4	gynecomastia, hyperkalemia, ataxia, alopecia	Spironolactone (Aldactone) 25 mg

Methyldopa can be used orally alone or in combination with other agents to chronically control blood pressure in children with severe hypertension. Major side effects include: somnolence which tends to lessen with time, drug fever, a Coombs positive hemolytic anemia, elevations in hepatic enzymes, nasal stuffiness, and gastrointestinal disturbances.(48)

Diazoxide (Hyperstat)R

Diazoxide(49) currently is our drug of choice to treat hypertensive emergencies. Diazoxide is a benzothiadiazine derivative similar in structure to the thiazide diuretics. It acts by acutely relaxing arteriolar smooth muscle throughout the body.(50) Although the baroreceptor response to diazoxide reflexively increases heart rate, stroke volume and cardiac output, the net effect on overall cardiac work is reduced. Systemic blood flow remains adequate in most circumstances because of the increased cardiac output.(49) Renal blood flow and GFR may fall transiently after an intravenous bolus of diazoxide but usually returns to normal within a few hours.(51) Only minimal effects on intrinsic cardiac function, autonomic reflexes and capacitance vessels occur with diazoxide.(49)

Diazoxide has been used three ways: 1) bolus doses, single or multiple; 2) continuous infusion or 3) repeated doses at fixed intervals. A significant linear log dose response relation between bolus diazoxide and the decrease in diastolic blood pressure was observed in 16 children ages 10 months to 13 years with secondary forms of hypertension.(52) Bolus doses of 2, 3 and 5 mg/kg of diazoxide resulted in mean drops of diastolic blood pressure of 23, 30 and 40 mm Hg respectively. In 5 patients, 2-3 repetitive intravenous bolus injections of 2 mg/kg of diazoxide at 10-15 minute intervals were as effective in lowering diastolic blood pressure as a single dose of 6 mg/kg. (52)

In a recently reported study involving adult patients,(53) a scheme was reported for giving diazoxide as a continuous infusion or repetitive doses aimed at a graded and predictable reduction in blood pressure. A loading dose of 7.5 mg/kg was given at a rate of 7.5 mg/min until the mean arterial pressure fell by 25%. If additional diazoxide was needed, it was infused at a rate of 3.75 mg/min. Once the desired reduction was achieved, a maintenance dose of 10% of the loading dose was given either every 6 hours or as a continuous infusion lasting 6 hours. Once blood pressure stabilized, oral antihypertensive therapy was instituted.

Although it is the free or unbound levels of diazoxide that determine its hypotensive effect, higher drug levels were required in continuous, as opposed to bolus, infusion of diazoxide to maintain a reduced blood pressure. The reason for this is unclear, but may reflect diazoxide induced stimulation of the renin angiotensin system or cardiovascular effects. In patients with renal failure, reductions in blood pressure following bolus diazoxide correlate well with BUN since diazoxide binding to serum protein is reduced in uremic patients.(54)

Major side effects include hyperglycemia, hyperuricemia, salt and water retention, and displacement of anticoagulants from albumin.(55) Cardiac arrhythmias, angina, headache and flushing can also occur. Expansion of extracellular volume has been shown to decrease the responsiveness to diazoxide.(56) Hyperglycemia results from the direct effect of diazoxide to lower insulin secretion by beta cells of the pancreas.(57) Nonketotic hyperglycemic coma may develop unless the patient is monitored. Therapy should be instituted to lower the blood sugar when it persistently exceeds 275-300 mg/dl. Hyperuricemia results from an inhibition of the tubular secretion of uric acid.(51)

Nitroprusside (Nipride)^R

Sodium nitroprusside acts as a direct vasodilator of both resistance arteries and capacitance veins.(58) The effect of nitroprusside on cardiac output is minimal and dependent upon changes occurring in venous return. The degree to which blood pressure falls during a nitroprusside infusion is dose dependent. Improvement in myocardial function can be anticipated when nitroprusside is used in patients with concomitant heart failure and hypertension.[59]

Blood pressure falls within seconds after beginning a continuous infusion of Nipride(R). In hypertensive crises, nitroprusside may be infused initially at a dose of 0.5 - 1.0 ug/kg/min and increased by 0.5 to 1.0 ug/kg/min every 2-3 minutes to a maximum rate of 8 ug/kg/minute or until the desired pressure is obtained. Blood pressure determinations should be taken every minute. Since the magnitude of the blood pressure fall is so critically dose dependent, the drug is best administered using a constant rate infusion pump. A microdrip chamber can be used if a constant infusion device cannot be obtained. Because sodium nitroprusside decomposes when exposed to either heat or light, intravenous solutions must be shielded from light.

In a group of twenty children 7 to 17 years of age with diastolic blood pressures exceeding 100 mm Hg, the average fall in systolic and diastolic blood pressures was 47 and 49 mm Hg respectively.[30] Desired control of blood pressure was usually obtained within five minutes while cardiac failure was reversed within 24 hours, and neurologic signs abated in 24-48 hours. Intravenous furosemide (5 mg/kg) was used as supplemental therapy in patients with congestive heart failure.[30] The infusate was prepared by dissolving Nipride 35 mg in 500 ml of 5% Dextrose in water (70 mg/ml) or 35 mg in 250 ml of 5% Dextrose (140 mg/ml) in children with oliguria. Nipride infusions have been used for up to 28 days in children without tachyphylaxis or significant toxicity developing.[60]

Major side effects of nitroprusside include psychotic reactions, seizures, coma, muscle spasm, bone marrow depression, anorexia, metabolic acidosis, and hypothyroidism. Thiocyanate inhibits the uptake and binding of iodine by the thyroid gland.[61] Less serious side effects include anorexia, nausea, fatigue, skin rashes, and minimal drops in renal function. Serum levels of thiocyanate should be monitored in children undergoing prolonged infusion of nitroprusside and therapy modified when levels exceed 10 mg/dl.

Nitroprusside is non-enzymatically metabolized to cyanogen and subsequently converted to thiocyanate by the enzyme rhodanase in liver and red cells.[62] Thiocyanate has a half-life of several days and is eliminated by the kidney. The renal clearance of thiocyanate is 2.2 ml/min [63,64].

The toxic effects of nitroprusside may be due to either thiocyanate or cyanide accumulation.[58] Thiocyanate can be rapidly removed by either peritoneal[58] or hemodialysis.[63,65] Hemodialysis removes thiocyanate from the body more rapidly than it is cleared by the kidney. Toxicity can be treated by discontinuing or lowering the rate of infusion, the use of dialysis to increase removal of drug, or by concomitantly infusing hydroxycobalamin which combines with cyanide to form cyanocobalamin, which is relatively nontoxic.[66]

Saralasin (Sarenin)[R]

Saralasin acetate is a specific competitive inhibitor of angiotensin II used primarily to diagnose renin mediated hypertension. It can only be given intravenously. A significant drop in blood pressure occurring in response to a saralasin infusion is considered diagnostic of hyperreninemia. Although not considered to be an antihypertensive agent per se, a continuous infusion of saralasin in a few patients unresponsive to other drugs has been shown to adequately lower blood pressure without major adverse effects.[67,67A] In two children, one weighing less than 1000 gm and an 8 year old, a continuous infusion of saralasin ranging between 0.05 to 15 mcgm/kg/min was used for as long as 13 days to control blood pressure [67A].

Based on very limited experience, it seems that saralasin may be an effective new agent for temporarily controlling severe hypertension. Its ultimate role remains to be more clearly defined. Sarenin[R] has not been approved for this form of therapy by the FDA.

Oral Agents for Treating Severe Persistent Hypertension (Minoxidil, Captopril)

Although intravenous therapy remains the principal initial form of treatment for hypertensive emergencies, two potent oral vasodilators, minoxidil and captopril are currently available for use in children with severe hypertension. The judicious use of these agents may enable fewer drugs or tolerable doses of other agents to be used, permit long term control of severe hypertension to be achieved and prevent further hypertensive crises. Clear indications for initiating therapy in children with these agents remain to be defined.

Minoxidil, (Loniten[R]), a piperidino-pyrimidine derivative, acts as a vasodilator on systemic arteries without any effect on veins. Even though it has been widely used for a number of years to treat children with severe hypertension, it has not been formally approved for use in children. Because of significant side effects, its use is best reserved for children who remain severely hypertensive despite oral therapy with a combination of three or four antihypertensives and diuretic agents. Minoxidil is rapidly absorbed from the gastrointestinal tract, reaches peak plasma levels in approximately one hour, requires two to four hours for its maximal effect and exerts a hypotensive effect for 12-24 hours.[68]

Minoxidil has been shown to be an effective agent in treating severe hypertension in children.[69-73] Starting daily doses in children are 0.1 to 0.2 mg/kg/day given two to four times a day.[26] Each dose may be increased until the desired effect or a maximum dose of 40 mg/day is given. The maximum approved daily dose for use in adults is 100 mg.[69] In a report of 21 children ages 6 months to 16 years, minoxidil was begun at a dose of 1 mg with subsequent increases to 2, 3, 5, 7.5 and 10 mg at 12 hours intervals until the blood pressure fell to 130-140/90-100 mm Hg.[69] The mean and range of doses of minoxidil were 0.48 and 0.07 - 1.6 mg/kg/day respectively. Factors which limited its effectiveness were fluid retention and the use of prednisone to treat transplant rejection.

Although it was originally thought that most other antihypertensive agents should be discontinued when minoxidil was used, the addition of smaller doses of minoxidil to other antihypertensives has been shown to be effective in controlling blood pressure. Thus a lower dose of minoxidil can be used and its concomitant side effects, especially hypertrichosis, reduced.

Hypertrichosis reaches a maximum in 5-8 weeks. Generalized body hair growth which may become psychologically unacceptable occurs at the hairline above the eyebrow and over the temples. Depilatories or shaving can be used to remove undesired hair.[68] Discontinuation of minoxidil usually results in the disappearance of excessive growth of hair; it may take 4-5 months for the hypertrichosis to resolve.

Life threatening pericardial effusions may result from the use of minoxidil. Although pericardial effusions may result from minoxidil alone, such effusions tend to occur more frequently in patients with predisposing factors including uremia, congestive heart failure, and collagen vascular disorders.[74] The other major side effects of minoxidil including reflex tachycardia, salt and water retention, augmented renin release,[75] and sympathetic nerve discharge are best viewed as physiologic effects of the potent vasodilation and subsequent baroreceptor responses. The concomitant use of propranolol, a beta blocker,[76] or clonidine, a suppressor of sympathetic outflow from the brain,[77] together with a diuretic such as furosemide,is usually required to reduce these effects.

Rebound hypertension has been reported in children following the withdrawal of minoxidil. The occurrence of rebound hypertension correlates with the total cumulative dose in mg/kg/week, and the rapidity (4-8 weeks) of withdrawal of the agent.[78] Pretreatment with an alpha blocking agent (Prazosin) or discontinuation of a beta blocker (Propranolol) prior to withdrawal may prevent rebound.

Captopril, (Capoten(R)), is the first available oral agent which specifically inhibits the activity of the renin angiotensin system.[79] Captopril prevents the conversion of inactive angiotensin I to the potent vasoactive peptide angiotensin II through its action as a competitive inhibitor of the angiotensin-converting enzyme. Although the primary mechanism of captopril in lowering blood pressure is inhibition of angiotensin II generation, angiotensin converting enzyme is also bradykinase. Captopril may inhibit the degradation of bradykinin, a vasodepressor peptide, and lower blood pressure in part by limiting the rate of removal of vasodepressor kinins.[80] Captopril lowers peripheral arteriolar resistance without significantly altering cardiac output, heart rate or venous resistance.[81,82] Although the initial fall in blood pressure is proportional to the pretreatment plasma renin activity,[83] chronic therapy fails to show such a correlation.[79] Patients with normal, high and low levels of plasma renin activity have responded to captopril administration by lowering their blood pressure. Although captopril, in contradistinction to other vasodilators, does not lead to significant salt and water retention, the addition of a thiazide diuretic often enhances its blood pressure lowering effect.

Major side effects of captopril include proteinuria most often in patients with pre-existing renal diseases, and neutropenia, most often occurring in patients with lupus, immunologic disorders, or in patients with reduced renal function.[79] Consideration should be given to discontinuing captopril if proteinuria increases or develops in patients after the initiation of therapy. Membranous nephropathy similar to that occurring with other drugs such as gold, penicillin and trimethadione may develop. Transient elevations in serum creatinine and acute reversible renal failure have been noted during captopril therapy.(79) White counts should be monitored at two week intervals for the initial three months of therapy as neutropenia most often develops 3-12 weeks after starting therapy. After the third month of therapy, white counts can be monitored at less frequent intervals. Since captopril administration leads to a secondary decrease in aldosterone production, elevations in serum potassium may occur, especially in patients with advanced renal insufficiency. Serum potassium elevations during captopril therapy are inversely related to GFR.(83A)

Initial therapy in stable adults is 25 mg t.i.d., which is increased to 50 mg t.i.d. when the response is not satisfactory after one to two weeks. If an additional two-three weeks of therapy fails to lower blood pressure, a thiazide diuretic or furosemide may be added. Captopril subsequently may then be gradually increased at weekly levels to a maximum dose of 150 mg t.i.d. In adult patients with accelerated hypertension, the starting dose of captopril may be increased to a dose of 25 mg t.i.d. daily until the desired response occurs and then slowly individualized on the basis of blood pressure measurements.

A number of reports have shown captopril to be effective in treating severe hypertension in children.(84-88) In children, our initial dose of captopril is 0.9 mg/kg/day given as 0.3 mg/kg every 8 hours. If the GFR is less than 50% we begin with a dose of 0.3 mg/kg/day. Dose increments in both situations are 0.3 mg/kg per dose. The maximum dose used is 8 mg/kg/day. In two recently reported abstracts involving children undergoing regular hemodialysis or following transplant, successful control of blood pressure was achieved with doses of captopril ranging from 0.1 to 10 mg/kg.(89,90) Once adequate control of blood pressure is achieved, the dose of captopril may be slowly tapered until the lowest daily individual dose allowing blood pressure control is achieved. Captopril given on alternate days has been used to successfully control blood pressure in children on hemodialysis.(89)

Diuretics

Diuretics are helpful additions in treating severe hypertension for a number of reasons. They reduce extracellular volume by increasing sodium excretion thereby affecting the volume limb of the blood pressure formula. Although they are rarely used as the sole agent to treat severe hypertension, their major role is to counteract the sodium retaining action of many of the vasodilator agents. Diuretics may also lower blood pressure by nonrenal mechanisms including effects on ions within the walls of blood vessels, alteration of baroreceptor responses, and by direct and indirect effects on the many volume-hormonal-nervous system loops involved in blood pressure regulation. We focus here only on those agents useful in treating severe hypertension and hypertensive emergencies.

Loop diuretics, principally furosemide, are the agents used most often by us to aid in treating severe hypertension in children. The effect of furosemide (Lasix(R)) given either orally or intravenously, is dose dependent. Furosemide is both filtered and secreted into the proximal tubule and inhibits chloride transport in the ascending limb of Henle.[91] The degree of inhibition of chloride transport is related to the concentration of furosemide reaching that segment of the tubule. Approximately 70% of an oral dose of furosemide is absorbed. In normal subjects, 12% of intravenously administered furosemide is excreted in the bile. This percentage rises to 60% in patients with advanced renal failure.[92] The half-life of furosemide is increased in patients with renal insufficiency but not to the extent anticipated. Only 5-10% of plasma furosemide is removed by hemodialysis.

The major side effects of furosemide reflect its actions on salt and water balance. Rapid loss of sodium and water can lead to orthostatic hypotension, prerenal azotemia, syncope and shock. Preload is reduced because of an increase in venous capacitance[93] as well as extracellular volume depletion. The overzealous use of furosemide with its attendant intravascular volume depletion may result in both reductions and redistributions of blood flow to vital organs and perhaps also trigger the coagulation cascade.

Hypokalemia results from the increased delivery of sodium to the distal sodium-potassium exchange sites and volume induced secondary hyperaldosteronism. Less common electrolyte problems include hyponatremia, metabolic alkalosis[94] and hyperuricemia. Both inhibition of urate secretion and volume related enhancement of urate reabsorption lead to a diminished renal clearance of urate.[95] Nonketotic hyperglycemic coma has also been reported with furosemide.

Less commonly used is ethacrynic acid, another potent loop diuretic, because of its association with irreversible ototoxicity. Furosemide usage can also be associated with ototoxicity, usually reversible.[96] Irreversible loss of hearing has been observed in patients with severe renal insufficiency when large doses of furosemide were infused rapidly or used in conjunction with other ototoxic drugs such as aminoglycosides.[97]

Furosemide is given intravenously to inpatients unable to take it orally, when a rapid diuresis is needed, or when hypertensive emergencies exist. Diuresis following the intravenous administration of furosemide begins within 5 to 10 minutes, peaks during the next 20 to 30 minutes and abates by 2 hours. Because of the potential extrarenal toxicity of furosemide, it has been recommended that furosemide be infused at a rate less than 4 mg/min in adults.[92] Such a rate of infusion in adults enables serum levels of furosemide to remain below 30 mg/ml, a level which can avoid significant toxicity, especially ototoxicity. In children requiring intravenous furosemide, we start at a dose of 1 to 2 mg/kg. Doses are increased at increments of 1 mg/kg and repeated at 1-2 hour intervals until either an appropriate response occurs or a maximum dose of 6 to 8 mg/kg is reached.

Therapy with oral furosemide is started at a dose of 1 mg/kg 1-4 times a day. Most often, two smaller doses will achieve a more even control of fluid balance than a single large dose. We have used furosemide, depending upon the child's disease and compliance, at intervals ranging from four times a day to once every 2 to 3 days. Oral daily doses up to 2,500 mg per day have been used in adults.[92,98,99] We have used up to 8 mg/kg/day in children without toxicity other than that related to changes in electrolytes and fluid balance. The measurement of the patient's urine output is the best way to initially judge responsiveness and the need to alter further doses. Another way to gain insight into its efficacy is to weigh the patients prior to, and 3 to 4 hours after taking the drug. Following the oral administration of furosemide, the onset of diuresis occurs within 1 hour, is maximal within the first to second hour and persists for 6 to 8 hours.

Other diuretic agents may be used to further modify the diuretic effect of furosemide. We have successfully added thiazides and aldosterone blocking agents, which inhibit sodium transport at sites in the nephron beyond those blocked by loop diuretics, to the therapeutic regime in refractory patients and observed both an increase in urine output and a further decrease in blood pressure. It has recently been demonstrated that thiazides may potentiate the effect of furosemide in adult patients with a low GFR, creatinine in the range of 2.3 - 4.9 mg/dl.[100] Once an adequate blood pressure response has occurred in a severely hypertensive child, diuretic agents less potent than furosemide, usually in combination with antihypertensive agents, may be effective and may be tried prior to beginning furosemide in the asymptomatic child with severe hypertension.

REFERENCES

1. Pascual, A.V.: Hypertensive Crises: Diagnosis and Strategies in Treatment, Hospital Medicine, January 1981, pp 43-59.

2. Byron, F.B: The pathogenesis of hypertensive encephalopathy and its relation to the malignant phase of hypertension-experimental evidence from the hypertensive rat. Lancet 2: 201, 1954.

3. Reinmuth, O.M., Beteta. E., and Scheinberg, P.: Total cerebral blood flow in cerebral vascular disease in relation to hypertension. Neurology 16:815, 1966.

4. Strandgaard, S., MacKenzie, E.T., Sengupta, D., et al.:Upper limits of autoregulation of cerebral blood flow in the baboon. Circ. Res. 34: 435, 1974.

5. Cuneo, R.A., and Caronna, J.J.: The neurologic complications of hypertension. Med. Clin. North Am. 61: 565, 1977.

6. Calhoun, J.: Ocular manifestations in disorders of the blood, blood vessels, heart, and lungs, and in the histiocytosis syndrome. In: Harley, R.D. (ed) Pediatric Ophthalmology. W.B. Saunders, 1975, p 656.

7. Kincaid-Smith, P.: Malignant Hypertension, Cardiovascular Reviews & Reports, 1: 41, 1980.

8. Leuman, E.P.: Blood pressure and hypertension in childhood and adolescence. In: Frick, H. von P., von Harnack, G.A., Martini, G.A., Prader, A., Schoen, R. and Wolff, H.P. (eds): Advances in Internal Medicine and Pediatrics. Bd 43 Springer-Verlag 1979, p 111.

9. Volhard, F., Fahr, K.T.: Die Brightsche Nierenkranheit. Springer-Verlag, 1914.

10. Keith, N.M., Wagener, H.P., Parker, N.W.: Some different types of essential hypertension: Their course and prognosis. Am. J. Med. Sci. 197:332, 1939.

11. Kincaid-Smith, P., McMichael, J., Murphy, E.A.: The clinical course and pathology of hypertension with papilledema (malignant hypertension). J. Med. 105 (new series 27): 117, 1958.

12. Keith, T.A. III: Hypertension Crisis - Recognition and Management. JAMA, 237: 1570, 1977.

13. Report of the Task Force on Blood Pressure Control in Children; Prepared by the National Heart, Lung, and Blood Institute's Task Force on Blood Pressure Control in Children. Pediatrics, 59: 797, 1977.

14. Guidelines for the Evaluation and Management of the Hypertensive Patient: U.S. Department of Health, Education, and Welfare, U.S. Public Health Service, National Institutes of Health, DHEW Publication no. (NIH) 74-593, Sept. 1, 1973.

15. Laragh, J.H.: Vasoconstriction-volume analysis for understanding and treating hypertension: the use of renin and aldosterone profiles. Am. J. Med. 55: 261, 1973.

16. Hiner, L.B., and Gruskin, A.B.: The physiology of blood pressure regulating normal and abnormal. Pediatr.Ann.6: 373, 1977.

17. Moser, M.: Management of Hypertensive Emergencies. Drug Therapy, May 1974, pp 143-157.

18. Bailie, M. D., Mattiolo, L. F.: Hypertension: Relationships between pathophysiology and therapy, J.Pediatr.95: 789, 1980.

19. Naranjo, G., Somani, P., and Elberg, A.J: The challenge of a pediatric hypertensive crisis. Drug Therapy, April 1979, pp 130-141.

20. McLain, L.G.: Therapy of Acute Severe Hypertension in Children, JAMA, 239: 755, 1978.

21. Rance, C.P., Arbus, G.S., Balfe, J.W., Kooh, S.W.: Persistent Systemic Hypertension in Infants and Children, Pediatr.Clin.North Amer.21: 801, 1974.

22. Perry, H.M.: The Management of Malignant Hypertension. Drug Therapy, October 1971, pp 33-43.

23. Finnerty, F.A.: Hypertensive Crisis. JAMA 229: 1479, 1974.

24. AMA Committee on Hypertension: The Treatment of Malignant Hypertension and Hypertensive Emergencies. JAMA, 228: 1673, 1974.

25. Mendlowitz, M.: Management of Hypertensive Emergencies. Hospital Medicine, December 1979, pp 63-67.

26. Reisman, L. and Selden, R.V: Management of Systemic Hypertension in Children. Pediatr. Ann. 11: 604, 1982.

27. Loggie, J.M.H.: Hypertension in Children and Adolescents. J. Pediatr. 74; 640, 1969.

28. Powell, H.R., Rotenberg, E., Williams, A.L., et al.: Plasma renin activity in acute poststreptococcal glomerulonephritis and the haemolytic-uremic syndrome. Arch. Dis. Child. 49: 802, 1974.

29. Repetto, H.A., Lewy, J.E., Brando, J.L., et al.: The renal functional response to furosemide in children with acute glomerulonephritis. J. Pediatr. 80:660, 1972.

30. Gordillo-Paniagua, G., Velasquez-Jones, L., Martini, R., et al.: Sodium nitroprusside treatment for severe arterial hypertension in children. J. Pediatr. 87:799, 1975.

31. Etteldorf, J.N., Smith, J.D., and Johnson, C.: The effect of reserpine and its combination with hydralazine on blood pressure and renal hemodynamics during the hypertensive phase of acute nephritis in children. J. Pediat. 48: 129, 1956.

32. Lowenthal, D.T, Pennock, R., Likoff, W. and Onesti, G: Therapy of Hypertension in the Dialysis Patient, in Management of the Cardiac Patient with Renal Failure. SA Davis Co., 1981, p 155.

33. Vidt, D.G.: The Management of Hypertension in Renal Failure. The Kidney 9: 15, 1976.

34. Garrett, B.N.: Treatment of Hypertension in Patients with Chronic Renal Failure. Contemporary Dialysis, pp 21-33, April, 1981.

35. Onesti, G., Swartz, C., Remirez, R. and Brest, A.N.: Bilateral nephrectomy for control of hypertension in uremia. Trans. Amer. Soc. Artif. Intern. Organs 14: 361, 1968.

36. Vertes, V., Cangiano, J.L., Berman, L.B., Gould, A.: Hypertension in end-stage renal disease. New Eng. J. Med. 280: 978, 1969.

37. Weidmann, P., Maxwell, M.H., Lupu, A.N., Lemin, A.J., and Massry, S.G.: Plasma renin activity and blood pressure in terminal renal failure. New Eng. J. Med. 285: 757, 1971.

38. Gruntzig, A., Vetter, W., Meier, B.: Treatment of Renovascular Hypertension with Percutaneous Transluminal Dilation of a Renal Artery Stenosis. Lancet. 1: 801, 1978.

39. Vaughan, E.D., Jr., Sos, T.A., Sniderman, K.W., Pickering, T.G., Case, D.B., Sealey, J.H., Laragh, J.H.: Renal Venous Renin Secretory Patterns Before and After Percultaneous Transluminal Angioplasty. In: Laragh, J.H., Buhler, F.R., Seldin, D.W. (eds). Frontiers in Hypertension Research. New York: Springer-Verlag, 1981, p 173.

40. Vaughan, E.D., Jr., Buhler, F.R., Laragh, J.H., Sealey, J.E., Baer, L., Bard, R.H.: Renovascular Hypertension: Renin Measurements to Indicate Hypersecretion and Contralateral Suppression, Estimate Renal

Plasma Flow and Score for Surgical Curability. Am. J. Med., 55: 402, 1973.

41. Ehrlich, R.M.: Vesicoureteral Reflux: A surgeon's perspective. Pediatr. Cl. N.Amer. 28: 827, 1982.

42. Koch-Weser, J., Hydralazine: N.Engl.J.Med.295:320, 1976.

43. Freis, E.D., Rose J.C., Higgins, T.F., et al: The hemodynamic effects of hypotensive drugs in man. IV. 1-hydrazinophthalazine. Circulation 8:199, 1953.

44. Perry, H.M., Jr: Late toxicity to hydralazine resembling systemic lupus erythematosus or rheumatoid arthritis. Am.J.Med.54:58, 1973.

45. Sinaiko, A.R., Mirkin, B.L.: Clinical pharmacology of antihypertensive drugs in children. Pediatr.Clin.North.Am.25(1): 146, 1978.

46. VanZwierten, P.A.: The central action of antihypertensive drugs mediated via central alpha receptors. J.Pharm.Pharmacol.25:89, 1973.

47. Mohammed, S. et al.:Effect of methyldopa on plasma renin activity in man. Cir.Res.25:543, 1969.

48. Furhoff, A: Adverse reactions with methyldopa. Acta Med.Scand. 203:425, 1978.

49. Koch-Weser, J.: Diazoxide. N.Engl.J.Med. 294:1271, 1976.

50. Powell, W.J. Jr., Green, R.M., Whiting R.B., et al.:Action of diazoxide on skeletal muscle vascular resistance. Circ.Res.28:167, 1971.

51. Johnson, B.F.: Diazoxide and renal function in man. Clin.Pharmacol.Ther. 12:815, 1971.

52. Boerth, R.C. and Long, W.R.: Dose-Response Relation of Diazoxide in Children with Hypertension. Circulation, 56, 1062, 1977.

53. Ogilvie, R.I., Nadeau, J.H., Sitar, D.S.: Diazoxide Concentration-Response Relation in Hypertension. Hypertension 4: 167, 1982.

54. O'Malley, K., Vesasco M.,Pruitt, A., et al.: Decreased plasma protein binding of diazoxide in uremia. Clin. Pharmacol. Ther. 18:53, 1975.

55. Sellers, E.M., Koch-Weser, J: Displacement of warfarin from human albumin by diazoxide and ethacrynic, mefenamic, and nalidixic acids. Clin. Pharmacol. Ther. 11:524, 1970.

56. Finnerty, F.A.,Jr., Davidov, M., Mroczek, W.J., Gavillovich, L.: Influence of extracellular fluid volume on response to antihypertensive drugs. Clin. Res. 27 (suppl 1): 71, 1970.

57. Charles, M.A., Danforth E. Jr: Nonketoacidotic hyperglycemia and coma during intravenous diazoxide therapy in uremia. Diabetes 20:501, 1971.

58. Palmer, R.F., and Lasseter, K.C.: Sodium nitroprusside. N. Engl. J. Med. 292: 294, 1975.

59. Cohn, J.N.: Blood pressure and cardiac performance. Am.J.Med.55:351, 1973.

60. Luderer, J.R., Hayes, A.H., Dubynsky, O., et al.: Long-term administration of sodium nitroprusside in childhood. J. Pediatr. 91:490, 1977.

61. Novak, D.S., Glassock, R.J., Solomon, D.H., and Maxwell, M.H.: Hypothyroidism following prolonged sodium nitroprusside therapy. Am.J. Med.Sci.248: 129, 1964.

62. Page, I.H., Corcoran, A.C., Dustan, H.P., and Koppanyi, T: Cardiovascular actions of sodium nitroprusside in animals and hypertensive patients. Circulation 11:188, 1955.

63. Danzig, L.E.: Dynamics of thiocyanate dialysis. N. Engl. J. Med. 252: 49, 1955.

64. Goldstein, F., and Rieders, F.: Conversion of thiocyanate to cyanide by an erythrocytic enzyme. Am.J.Physiol.173: 287, 1953.

65. Elberg, A.J., Gorman, H.M., Baker, R., et al.: Prolonged nitroprusside and intermittent hemodialysis as therapy for intractable hypertension. Am. J. Dis. Child 132:988, 1978.

66. Posner, M.A., Rodkey, F.L., and Tobey, R.E.: Nitroprusside-induced cyanide poisoning: Antidotal effect of hydroxycobalamin. Anesthesiology 44:330, 1976.

67. Zawada, E.T., Maxwell, M.H., Marks, L.S., Lee, D.B., and Kaufman, J.J: The diagnostic and therapeutic uses of saralasin in renal transplant hypertension. J.Urol.123: 148, 1980.

67A. Ruley, E.J., Bock, G.H., and Smith, D.: Use of continuous saralasin infusion to control hypertension. J. Pediatr.101: 1013, 1982.

68. Pettinger, W.A.: Minoxidil and the Treatment of Severe Hypertension. N.Engl.J.Med, 303:922, 1980.

69. Lewy, P.R.: The Management of Resistant Hypertension - The Role of Minoxidil, (eds) Gruskin, A.B., and Norman M.E., In: Developments in Nephrology 3. Pediatric Nephrology. Boston: Martinus Nijhoff, 1981, p. 416.

70. Sinaiko, A.R., O'Dea, R.F., Mirkin, B.L.: Clinical response of hypertensive children to long-term minoxidil therapy. J Cardiovasc. Pharmacol. 2: Suppl: 181, 1980.

71. Sinaiko, A.R., and Mirkin, B.L.: Management of severe childhood hypertension with minoxidil: a controlled study. J.Pediatr.91:138, 1977.

72. Pennisi, A.F., Bernstein, B.H., Takahashi, M., et al.:Minoxidil therapy in children with severe hypertension, J.Pediatr.90: 813, 1977.

73. Puri, H.C., and Potter, D.E.: Long Term Minoxidil Therapy in Children with Refractory Hypertension. Pediatr.Res.14: 1009, 1980.

74. Martin, W.B., Spodick, D.H., Zins, G.R.: Pericardial disorders occurring during open-label study of 1,869 severely hypertensive patients treated with minoxidil. J.Cardiovasc.Pharmacol. 1980; 2: Suppl: 227, 1980.

75. O'Malley, K., Velasco, M., Wells, J., McNay, J.L.: Control plasma renin activity and changes in sympathetic tone as determinants of minoxidil-induced increase in plasma renin activity. J.Clin.Invest. 55: 230, 1975.

76. Pettinger, W.A., Mitchell, H.C.: Renin release, saralasin and the vasodilator-beta-blocker drug interaction in man. N.Engl.J.Med. 292: 1214, 1975.

77. Mitchell, H.C., Pettinger, W.A.: The hypernoradrenergic state in vasodilator drug-treated hypertensive patients; effect of clonidine. J.Cardiovasc.Pharmacol. 2: 1, 1980.

78. Makker, S.P., and Moorthy, B.: Rebound hypertension following minoxidil withdrawal. J.Pediatr.96: 762, 1980.

79. Vidt, D.G., Bravo, E.L., and Fouad, F.M.: Captopril, N.Engl.J.Med.306: 214, 1982.

80. Murthy, V.S., Waldron,T.L., Goldberg, M.E.: The mechanism of bradykinin potentiation after inhibition of angiotensin-converting enzyme (SQ 14,225) in conscious rabbits. Circ.Res. 43: Part 2: I-46-5, 1976.

81. Sullivan, J.M., Ginsburg, B.A., Ratts, T.E., et al.: Hemodynamic and antihypertensive effects of captopril, an orally active angiotensin converting enzyme inhibitor. Hypertension. 1:397, 1979.

82. Tarazi, R.C., Bravo, E.L., Fouad, F.M., Omvik, P., Cody, R.J. Jr.: Hemodynamic and volume changes associated with captopril. Hypertension. 2:576, 1980.

83. Case, D.B., Atlas, S.A., Laragh, J.H., et al.: Clinical experience with blockade of the renin-angiotensin-aldosterone system by an oral

converting enzyme inhibitor (SQ 14,225, captopril) in hypertensive patients. Prog.Cardiovasc.Dis.21:195, 1978.

83A. Textor, S.C., Bravo, E.L., Fouad, F.M., and Tarazi, R.C.: Hyperkalemia in azotemic patients during angiotensin converting enzyme inhibition and aldosterone reduction with captopril. Amer.J. Med.73: 719, 1982.

84. Oberfield, S.E., Rapaport, R., Levine, L.S., New, M.I.: Long-Term Treatment of Childhood Hypertension with Captopril. Pediat. Ann. 11: 614, 1982.

85. Waeber, B., Guignard, J.P., Brunner, H.R. et al.:Treatment of severe renal hypertension in a child with an inhibitor of the angiotensin converting enzyme (SQ 14225). Helv.Paediatr.Acta.40(suppl):10, 1978.

86. Oberfield, S.E., Case, D.B., Levine, L.S., et al.:Brief clinical and laboratory observations: Use of the oral angiotensin I-converting enzyme inhibitor (captopril) in childhood malignant hypertension. J. Pediatr.95:641, 1979.

87. Bacri, J.L., Dechaux, M., Gingnadoux, M.F., et al.:Short term response and long term management with captopril in severe hypertention (HT) of children. Pediatr.Res.14: 1009, 1980.

88. Friedman, A., Chesney, R.W., Ball, D., et al.:Effective use of captopril (angiotensin I-converting enzyme inhibitor) in severe childhood hypertension. J.Pediatr.97:664, 1980.

89. Callis, L., Vila, A., Vilaplana E., and Castello, F.: Effect of Captopril in patients on chronic hemodialysis. Int. J. Pediatr.Neph. 3: 111, 1982.

90. Ploos van Amstel, S.L.B. and Abbad, F.C.B.:Long-term treatment of severe hypertension with Captopril. Int. J. Pediatr.Neph. 3: 107, 1982.

91. Chennavasin, P., Sciwell, R., Brater, D.C. and Liang, W.M.M.: Pharmacodynamic analysis of the furosemide-probenecid interaction in man. Kid. Int. 16: 187, 1979.

92. Rubb, W.: Pharmacokinetics and Pharmacodynamics of Lasix. Scot. Med. J. 19: 5, 1974.

93. Dikshit, K., Vyden, J.K., Forrester, J.S., et al.:Renal and extrarenal hemodynamic effects of furosemide in congestive heart failure after acute myocardial infarction. New.Eng.J.Med.288: 1087, 1973.

94. De Rubertis, F.R., Michells, M.F., Beck, N., Davis, B.B.: Complications of diuretic therapy: Severe alkalosis and syndrome resembling inappropriate secretion of antidiuretic hormone. Metabolism 19: 709, 1970.

95. Steele, T.H., Rieselbach, R.E.: Renal handling of urate and other organic anions, (eds) Brenner, B.M., and Rector, F.C., In: The Kidney. WB Saunders, 1976, p 460.

96. Schwartz, G.H., David, D.S., Riggio, R.R., et al.: Ototoxicity Induced by Furosemide, New.Engl.J.Med. 282: 1413, 1970.

97. Mudge, G.H.: Diuretics and other agents employed in the mobilization of edema fluid. (eds) Gilman, A.G., Goodman, L.S., and Gilman, A. In: The pharmacological basis of therapeutics, 6th edition. McMillan Co., 1980, p. 906.

98. Seedat, Y.K.: High-Dose Furosemide (Lasix) in Renal Insufficiency. S. Arf. Med. J. 46: 1371, 1972.

99. Huang, C.M., Atkinson, A.J., Levin, M., et al.: Pharmacokinetics of furosemide in advanced renal failure. Clin. Pharmacol Ther. 16: 659, 1972.

100. Wollam, G.L., Tarazi, R.C., Bravo, E.L. and Dustan, H.P.: Diuretic potency of combined hydrochlorothiazide and furosemide therapy in patients with azotemia. Amer. J. Med., 72: 929, 1982.

Supported in part by Hoechst Roussel Corp., General Clinical Research Center Grant RR 75, and NIH Grants, HL 23511 and HL 19869.

Mailing Address: A. Gruskin, Section of Pediatric Nephrology, Department of Pediatrics, Temple University School of Medicine, St. Christopher's Hospital for Children, 5th & Lehigh Avenue, Philadelphia, PA. 19133.

PANEL DISCUSSION: RENAL EMERGENCIES

Moderator: José Strauss, M.D.

COMMENT: I don't quite follow your point regarding treating hypertension in patients with nephrotic syndrome, knowing that the majority of them are relatively hypovolemic.

RESPONSE: What I was referring to is the individual with rapidly progressive glomerulonephritis who has a nephrotic component to his disease.

QUESTION: You mentioned two of your three patients who underwent transluminal angioplasty? They responded. What is the period of follow-up?

RESPONSE: Six to eighteen months.

QUESTION: One of the problems that we have most of the time in the process of measuring the blood pressure in infants, is that it changes significantly in accordance with their state of alertness. Sometimes it can be very high, perhaps even 50% higher that the 95th percentile and in another hour or so, be within normal limits. Have you experienced the same?

RESPONSE: Not personally. Basically, what I am referring to, are children beyond the first year of age. If you are talking about hypertension in the newborn nursery, I don't think we know enough about it to make any specific recommendations.

QUESTION: I have two questions for two different faculty. You mentioned that nephrotic syndrome may be a complication of renal ischemia secondary to asphyxia in the newborn. Could you elaborate on that?

RESPONSE: I really can't elaborate very much. There was one report which I can try and get the reference for you. I haven't personally seen that as a complication but it has been reported in the literature.

COMMENT-QUESTION: A question which came out of your comment about the role of edema in brain ischemia, I wonder if it would be useful to differentiate the role of brain cell swelling within a rigid cranium versus the role of endothelial cell swelling in vessels in terms of the no reflux phenomenon. Might not these be two separate mechanisms? Might not that be the reason why cell swelling of the brain itself in the newborn with an expanding skull is perhaps less important than in older children?

RESPONSE: I think that is very important. What I was referring to is that there have been a number of studies that have looked at edema in the newborn and in the primate. In fact, when actual cell water is measured, there is no difference. There is no increase in cell water. I think that is the basis for the questions regarding the role of intracellular water in the newborn because the data, when you examine them more carefully, are not that clear. Certainly, the differences between the cytogenic versus the vasogenic edemas are extremely important but this has not been worked out in the neonate at all.

COMMENT-QUESTION: My second question. You said that one of the complications of the use of captopril was proteinuria and membranous nephropathy. Yet, I believe that a combined study, reported in the Lancet about a year ago, looked at this very carefully and was unable to corroborate the previous report from Holland that there was epimembranous GN. I wonder if you could comment on the isolated reports on acute renal failure occurring in association with the use of captopril?

RESPONSE: As far as the Lancet article is concerned, I'm aware of it. The package drug insert which I was referring to I believe does mention proteinuria and membranous nephropathy - at least some of the material that the company has published does. I think it still remains an open question, obviously. As far as acutely deteriorating renal function associated with the use of captopril, yes, this has been reported. We currently - and I don't know what is going to happen - are in the process of following a child who has polycystic kidney disease with hepatic fibrosis syndrome who had a creatinine of about 1.4 mg/dl, and was having GI bleeding. We went through a whole rearrangement of her medications, gave her captopril, and within about ten days, her creatinine went up to 4.5 mg/dl. We've stopped it; this was about eight days ago. When she was seen in clinic a few days ago, the creatinine was down to about 4.1 mg/dl. I think it's probably a real entity. The question which of course arises is, is it a functional change in GFR or is it something that is irreversible? There are two schools of thought about acutely lowering blood pressure as I'm sure some of you are aware. The first is that when you acutely lower blood pressure, you acutely lower GFR, and you may suffer irreversible consequences. The second is, when you lower blood pressure there is an associated drop in GFR; however, over time that GFR comes back to the same level or improves. And there are a number of patients reported who have been started on dialysis who have subsequently been able to discontinue dialysis perhaps because their blood pressure has been impacted upon, whatever that may mean. It's a fascinating issue and still one that is not clear, at least in my own mind.

COMMENT: I'll add my comment about captopril. We have a young infant with bilateral renal stenosis that we put on captopril who also had an elevation in her serum creatinine, though not as dramatically as the patient described by the speaker. I also believe that this is a renal phenomenon. Considering the small numbers of patients treated with captopril, this small experience - we're talking about two patients - I don't know how many altogether you have treated but that's a large proportion of the numbers we have treated with captopril. So, I respect this problem of acute renal failure though I have no idea of its pathophysiology.

COMMENT: Just one other comment. We had a 16 year old child with the hemolytic uremic syndrome who had uncontrollable hypertension a few years ago and went through a number of drugs and finally I put her on captopril. It was then an experimental protocol. She was on hemodialysis for six months; she now has a GFR of 33% of normal and she's come off of dialysis. So, it works both ways . . . maybe.

COMMENT-QUESTION: We've seen that with a different drug. It also is a part of the natural history of the disease. I wanted to make a comment about another presentation we just heard and then ask a question. The comment is that I am going to plead for an NIH grant or for the speaker to be sent to Hollywood and give his lecture there because he has educated me. I have fallen prey to the folklore of Hollywood where a victim is always neatly plucked out of the water and upon receiving resuscitation, spits out a half a quart of fluid from his lungs. I gather from what you are trying to teach us, that this really doesn't happen.

COMMENT-RESPONSE: I want to comment specifically on the, I guess at this point, about 150 odd patients we have seen personally. In fact, it does not occur in children. We have a special opportunity here in Miami because of two things: one, we get a tremendous number of patients. We're averaging somewhere on the order of 30 to 40 near-drowning victims a year. The other very significant advantage is that our fire-rescue service is superb, certainly better than any other I am familiar with personally. We do get our victims within minutes of being removed from the water. This gives us a unique opportunity to observe patients as close to the actual incident as possible. Many of the other studies reported in very nice articles, unfortunately, had fire-rescue services and transport services available to them with averages somewhere on the order of half an hour. So, you're getting a somewhat skewed population that arrives at the hospital or other centers under different conditions than ours. I think we're getting a broader based population. The other comment I'd like to make - I do appreciate your comment on my opportunity to work in Hollywood but I don't think the weather could be as nice there as it is here in Florida - the vast majority of the literature in drowning is published out of adult-based services by adult-based physicians. There is a separate set of occurrences that happen with the adults. I didn't present the data that we have on the system involvement but, clearly, the adult survivors present to the emergency room with lung disease and almost no central nervous system disease while the children, diametrically opposite, present with central nervous system disease and virtually no lung disease. In our retrospective which I showed you briefly, there were 99 children that we had completed when that slide was made. Nine of them had some pulmonary symptoms; only two of those nine had any significant pulmonary disease beyond 48 hours. In those 99 children, there were 36 or 37, as I remember, who had specific central nervous system disease, hypoxic encephalopathy. And now that we have increased the number of patients upwards of 250, that same percentage is holding up. It's my very distinct impression, not only from the retrospective but in the patients I have personally taken care of, that the lungs are rarely involved in children.

COMMENT-QUESTION: With the predominance of central nervous system involvement just described, I would like to share with the audience something to which I was recently exposed myself. That is that sensory evoked potentials which are being used more and more to evaluate the neurologic status of patients and their rate of recovery, are affected by hypothermia. One gets distorted results if one is using hypothermia as one would in the treatment of these patients.

The question I want to ask is whether or not my other colleague is as reluctant as we are to do bilateral nephrectomies on patients with chronic renal failure and particularly those on dialysis. Our experience has been that the anemia is more pronounced in the nephrectomized patients. Our group, using radio-immuno-assay identification of erythropoietin, has demonstrated that the patients with chronic renal failure have normal erythropoietin levels although they are inappropriately low for the degree of anemia. Also, there is good erythropoietin and hematocrit response in acute situations such as those in patients who come in with pulmonary edema and hypoxemia. This can help the patient that has diseased kidneys but needs to elevate his blood hematocrit. The other instance where I find that having the kidneys in place, of course, is valuable is in a patient who has some degree of urine output, despite being on dialysis; he then can be helpful in maintaining a desirable fluid balance.

Another point I want to make pertains to dialyzing patients to true dry weight. I must say this is something I've learned from the internists. When I was surrounded by pediatric nephrologists I never had this fetish that I have now for getting the patient to dry weight. It's remarkable how when I think I have reached dry weight, I really haven't, and by pushing and pushing, we can control the blood pressure in these patients almost invariably. When we can't, usually we add some medication and we succeed in controlling the blood pressure in patients in whom we failed with medications alone. So we are very reluctant to use nephrectomy. I wanted your comment on this.

RESPONSE: Everyone has moved away from doing as many nephrectomies as we used to do. I would offer a few comments though. One, granted, you will need more transfusions with bilateral nephrectomy. I don't think there is any doubt about that but I'm not so sure, given the current thinking about transfusions prior to transplant, that that in itself is bad because we no longer transplant anyone immediately. We put them on our list until they've had at least five transfusions, and we're moving toward ten. I'm not sure that that in itself is an issue. Secondly, the issue of volume. If I were going to have an option to do a nephrectomy, obviously I would want to wait until the urine output became fairly low, where it is not 1,000 cc's a day but around a couple of hundred of cc's; this is not as much of a problem. Thirdly, there are some data showing that for any adult patient with chronic renal disease, for any given level of blood volume, removing the kidneys lowers the blood pressure somewhat. So, a bilateral nephrectomy theoretically will lower the blood pressure wherever they happen to be on the blood volume. Because bilateral nephrectomy may not correct hypertension, that does not make it good or bad per se.

The ability to get children down to dry weight, that's a double issue. It's not <u>getting</u> them down to dry weight because you can lock them in a room, and dialyze them, and get them down to dry weight. It is <u>keeping</u> them at that dry weight, sustained over time, where obviously the problem arises, as in two patients we have and we absolutely do not understand. We have gotten them down to dry weight with nephrectomies but their blood pressures are still high and will not come down. So, the question that comes up is, if he's had his hypertension long enough before you get around to a nephrectomy, what happens thereafter? Has he reached a stage of end-organ damage? The final point I would make about bilateral nephrectomy is philosophy, not fact. What do you do in this patient population when you are looking for end-organ changes, myocardial function and left ventricular hypertrophy. What are we trading off in a child who we hope is going to survive five, ten, 30 years? Again, I don't know. It worries me. In our gestalt we tend to add into the decision whether or not someone has myocardial dysfunction or whatever you want to call it. There are no absolute rules.

MODERATOR: Our experience here with a very aggressive transplantation program may be of interest to you. Nephrectomies are performed whenever possible in the pre-transplant period. Practically, we must have indicators not to take out the kidneys; otherwise, all patients have a BNS (bilateral nephrectomy and splenectomy). The rationale expressed in the last comment is basically what we use. We try to protect the whole patient, not the obsolete kidneys. Anytime we have infection or hypertension, any possible problems that could come from those end-stage kidneys being left in place, we don't hesitate to do a bilateral nephrectomy, probably more readily than most groups. When we have one kidney with good function and the other with congenital problems, then we become the strongest defenders of saving the abnormal one and agree on its removal only if there are complications obviously due to that kidney. I must clarify that we don't take out a normal kidney either.

COMMENT: Just to comment on the two patients referred to earlier. We had an experience in two patients that were anephric, on dialysis, and severely hypertensive to the point that we believed they were under dry weight. In these two patients we measured catecholamines several times and they were very elevated. One patient had sickle cell disease and the other one had lupus. In this latter patient, when she received a transplant, blood pressure normalized completely.

COMMENT: There is a point I must clarify. We do not tolerate hypertension in our patients. I didn't mean to imply that at all. What I am saying is that we have been able to control hypertension in patients without doing bilateral nephrectomies. The armamentarium of medications now available has allowed us to control it. Only in one instance have we had to do a bilateral nephrectomy and perhaps some post-operative complications in that child have tinted my view to being very conservative on that score. I might say that the internists are now by and large much more conservative than what you are describing. I would have to disagree with the position that you are taking. Although, I could be wrong.

MODERATOR: Let's clarify that we are talking about the end-stage disease and the pre-transplant patients only. Is the patient going to maintain his or her own kidneys after transplantation? Regarding the treatment of a hypertensive crisis of renal origin, we did go through a period when a bilateral nephrectomy was recommended under extreme circumstances but that has been superceded in the last eight to ten years by the potent antihypertensive agents available. So what we are talking about, really, is the pre-transplant period.

COMMENT: If I may add a comment in that respect, with the introduction of CAPD on the horizon of therapy, what was said about getting patients to true dry weight has been substantiated time and again and I should again state that we have the unique opportunity of dealing with a population which is being regularly nephrectomized pre-transplantation. Two of our patients on CAPD were nephrectomized and entered CAPD with quite prominent hypertension. Within a week or two, they were off their antihypertensive medication because what we felt was that their dry weight was far from the dry weight, and they lost two or three liters. Obviously, volume plays a predominant role in probably the bulk of hypertensive patients in end-stage renal disease.

COMMENT: I believe there is some evidence that CAPD even in "dry patients" removes something that elevates blood pressure. Middle molecules, who knows what. Obviously, volume is important but there seems to be still something else going on.

COMMENT: That might be applied to the fact that despite nephrectomy, our CAPD patients require less transfusions than patients on hemodialysis. By the same token, maybe erythropoietin is not the whole story but something is being removed by CAPD.

COMMENT-QUESTION: I have a comment and a question, please. I have one comment concerning one of the manifestations of hypertensive crisis in pediatrics that was not mentioned and I think that sometimes might represent difficulty with the differential diagnosis. It pertains to the patient who has severe hypertension and presents to us with renal dysfunction, thrombocytopenia, schistocytes and severe CNS involvement; in him, the diagnosis of HUS might be made. Really, the manifestations are secondary to malignant hypertension. Once we control hypertension, the whole clinical picture disappears.

COMMENT: I would agree; we have seen it.

QUESTION: The other provocative question is, as we know, recent studies have shown that the renin-aldosterone system is suppressed in post-streptococcal acute GN. I wonder why should the renin be increased in rapidly progressive glomerulonephritis and suppressed in AGN?

RESPONSE: I don't have the answer except to say that in post-infectious nephritis perhaps you don't get as much ischemia, infarction in the glomeruli, etc. and that what you get is a rapid fall in GFR, volume retention and renin suppression. Even though renin is stated to be reduced in post-infectious nephritis, if you look at some of those articles, there are a number of patients whose renin levels are "normal". The question arises for their state of volume balance, isn't their renin relatively elevated? Leave that as it may be. As far as the rapidly progressive patient who gets a fair amount of renin release, I believe it's related to ischemic changes, blood flow distribution, changes that are acute, that just result in increased renin release.

MODERATOR: We are running short of time; so, if the questions and answers are rather brief, I would appreciate it.

QUESTION: This is a rather broad question: patients that present with high blood pressure and have a normal physical examination, normal urinalysis, how far do you go in investigating them?

RESPONSE: If you are talking about somebody who has moderate or severe hypertension you'd better do something about it. We tend to go until we can find an answer, whatever that may mean. You just see very few people below 21 years old who have severe hypertension, who do not have a secondary cause. On the other hand, I think the most common type of hypertension in an adolescent population is probably mild essential hypertension. I don't think they have much in the way of severe hypertension. So, I think if you are talking about severe hypertension, we will go the whole gamut of testing. We talked about this a couple of years ago when I was here. We use renin profiling in most of our children with hypertension as a clue to where to go diagnostically.

COMMENT: A response to the question posed about erythropoietin levels, CAPD vs hemodialysis. My associate has demonstrated that the immunoreactive erythropoietin levels are higher in CAPD patients though not as high as should be for the level of anemia. We've had the unique opportunity to evaluate one patient who, because of lack of access, switched from hemodialysis to CAPD and we showed that the hematocrit went up to 41% from levels of 15% associated with increase in erythropoietin.

QUESTION: What are your feelings about and experience with captopril, on transplant patients?

RESPONSE: We haven't used it. Other people have and have reasonably good success. I think you do much better if you lower the steroid dose.

RESPONSE: When I trained at Alabama, we had four patients who had later documented renal artery stenosis. Lots of patients were treated with captopril, but those four patients, in fact, lost function on captopril-which was reversible. It was apparent that their hypertension was pressor-mediated and the captopril locked the pressor and blocked their hypertension but caused loss of function. They went on later to have either correction or complications and a surgical approach to correction for transplant renal artery stenosis.

COMMENT: We have a patient in the hospital now who has a creatinine of about one post-transplant, just found to have renal artery stenosis, who came with a seizure a few weeks ago. As yet we have not been able to bring his blood pressure down with Captopril.

QUESTION: What do you think are the dangers for the brain when you quickly lower high blood pressure? You mentioned the problems with GFR if you acutely lower the blood pressure but there are opinions that when you acutely lower very high blood pressure, the result may be some brain damage. When you are left with children after hypertensive encephalopathy-children with some cerebral sequellae, you really don't know whether the sequellae are the result of the hypertension or of your acute use of treatment. Can you please comment on that.

RESPONSE: I don't know that the answer to that question is known in children. The information that you may be referring to is from extensive experience with malignant hpertension in adults. These, of course, are generally patients who have had chronic hypertension, have severe atherosclerosis, and have problems with regulatory mechanisms of vessels. If their pressure is reduced too rapidly, they certainly will suffer ischemia from it with major neurological sequellae. I'm not aware of that in children but perhaps it has been documented.

COMMENT: People also discuss the situation of a hypertensive patient who has had a hemorrhagic infarction. In that case, the drug of choice may be sodium nitroprusside as opposed to something like Hyperstat. With the latter, the pressure goes down and up and down; and therefore, to use an agent (like sodium nitroprusside) which allows a smooth, gradual drop in pressure and which can maintain it down, should be preferable. I'm not aware of any information in children that would suggest that these kinds of changes in blood pressure have produced irreversible kinds of problems. I would expect it to happen sooner or later.

COMMENT: In a recent (not yet published) study, I was told that there is evidence of the appearance of brain damage after the use of diazoxide.

MODERATOR: Someone wants to make a comment. Is that a continuation of the same point?

COMMENT: Yes. There are data in an adult population that I want to point out, cases with rapid reduction of blood pressure. Most of those patients were not of an age where one could invoke cerebral atherosclerosis as the reason for their problems.

MODERATOR: I particularly want to ask about the oliguria that seems to occur in the acute stage of the hypoxic episode. There seems to be a discrepancy between that type of reaction in the human and the results of hypoxic studies which Marc Rowe and I did a number of years ago and that have been done now in collaboration with the neonatology group at the Medical School and Columbia University. We see a polyuria occurring in the piglet regardless of whether the piglet becomes hypoxic and hypocarbic or hypoxic and normocarbic. Do you have any thoughts on the cause of discrepancies, what may be the explanation for those different urine volumes?

RESPONSE: What I was referring to before was in our study population now which I find surprising that within about 15 hours we have passage of urine and it seems to persist at least a cc or greater per kilo/hour which is high urine output for a stressed neonate. Most of these children are, if anything, hypocarbic, mainly because their course is complicated by persistent pulmonary hypertension. One approach towards treatment is hyperventilation. I would say that the majority of our babies are hypocarbic. We haven't really seen the renal complications that I thought we would with a fairly large group of asphyxiated infants.

MODERATOR: Thank you. Changing the subject and speaker, how do you explain the problems that we have with a BUN of 150 mg/dl while you say that with a BUN of up to 400 mg/dl - if I interpreted your presentation correctly - there is no actual correlation with CNS manifestations? Are we seeing a different population or are we talking about different manifestations? Probably our problems come up at the time when we dialyze one of those patients with a BUN of 150 mg/dl or thereabouts. Do you have any thoughts on that?

RESPONSE: I really don't. I would guess that the occasional patient with a BUN of 200 or 300 or 400 mg/dl without neurological problems must be very unusual. I have not personally seen such a patient but they have been reported. I was really reflecting on the literature which is obviously more adult than child, too, suggesting that neurological syndromes related presumably to renal disease and/or dialysis are not tightly correlated with BUN.

MODERATOR: One of the reasons why I invited my colleague to join us was because he has been very helpful, at least in keeping us from doing too much, or at least me from doing too much. Some of the people in our group I think don't quite agree with that approach. It might be interesting to discuss what should we do with the patient that goes to hemodialysis and has a convulsion? Would you care to describe what your approach would be or what your recommendation would be? A "simple" seizure at the beginning, middle, end, next day, first dialysis, second dialysis. What are the dangers of treating, not treating, and how could you handle it?

RESPONSE: I'm not sure what I've said in the past. I claim ignorance about that. Probably what you are referring to is my reluctance to be very aggressive with intravenous barbiturates and Valium. Certainly that is my position because an awful lot of the kids have rather brief seizures, and I think the epileptiform event itself is rarely brain injuring. This is a general statement for epilepsy as a whole, regardless of the pathogenesis. It's the cause of the seizure, not the seizure itself that kills cells, at least not enough to result in a disabled patient. So, probably I have been the one that has something to do with a nihilistic attitude. Dilantin I favor strongly, if you feel that you have to be aggressive; we know the most about it, the effect that renal disease and dialysis have upon the kinetics of Dilantin and it can be used intravenously if the seizure persists. It can be used very nicely for effective control of status epilepticus, if that's what you are dealing with - if status epilepticus in that case is treatable at all; of course, many of them are not. The people in the Pediatric Intensive Care Unit know that story all too well. We have our fair share of kids who cannot, do not respond to anything and finally just stop seizing. I would favor intravenous Dilantin as the drug that we know the most about, and is a known, effective drug for repeated seizures. But I'm talking now about status which is one seizure after another without the patient awakening in between and/or a continuous epileptiform EEG.

MODERATOR: What would you do with one seizure? A patient's vital signs otherwise are stable, surrounded by doctors, nurses, and equipment. Let me make it more dramatic. Would you agree with one occurrence we had not too long ago where code blue was called because one of those patients had a seizure. What would be your approach? Could I put words in your mouth? You would not treat the patient?

QUESTION: Are we talking about chronically or acutely?

MODERATOR: An acute patient.

RESPONSE: First of all, obviously you do oxygenate the patient, right? That would be the beginning. The seizure phenomenon may not be what you are stuck with on a long term basis. That may be over before you can find the Dilantin file. Obviously, you'd like to know what the patient's fluid and electrolyte status is like. In all likelihood, you do know because I know the way you take care of your patients; so clearly in a case of "severe seizures", the most important method of treatment is to treat the origin. So, if you can possibly find the source, go for that rather than anticonvulsant management.

MODERATOR: The patient is having hemodialysis and you are removing whatever solutes, water, and whatnot, and the patient has a seizure. What would you do if you are there having coffee with us and the patient happens to have a seizure?

RESPONSE: Well, I'd wait a minute before I did anything. Then if I felt I had to use a drug, I'd go back to the same one. I'd use intravenous dilantin, if you feel like you have to do something for the patient. I would hope the seizure is going to be over in 30 to 60 seconds. We're all going to breathe a sigh of relief that we haven't poisoned the patient.

COMMENT: Since his office currently is two blocks from the hospital, and mine tends to be somewhat closer,in those situations you have described I would suggest that the members of the audience who would be responding read a book called House of God. The first rule is to take your own pulse. More often than not if we don't intervene acutely, just make sure that patient is ventilating and oxygenating adequately, a lot of these seizures will stop on their own and the cause or other problems will be a lot more detectable than if the patient is loaded up on phenobarbital or other drugs, anticonvulsants.

COMMENT: The other issue, of course, talking about the first or second dialysis that this child has ever had is different from the one who has been on dialysis for three years. In the former situation, you are talking about some manifestation of acute dialysis disequilibrium which we try to prevent: one, by giving some mannitol for the first couple of dialyses; two, dialyzing the first couple of treatments shorter; three, if you do have a seizure, cutting down the blood flow rate or adding some mannitol. I think that's a separate and distinct issue from someone who is chronic and stable and now has a new seizure. The question then is, what is the etiology of that seizure in someone who has been on dialysis for a year? Does it represent some other kind of a problem, focal bleeding, subdural, whatever. We approach them somewhat differently but we walk slowly. Take our pulses; call the neurologist...

MODERATOR: We are talking about the one that is presumably predictable and we take the necessary steps and give mannitol and this and that. Still we see an occasional seizure. It was that type of reassurance that I wanted to convey to the group. Some of the people in practice with that type of minor seizure apparently take an extra ride around the block before getting to the patient. By the time they get to see the patient, the seizure has stopped.

COMMENT: In terms of management of the acute convulsive episode, what mostly preoccupies the nurses is the possible loss of the access. We have to remember that these patients are connected to the lines of the dialysis machine. So one of the things they have to do in the treatment of those patients, of course, is hold the arm or leg.

MODERATOR: No questions or disagreements with that. That's a part of the practical life that we all have to face. Our time has run out. I want to thank everyone for being here and for participating so actively in a very exciting discussion.

III

ACUTE RENAL DISEASES

A THERAPEUTIC UPDATE OF SUPERFICIAL SKIN INFECTIONS

Lawrence Schachner, M.D., David Taplin, Gwendolyn B. Scott, M.D.
and Michael Morrison, M.D.

BACTERIAL INFECTIONS

The most common skin infection found in children is simple superficial impetigo. It occurs so commonly that it is usually treated on clinical grounds. It is generally considered that there are two basic forms of the disease which may be distinguished clinically, bacteriologically, and histologically. The first is considered to be primarily of streptococcal origin and is characterized by thick, crusted lesions; the second is of staphylococcal origin and is associated with fluid-filled bullae.

In the United States, it has been well established that common skin infections among low income populations in warm climates are almost entirely due to a group A β-hemolytic S. *pyogenes* (8,11,29). Summertime studies in northern areas of the country have also shown a predominance of group A β-hemolytic S. *pyogenes* (1,6). These latter studies found a distinct predominance of streptococcal pyoderma as the morphologic type of superficial skin infection, and a distinct predominance of β-hemolytic S. *pyogenes* or mixed infections of S. *pyogenes* and S. *aureus* in cultures from patients studied. The authors concluded that S. *pyogenes* was the primary organism in these infections and that when S. *aureus* existed in these mixed infections,it was as a secondary invader. Thus, treatment was aimed at the S. *pyogenes*, and even the presence of penicillin-resistant S. *aureus* did not inhibit healing in those patients treated with penicillin (7,8,11,16,29).

Literature from Europe often reports a predominance of S. *aureus* grown from superficial skin infections (Table 1); this is not found in previous studies emanating from the United States.

Staphylococcal bullous impetigo is a superficial skin infection characterized by the eruption of bullae on previously untraumatized skin. The flaccid bullae rupture in one to two days, leaving a superficial erosion with a varnished appearance and scant crusting. The usual distribution described for this superficial skin infection involves the face, buttocks, trunk and perineum. Streptococcal pyoderma involves an eruption on previously traumatized skin, be it by scratch, insect bite, or other micro-trauma. The lesions may start as small vesicles, but quickly become pustular and feature the emergence of thick crust. If the crust is removed, the erosion is significantly deeper than that seen in the staphylococcal bullous impetigo. These pyodermas are often found to grow S. *aureus* as well as S. *pyogenes* upon culture. The predominant site of streptococcal pyoderma is the extremities.

Table 1. Reports of Epidemiology of Impetigo*

AUTHOR	SITE/YEAR OF REPORT	NO. OF PATIENTS	STAPH (%)	STREP (%)	MIXED (%)	NO GROWTH OR OTHER(%)
Parker [28]	England, 1941	298	53	0.7	45	1.3
Parker [28]	England, 1955	190	44	13	39	4
Barrow [2]	England, 1955	119	72	5	10	13
Burnett [4]	Maryland, USA, 1962	60	32	23	27	18
Markowitz [25]	Maryland, USA, 1965	303	34	17	6	43
Shuler [33]	Louisiana, USA, 1966	100	49	26	24	1
Hughes [21]	Kentucky, USA, 1967	62	23	18	30	29
Anthony [1]	Minnesota, USA, 1967	270	10	25	57	8
Dillon [8]	Alabama, USA, 1968	497	11	32	54	3
Taplin	Florida, USA, 1968	40	5	12.5	82.5	0
Esterly [16]	Maryland, USA, 1970	166	37.3	27.2	35.5	0
El Zawahry [14]	Egypt, 1972	131	41	9	36	14
Mobacken [26]	Sweden, 1972	200	72	10	15	3
Conner [5]	England, 1972	72	69	3	18	10
Dajani [6]	Minnesota, USA, 1973	150	13	24	58	5
Linder [24]	Georgia, USA, 1978	127	23	53	19	5
Schachner	Florida, USA, 1980	101	77	1	9	13

*Several studies had small numbers of non-group A *streptococcus* or *staphylococcus epidermis* included.

Our more recent experience suggests that the predominant pathogen that causes superficial pyodermas may be changing. In the summer of 1978, an apparent change was noted in superficial skin infections seen at the Jackson Memorial Hospital pediatric out-patient department. There had been a marked predominance in streptococcal pyoderma among children attending our ambulatory care facilities. An apparent increase in staphylococcal bullous impetigo suggested that a reevaluation of the etiology and therapeutic approach to superficial skin infections in our population was warranted. S. *pyogenes* was long considered the much predominant superficial skin infection, and penicillin the conventional first-line treatment in our clinic, as well as the community at large.

We evaluated 101 children with pyoderma. Microbiology was evaluated at the initial visit and after one week of treatment. Following the initial culture, children were randomly assigned to receive either penicillin V potassium or cloxacillin sodium. Any child considered to be a treatment failure at one week was switched to the other antibiotic and was reevaluated after two weeks of therapy. The predominant age of our patients was six months to three years. Table 2 demonstrates the clinical frequency of the different morphologic lesions and secondary changes seen in our patients with cutaneous infections. Although most patients had vesicular bullous lesions, the predominant lesions seen with staphylococcal impetigo were pustules. The leading site of the lesions was the extremities followed by the truncal lesions and facial lesions. This is in counterdistinction to the conventional wisdom that tells us that staphylococcal bullous impetigo predominates on the face and genitalia.

Table 2. Clinical Lesions: Physical Examination

Vesicular Bullous (59)	
50 *Staphylococcus aureus*	11 treatment failure
6 No growth	
3 Both	1 treatment failure
Pustular (74)	
55 *Staphylococcus*	12 treatment failure
10 No growth	1 treatment failure*
8 Both	1 treatment failure
1 *Streptococcus pyogenes*	
Ecthymatous (59)	
42 *Staphylococcus aureus*	12 treatment failure
10 No growth	1 treatment failure
6 Both	1 treatment failure
1 *Streptococcus pyogenes*	
Erosions (14)	
14 *Staphylococcus aureus*	2 treatment failure

*Grew *Staphylococcus aureus* at second visit.

Table 3. Results of Bacteriologic Cultures at First Visit

	PERCENTAGE OF PATIENTS	NUMBER OF PATIENTS
Staphylococcus aureus	77	78
Staphylococcus aureus and group A β-hemolytic *streptococcus*	9	9
Group A β-hemolytic *streptococcus*	1	1
No growth	13	13

Table 3 shows the results of bacteriologic cultures taken on the enrollment day of the study. Seventy-seven per cent of the patients grew a pure culture of S. *aureus*. Nine per cent grew both S. *aureus* and group A β-hemolytic S. *pyogenes*. Thirteen patients had no growth.

Of 29 patients who grew S. *aureus* and who were treated with cloxacillin, there were no treatment failures at one week. Of 38 patients who grew S. *aureus* and were treated with penicillin V potassium, 18, or 47 per cent, were treatment failures at one week. Of the nine patients who grew both S. *aureus* and *S. pyogenes*, four had been placed on cloxacillin sodium and five had been placed on penicillin V potassium. There were no treatment failures among the four patients treated with cloxacillin sodium. Two of five patients, 40 per cent, with mixed infections were treatment failures on penicillin V potassium.

Dillon's studies 10 years ago revealed a penicillin resistance in staphylococcal bullous impetigo approximating 50 per cent. While an increasing degree of resistance has been noted by several authors (9,10, 24),our degree of resistance has been the most overwhelming, with greater than 98 per cent of all *S. aureus* grown from these superficial skin infections resistant to penicillin.

The appropriateness and the effectiveness of oral and intramuscular penicillin in childhood pyoderma has been considered conventional wisdom. The confirmation of our suspicion that an increase in staphylococcal bullous impetigo had taken place in our clinic presented a much more dramatic change than we had expected. Since our study, however, several recent reviews suggest that our experience is similar to that noted in other communities. A significant increase in staphylococcal bullous impetigo in children in Alabama (9) and in an adult population seen by private dermatologists in Boston (17) indicates that these investigators were also seeing a predominance of *S. aureus* in their patients with superficial skin infections.

It has long been felt that in mixed infections of *S. pyogenes* and *S. aureus* effective therapy for the *S. pyogenes* would eradicate the infection. Although it is hard to draw statistically significant results from this small number of patients with mixed infections, our data suggest that penicillin was not appropriate for mixed streptococcal and staphylococcal pyoderma.

Our experience along with that reported from other centers suggests that a reevaluation of the empiric therapy for superficial pyoderma is in order. Therapeutic approaches directed at both the staphylococcal and streptococcal pathogens must be espoused. In choosing alternatives to penicillin V potassium, factors such as local antimicrobial sensitivity patterns, patient acceptability (especially with liquid preparations), and cost must be considered.

To date the only drug compared in a randomized fashion with penicillin V potassium has been cloxacillin sodium. More than 98 per cent of the *S. aureus* isolates at the University of Miami show in vitro sensitivity to cloxacillin. Moreover, in mixed infections of streptococcal pyoderma secondarily colonized with *S. aureus*, cloxacillin would be an appropriate antibiotic to eliminate both organisms.

Alternative choices may include erythromycin, dicloxacillin, or cephalexin. In our experience erythromycin resistance is present in approximately 10 per cent of clinical *S. aureus* isolates and there is a high frequency of gastrointestinal side effects. Dicloxacillin, which should be as effective as cloxacillin, may not be useful for young children. The oral suspension is very bitter and is formulated at only 62.5 mg/5 ml, thus requiring that large volumes be administered with each dose. Cephalexin is effective, palatable, and a well tolerated alternative.

This shift in the epidemiology of superficial skin infections from streptococcal predominance to staphylococcal predominance had an interesting correlation with pediatric-nephrological disease. During the two years following this study, pediatric-nephrology service reported their smallest number of new cases of acute glomerular nephritis in over a decade. We feel this is a direct correlation with the decrease in childhood streptococcal pyodermas in the community.

REFERENCES

1. Anthony, B.F., Perlman, L.U., and Wannamaker, L.: Skin infections and acute nephritis in American Indian children. Pediatrics, 39: 263-279, 1967.
2. Barrow, G.: Clinical and bacteriological aspects of impetigo contagiosa. J. Hygiene, 53:495-508, 1955.
3. Borelli, D.: Treatment of pityriasis versicolor with ketoconazole. Rev. Infect. Dis. 2:592-595, 1980.
4. Burnett, J.W.: Management of pyogenic cutaneous infections. N. Engl. J. Med., 266:164-169, 1962.
5. Conner, B.: Impetigo contagiosa in the United Kingdom. Br. J. Dermatol., 86:48-54, 1972.
6. Dajani, A., Ferrari, P., and Wannamaker, L.: Endemic superficial pyoderma in children. Arch. Dermatol., 108:517-522, 1973.
7. Derrick, C., and Dillon, H.: Impetigo contagiosa. Am. Fam. Physician, 4:75-81, 1971.
8. Dillon, H.: Impetigo contagiosa: Suppurative and non-suppurative complications. Am. J. Dis. Child., 115:530-541, 1968.
9. Dillon, H.: Topical and systemic therapy for pyoderma. Int. J. Dermatol., 19:443-451, 1980.

10. Dillon, H., and Derrick, C.: Clinical experience with clindamycin hydrochloride. Pediatrics, 55:205-212, 1975.
11. Dillon, H., Moody, M., Maxted, W., et al.: The epidemiology of impetigo and acute glomerulonephritis. Am. J. Epidemiol., 86: 710-723, 1967.
12. Drouchet, E., and Dupont, B.: Chronic mucocutaneous candidosis and other superficial and systemic mycoses successfully treated with ketoconazole. Rev. Infect. Dis., 2:606-619, 1980.
13. Eaglstein, W., Feinstein, R., et al.: Systemic antibiotic therapy of secondarily infected dermatitis. Arch. Dermatol., 113:1378-1379, 1977.
14. El-Zawahry, M., Azia, A., and Soliman, M.: The etiology of impetigo contagiosa. Br. J. Dermatol., 87:420-424, 1972.
15. El-Zawahry, M., Aziz, A., Soliman, M., et al.: Clinical and bacteriological evaluation for the treatment of skin infections. Br. J. Dermatol., 95:177-180, 1976.
16. Esterly, N., and Markowitz, M.: The treatment of pyoderma in children. J.A.M.A., 212:1667-1670, 1970.
17. Finnery, E., and Folan, D.: Changing antibiotic sensitivities of bacterial skin diseases. Cutis, 23:227-230, 1979.
18. Hall, W., Blumberg, R., and Moody, M.: Studies in children with impetigo. Am. J. Dis. Child., 125:800-806, 1973.
19. Hay, R.J., Wells, R.S., Clayton, Y.M., et al.: Treatment of chronic mucocutaneous candidosis with ketoconazole: A study of 12 cases. Rev. Infect. Dis., 2:600-605, 1980.
20. Heel, R.C., Brogden, R.N., Carmine, A., et al.: Ketoconazole: a review of its therapeutic efficacy in superficial and systemic fungal infections. Drugs, 23:1-36, 1982.
21. Hughes, W.T., and Wan, R.: Impetigo contagiosa. Am. J. Dis. Child., 113:449-453, 1967.
22. Jones, H.E., Simpson, J.G., and Artis, W.M.: Oral ketoconazole, an effective and safe treatment for dermatophytosis. Arch. Dermatol., 117:129-134, 1981.
23. Legendre, R., and Steltz, M.: A multi-center, double-blind comparison of ketoconazole and griseofulvin in the treatment of infections due to dermatophytes. Rev. Infect. Dis., 2:586-591, 1980.
24. Linder, C.: Treatment of impetigo and ecthyma. J. Fam. Pract., 7:697-700, 1978.
25. Markowitz, M., Bruton, D., Kuttner, A., et al.: The bacteriological findings, streptococcal immune response and renal complications in children with impetigo. Pediatrics, 35:393-404, 1965.
26. Mobacken, H., and Holst, R.: Epidemiological aspects of impetigo contagiosa in western Sweden. Scand. J. Infect. Dis., 7:39-44, 1975.
27. Negroni, R., Iglesia, M.R., and Casala, A.M.: The activity of ketoconazole in the treatment of onychomycosis. Rev. Infect. Dis., 2:596-598, 1980.
28. Parker, M., Tomlinson, A., And Williams, R.: Impetigo contagiosa. J. Hygiene, 53:458-473, 1959.
29. Peter, G., and Smith A.: Group A streptococcal infection of the skin and pharynx. N. Engl. J. Med., 297:311-317, 1978.
30. Peterson, E., Alling, D., and Kirkpatrick, C.H.: Treatment of chronic mucocutaneous candidosis with ketoconazole: A controlled clinical trial. Ann. Intern. Med., 93:791-795, 1980.

31. Robertson, M.H., Hanifin, J.M., and Parker, F.: Oral therapy with ketoconazole for dermatophyte infections unresponsive to griseofulvin. Rev. Infect. Dis., 2:578-581, 1980.
32. Rosenblatt, H.M., Byrne, W., Ament, M.E., et al.: Successful treatment of chronic mucocutaneous candidiasis with ketoconazole. J. Pediatrics, 97:657-660, 1980.
33. Shuler, S.E.: Impetigo. Calif. Med., 105:113-116, 1966.
34. Singh, G.: Pathogenesis of staphylococcal infections of the skin. Int. J. Dermatol., 14:755-760, 1975.
35. Welsh, O., Rodriguez, M.: Treatment of dermatomycoses with ketoconazole. Rev. Infect. Dis., 2:582-585, 1980.

Revised with permission from *Pediatric Clinics of North America*, Vol. 30, No. 2, April 1983, pp. 397-404.

GLOMERULONEPHROPATHIES CAUSING THE ACUTE NEPHRITIC SYNDROME: SIMILARITIES AND DIFFERENCES

MELINDA MC VICAR, M.D.

The acute nephritic syndrome (Table 1) as it is encountered in childhood encompasses a wide variety of clinical entities, frequently of unknown etiology with diverse histologic manifestations (Table 2) and with variable prognoses. Strictly speaking, "acute" nephritis is a self-limited disease with an excellent outcome and the majority of patients which present with the acute nephritic syndrome (ANS) follow this pattern.

The individual components which comprise the ANS, however, may be encountered as a phase of many conditions, both systemic and primary renal, which result in chronic progression. In addition, hematuria, the most frequently encountered common denominator in the ANS has on occasion been reported to be absent in acute nephritis while isolated hematuria can occur in benign essential hematuria (not usually considered a nephritis) or as the sole manifestation of acute nephritis. The subject must, therefore, be approached on multiple levels simultaneously considering the epidemiology, clinical manifestations, pathogenic mechanisms and renal histology. A reasonable assessment of prognosis and potential therapeutic intervention may then be made.

The following discussion will emphasize the features of different entities which share in common their presentation as the acute nephritic syndrome (ANS). Emphasis will be placed on the most frequently encountered primary glomerulopathies. These are acute post-infectious glomerulonephritis, membranoproliferative glomerulonephritis, and IgA nephropathy (Berger's disease). A brief description, however, of some of the systemic disorders which must be differentiated from the primary causes of the ANS is in order.

SECONDARY ACUTE NEPHRITIC SYNDROME

The most common systemic diseases which result in ANS are systemic lupus erythematosus (SLE), anaphylactoid purpura, or Henoch-Schönlein purpura (HSP), and the hemolytic uremic syndrome (HUS). The proposed revised ARA criteria for clinical diagnosis of SLE with the addition of anti-DNA antibodies, and

Table 1. Acute nephritic syndrome

Hematuria +	Proteinuria Hypertension Decreased GFR Oliguria Edema

hypocomplementemia, which tend to be prominent during clinical activity, have greatly facilitated the diagnosis of SLE.

Briefly, the criteria are fulfilled when any four or more of the following eleven conditions are found in any sequence of time: 1) Malar rash, 2) Photosensitive rash, 3) Discoid lupus, 4) Oral or nasopharyngeal ulceration, 5) Arthritis without deformity, 6) Proteinuria greater than .5g per day or cellular casts, 7) Pleuritis or pericarditis, 8) Psychosis or seizures, 9) Antibody to DNA or SM antigen or LE cells or false positive biologic test for syphilis, 10) Positive FANA, 11) Leukopenia, lymphopenia, decreased platelet count, or hemolytic anemia (1). A modification of these criteria which would include all patients with diffuse proliferative lupus nephritis by the addition of low C4 to the criteria has recently been suggested but must be tested further (2).

Patients with SLE who have no clinical renal manifestations will almost invariably have some evidence of renal involvement on kidney biopsy. In fact, even the more severe diffuse proliferative nephritis has been found in patients lacking laboratory evidence of renal involvement and some investigators advocate renal biopsy in all patients with SLE(3).

When the presenting finding of SLE is an ANS without any evidence of systemic manifestations, observation over a period of time will eventually reveal the multisystem involvement of the disease. The marked predominance of females afflicted with SLE (approximately 90%) is in contrast to other nephropathies. Renal biopsy findings may not distinguish SLE from several of the other entities which cause ANS since virtually any histologic picture can be found in SLE. The presence of IgA immune deposits as well as other immunoglobulins and complement in the glomeruli is characteristic of SLE, but is also characteristic of Henoch-Schönlein purpura and IgA nephropathy. IgA deposits are present far less frequently in mesangiocapillary glomerulonephritis and rarely in post-infectious glomerulonephritis.

The systemic manifestations of Henoch-Schönlein purpura (HSP) are also the features which distinguish it from other causes of ANS. The most characteristic of these is a purpuric rash which is usually symmetric and most prominent over the extensor surfaces and in the dependent areas. The purpura is vasculitic and platelet counts as well as coagulation factors are normal. The rash is sometimes accompanied by systemic complaints of malaise and rarely fever and may be associated with edema without hypoalbuminemia or circulatory congestion(4). A peculiar edema of the scalp and forehead has been noted especially in younger children. Arthralgias, especially of the knees and ankles, which are non-migratory and non-deforming are a relatively common finding. Abdominal manifestations, especially colicky abdominal pain which has led to exploratory abdominal laparotomy and may be associated with melena, complete the clinical triad of this syndrome.

Henoch-Schönlein purpura is accompanied by clinical nephritis in approximately 50% of cases and a wide variation in incidence is found according to the criteria used. In one study, abnormal renal histology was found on biopsy in a series of children with normal routine urinalysis (5). The renal as well as the joint, skin and abdominal findings may occur in any sequence over a period spanning up to several months (6).

An ANS tends to occur in the more severe cases and nephrotic syndrome, when it occurs, is usually a progression from the ANS. Recurrent bouts of ANS have been reported and sometimes HSP may mimic acute post-streptococcal glomerulonephritis (7). However, no good evidence for association with streptococcal infections has been found. Serum complement levels are almost always normal (8). Recently, some investigations have advanced the thesis that HSP and mesangial IgA nephropathy (Berger's) share the same pathogenic mechanism and are merely two ends of a single spectrum. This concept will be discussed in greater detail in the section on IgA nephropathy.

Table 2. Types of histologic lesions most often encountered in the acute nephritic syndrome

Diffuse exudative and proliferative glomerulonephritis
Membranoproliferative (mesangiocapillary) glomerulonephritis
Focal proliferative glomerulonephritis
Mesangial IgA (Berger's) nephropathy
Lupus nephritis
Necrotizing glomerulonephritis
Crescentic glomerulonephritis

The hemolytic uremic syndrome (HUS) is the focus of discussion in other sections of this text and will be described here in the briefest terms as it comprises part of the differential diagnosis of the ANS. Children under the age of 5 years are the most frequently affected in contrast to other common causes of ANS (9). In its more severe form, HUS is more readily diagnosed as it frequently presents with acute renal failure and a predominant anemia which can be established as the result of microangiopathy with hemolysis by the findings of fragmented and distorted erythrocytes on smear and decreased serum haptoglobin levels. Platelet counts are almost always decreased but may be high in the rebound phase (10). Hypertension occurs in 30-60% of cases and although hypocomplementemia is indeed extraordinary, it is known to occur (11). The milder forms may especially mimic acute nephritis, if the hematologic manifestations are not diligently sought. Recurrent episodes of the entire syndrome may occur (12).

These three entities, SLE, HSP and HUS should always be considered and carefully excluded in patients who are being evaluated for the ANS. Their diagnosis may alter prognosis, management considerations, and plans for therapeutic intervention.

When the diagnosis remains in question, a renal biopsy may be performed to further categorize the process. The various types of histologic lesions which may be encountered in cases of the acute nephritic syndrome are listed in Table 2. The histologic correlate for HUS, in the rare instances in which it is not clinically apparent, is a thrombotic microangiopathy which is quite characteristic. It does not overlap with any of the lesions cited in Table 2 except, occasionally, crescentic glomerulonephritis. Varying degrees of cortical necrosis are also characteristic of HUS, particularly in infants.

PRIMARY ACUTE NEPHRITIC SYNDROME

Several primary glomerular diseases have in common features of the ANS which are typically present at the time of onset. Among these are acute post-streptococcal and other forms of post infectious glomerulonephritis, membranoproliferative glomerulonephritis, IgA nephropathy (Berger's disease), focal and segmental proliferative glomerulonephritis and mesangial proliferative glomerulonephritis. In addition, it must be appreciated in the differential diagnosis of acute glomerulonephritis that approximately 20% of patients with chronic progressive glomerulonephritis experience exacerbations resembling acute nephritis, usually at the time of an upper respiratory infection (13). The group of disorders known as rapidly progressive glomerulonephritis characterized by a fulminant course and usually terminating in end-stage renal failure within a three month period must also be considered in the differential diagnosis of ANS, especially when oligo-anuria is prominent.

Although the incidence varies from center to center, acute post-infectious glomerulonephritis is still probably the most common form of acute nephritis encountered in childhood and is the standard against which other forms of ANS are measured. For this reason, it will be discussed in greater detail than the others. Other relatively common primary types of acute glomerulonephritis (AGN) seen in children are mesangial IgA nephropathy (Berger's) and membranoproliferative (mesangiocapillary) glomerulonephritis. Similarities and differences among these three forms of AGN are outlined in Table 3.

Table 3. Primary acute nephritic syndrome: similarities and differences

	APSGN	Berger's IgA nephropathy	MPGN I	MPGN II
Clinical				
Recent streptococcal infection	+++	+	+	+
Gross hematuria	+++	+++	+	+++
Hypertension	++	+	++	+++
Proteinuria < 1 g	+++	+++	++	+
Nephrotic syndrome	0	0	++	+++
Decreased GFR	+++	+	+++	+++
Oliguria	++	0	++	+++
Edema	+++	0	++	+++
Decreased serum complement	+++	0	++	+++
C3NeF	0	0	+	+++
Recurrence in transplanted kidneys	0	+	+	+++
Histologic				
Diffuse exudative and proliferative GN	+++	0	++	+
MPGN	++	0	+++	+++
Subendothelial deposits	+	+	+++	0
Intramembranous deposits	0	0	0	+++
Crescentic GN	++	+	++	+++
Mesangial IgA	0	+++	+	+
Normal or mildly proliferative	++	+++	+	0

0 Absent or rare
\+ Infrequent
++ Moderately frequent
+++ Frequent

Acute post-streptococcal glomerulonephritis

Acute post-strep glomerulonephritis (APSGN) which is representative of the group designated as post-infectious nephritis is the prototype for the ANS. Post-infectious nephropathies are characterized by low serum complement. Examples of post-infectious nephritis in which the antigens have been demonstrated in the glomeruli are pneumococcal (14), staphylococcal (15) and streptococcal (16). Only the latter is common and extensive references of specific causes may be found in basic textbooks (17).

It is important to accurately diagnose patients with APSGN and other post-infectious nephritis because, although there is some controversy about the ultimately good prognosis of this disease (18), the most carefully documented reports indicate an excellent prognosis for full recovery in the majority of patients (19). Specific diagnosis is hence more important for prognostic reasons than for therapeutic intervention, since after treating the infection, therapy for the nephritis is symptomatic and supportive.

The diagnosis can be made with most accuracy early in the course of the disease when the streptococcal etiology can be documented and serum complement is almost invariably low.

Incidence and epidemiology. It appears that APSGN is less frequently encountered than in the past and may even have become a rare cause of nephritis (20). The incidence is variable and depends on infection with certain nephritogenic strains of Group A, B-hemolytic streptococci. These are typed according to M-proteins and type 12 has been the most commonly encountered nephritogenic strain(21). Many other types have also caused APSGN, including types 4, 25 and 49 (22).

Type 12 has been most commonly associated with upper respiratory infections which tend to occur in the winter and spring. Type 49 is most frequently associated with the sporadic form of APSGN which is seen secondary to skin infections most commonly in summer, especially in the southern states of the United States (23).

Many cases of APSGN are subclinical as shown, for example, by examination of urine in asymptomatic family members (24). This makes it difficult to arrive at an actual incidence of APSGN. Figures as high as 20% have been reported following an epidemic of streptococcal infection (25). Most studies however, report an attack rate of 1-2% symptomatic APSGN following skin infections (26). Patients with proven streptococcal disease followed prospectively have an abnormal urine after the latent period in 14% of cases with half of these having depressed serum complement as well (27). This is similar to the 15% incidence of nephritis and unexplained hematuria found in the Red Lake Indian Reservation epidemic of type 49 streptococcal infection (28).

Clinical presentation. A wide variety of clinical features may be found in APSGN ranging from virtually asymptomatic cases (24) to cases in which the course is fulminant with gross hematuria, oligo-anuria, hypertension (sometimes complicated by seizures), circulatory congestion, advanced uremia and even nephrotic syndrome (19).

In the typical case, a latent period of about 10 days occurs between the streptococcal infection and the onset of acute nephritis. An important consideration in the diagnosis is the duration of the latent period since shorter periods of only a few days are often indicative of an exacerbation of a pre-existent renal disease (13).

Edema. Edema is common and fluid retention of some degree is a normal constant finding which may only be appreciated by retrospective evidence of weight loss with diuresis. Edema or gross hematuria are the findings which usually bring the patient to the attention of the physician. A number of factors influence the amount of edema formation including the ingestion of fluid and salt, degree of proteinuria and level of renal insufficiency. The degree of fluid retention with its attendant complications can, to a large extent, be controlled by an understanding of the relationship of intake of salt and water to this problem.

Circulatory congestion. Volume overload may lead to symptoms of dyspnea, orthopnea and cough which can be accompanied by x-ray findings suggesting pneumonia, but which clear with diuresis (29). Apparent anemia which is dilutional and subsides with diuresis is primarily the consequence of expanded plasma volume (30).

Hematuria. Gross hematuria is present, usually at the onset, in about one-third of the patients and usually clears over several days or weeks. The brown color is caused by the release of hemoglobin which is converted to hematin in acid urine (31). Hematuria which persists up to a year after onset of the disease is compatible with a typical course and the meaning of urinary abnormalities which persist for longer periods is uncertain (32).

Hypertension. The pathogenesis of hypertension in APSGN is unknown and is probably related to multiple factors. It has been demonstrated that diuretic induced removal of fluid and sodium is not always accompanied by reduction in the level of blood pressure (33). Hypertensive encephalopathy is a severe complication of APSGN and is probably related to vasodilatation of the cerebral vessels with formation of brain edema secondary to leaking of plasma through the dilated vascular wall (34). Renin is generally not elevated in APSGN associated with hypertension (35).

Laboratory findings. Confirmatory lab findings for the diagnosis of APSGN are listed in Tables 3 and 4. Critical for the diagnosis is evidence of recent streptococcal infection. A single test which measures antibodies to streptolysin, streptokinase, hyaluronidase, DNAase, and NADase, the streptozyme slide test has been shown to be quite effective in detecting recent streptococcal infections (36). Decreased serum complement early in the course of the disease is so typical that the diagnosis should be questioned if complement is not depressed(37). The

Table 4. Features which indicate post-streptococcal glomerulonephritis and generally influence against renal biopsy *

A. Evidence of recent Group A, Beta hemolytic streptococcal infection:

Positive culture Group A, Beta hemolytic streptococcal infection

-within one month of apparent onset AGN
-at least five days prior to onset AGN

Increased single ASLO titer $\geq$ 1250 TU **
Increased serial antistreptococcal antibody titers by $\geq$ 2 tube dilutions

Positive streptozyme test

B. Typical clinical and laboratory features:

Absence of nephrotic syndrome
Absence of systemic disease
Negative family and personal history for renal disease
Serum complement decreased for up to 4 weeks
Normal stature and normal kidney size
Age 5 years or older
Gross hematuria or hypertension for $<$ 2 weeks
Normal or moderate decrease in GFR and urine volume
Recovery from proteinuria $<$ 6 mos; hematuria $<$ 12 mos

* Renal biopsy is not performed when the clinical diagnosis of APSGN seems definite and duration is $<$ 1 year.

**Administration of antibiotics will interfere with increase in antibody titers.

urine sediment most often demonstrates many RBC and WBC and RBC casts. There is usually qualitative proteinuria which rarely exceeds 20 $mg/M^2/hr$. Glomerular filtration rate may be normal, but is frequently decreased. A slight anemia is often detected but is dilutional and disappears when diuresis occurs.

Histology. By light microscopy, the glomeruli are usually enlarged and hypercellular. Polymorphonuclear leukocyte infiltration is very characteristic when it occurs, but is frequently absent. Epithelial crescents are sometimes found in the more fulminant cases. Immunofluorescent granular deposits are present along the capillary loops. The glomerular basement membrane is of normal thickness. This is an important distinguishing feature from membranoproliferative (mesangiocapillary) glomerulonephritis which can have virtually the same clinical presentation, except for well documented streptococcal etiology. The major electron microscopic finding is the presence of large discrete deposits in a subepithelial distribution.

MEMBRANOPROLIFERATIVE (MESANGIOCAPILLARY) GLOMERULONEPHRITIS

In 1965, West et al. (38) described a persistent form of glomerulonephritis in a group of children and adolescents which had distinctive histologic features and characteristic clinical and laboratory findings. The histologic findings have been further delineated and three types of membranoproliferative glomerulonephritis (MPGN) have been described. Although the clinical features in each are similar, certain differences have been emphasized. Type I MPGN has subendothelial deposits while Type II has dense intramembranous deposits and is also called dense deposit disease. A third type has been emphasized in which there are subendothelial, subepithelial and mesangial deposits associated with lamination and fraying of the GBM which is best appreciated on silver stain (39). Many authors, however, prefer to consider Type III as a variant of Type I (40).

Recently another subcategory of MPGN has been described which is associated with a considerably better prognosis (41). We have followed three patients with this variant. Two have been in complete remission for four years and two years while a third has had a mild clinical course with disappearance of hematuria and decreased proteinuria over the past year.

The classification of MPGN has been based principally on histologic findings with a wide range of clinical correlates. It must, therefore, be appreciated that both ANS and nephrotic syndrome, and sometimes both are encountered in typical MPGN and hypocomplementemia is another frequent finding. Table 3 outlines the typical features of MPGN.

Clinical features

Most patients with MPGN have the onset of their disease between the ages of 5-20 years (42). In studies of pediatric populations, the peak incidence is generally from about 8-16 years (43) and although we have followed a child with onset at two years who progressed to renal insufficiency, onset in children under 5 years is quite rare (43). There is a slight preponderance of females with Type I MPGN, especially among younger patients in some reported studies and in the group of patients followed prospectively in the International Study of Kidney Disease in Children (ISKDC)(44)although others point out a more equal distribution (43).

The onset of MPGN frequently mimics APSGN and it is possible that some of the cases of PSGN which follow a progressive course are actually MPGN. This may be especially true when cases which lack strict criteria to prove recent streptococcal infection are included under the diagnosis of APSGN because of clinical or histologic features which may be found in each. Furthermore, infections including streptococcal can provoke exacerbations of pre-existing renal disease as previously pointed out in the section on APSGN. Increased ASO titers have been reported in patients with MPGN (43) and URI is a frequent preceding event at apparent onset. There is, however, no clear evidence linking the respiratory infections to MPGN. Onset with ANS has been observed in as many as 50% of cases (45) but is more commonly observed in about one-fourth to one-third of cases and almost all have some hematuria at presentation(42) Gross hematuria has been found more commonly among patients with Type II MPGN (46) and is found mainly in the first year of the disease and patients may have an intermittent pattern (43). Patients may present with asymptomatic proteinuria. About half of the patients have nephrotic syndrome on presentation which may be persistent, transient or intermittent. Habib et al. (43) have found that most patients with persistent nephrotic syndrome developed renal failure and in the series of Cameron et al. (42) all of the patients with GFR < one-third of normal had nephrotic syndrome while among the 5 patients with normal GFR on follow up only 1 had nephrotic syndrome. Furthermore, 5 of 6 patients with both ANS and nephrotic syndrome required dialysis or had died.

Hypertension is common and is seen at the onset in approximately 30% of patients (43) while decreased renal function also occurs in approximately 30-50% of cases (42).

Laboratory features

Decreased complement. Decreased serum level of C3 is one of the most characteristic findings in MPGN and is usually present at onset (47). The levels tend to fluctuate in Type I MPGN whereas the concentration is more markedly and persistently reduced in Type II MPGN (48). In Type I disease early components of both the classical pathway (Cl_q, C4) and of the alternative pathway (factor B, properdin) are frequently reduced. In contrast, in type II MPGN Cl_q and C4 tend to be normal while factor B and properdin are decreased, suggesting a predominance of alternative pathway activation in this type of disease (49).

C3 nephritic factor. The presence of C_3 nephritic factor (C3NeF), an IgG autoantibody against C3 convertase ($C3_{bBb}$)of the alternative pathway, is found in almost all patients with Type II MPGN and is much less common in Type I (50). C3NeF activates the alternative pathway by stabilizing $C3_{bBb}$, similar to properdin. But, instead of being reversible by the action of BIH (one of the two plasma inhibitory proteins which displaces Bb and allows inactivation of $C3_b$) inactivation by this pathologic protein is irreversible, enhancing the function of C_3 convertase with a 30-fold increase in half-life. It allows continuous activation of the alternative pathway (51). Elevation in C3NeF per se, even when associated with hypocomplementemia, is not, however, invariably associated with renal disease as has been shown in some patients with partial lipodystrophy (52) and there is inconsistent correlation between serum levels of C3 or C3NeF and the outcome or activity of MPGN (53).

Cryoglobulins and immune complexes have also been described in the circulation in both Type I and Type II MPGN but their significance is unclear.

Anemia. A normochromic, normocytic anemia which is frequently noted to be more severe than would be expected for the degree of renal insufficiency, has been recognized (54), and is possibly related to lysis of RBC by terminal components of complement which may act upon the non-sensitized RBC (55).

Pathology

Several detailed descriptions of the histologic features of MPGN are available (56, 57). The major alterations in Type I MPGN are hypercellularity and thickening of the capillary walls with expansion of the mesangium, hence the synonym mesangiocapillary glomerulonephritis. When mesangial hypercellularity is pronounced there is accentuation of the lobular pattern. Sometimes polymorphonuclear leukocytes are found infiltrating the mesangium (56). The capillary walls are thickened and frequently demonstrate the characteristic "double contour" or "railroad track" appearance which is caused by interposition of the expanded mesangial portion of the glomerulus. Crescents may be seen initially as well as during progression. When crescents are numerous they usually indicate a poor prognosis, although this is not always true (58).

Treatment

MPGN is, in most circumstances, a relentlessly progressive disease. A wide variety of immunosuppressive regimens has been analyzed in uncontrolled retrospective reviews without clear implications for therapy (42,59,60). It appears that the experience reported by West and his colleagues and recently reviewed (61) has been the best for patients with this disease with cumulative kidney survival of nearly 80% over a 16 year period. These workers have used alternate day prednisone (2 mg/Kg/q alternate a.m. up to 80 mg/day) for one year with gradually tapering doses thereafter. Improvement of the complement profile and hematuria were used as end points for therapeutic adjustments after one year of high dose alternate day therapy. In view of the recentlv described probable role of filtered protein in the evolution of glomerulosclerosis (62) and confirmed by our group (63), proteinuria may be a more important parameter to utilize for dosage adjustment after the first year of high dose treatment. A similar, but lower dose, prednisone regimen was tested in a controlled prospective trial in 37 children with Type I

MPGN by the International Collaborative Study of Kidney Disease in Children (64). It was concluded that the overall five year success rate was no different between the patients treated with alternate day prednisone and placebo. This conclusion, however, does not seem valid since the five year success rate in the alternate day prednisone group was 95% versus 57% in the placebo group when a 50% decrement in GFR was used as the sole end point. It was only after severe hypertension was added as a part of the definition of treatment failure that the difference became insignificant.

Our current practice is to treat MPGN with the regimen proposed by West et al. and treat hypertension vigorously with diuretics (to counteract the sodium and water retention induced by steroids) as well as with the expanded armamentarium of other effective antihypertensive medications now available. It has been folklore that daily prednisone therapy in MPGN may be accompanied by rapid deterioration of GRF, probably when associated with poorly controlled hypertension (65).

MESANGIAL IGA NEPHROPATHY (BERGER'S DISEASE)

Berger's Disease is a glomerulopathy distinguished by predominance of mesangial IgA deposits. The characteristic clinical features are reported in adults and in children. The typical features are: a male preponderance (2:1), intermittent gross and persistent or intermittent microhematuria, absent or mild proteinuria (usually less than 1g/day), and normal glomerular filtration rate. Most of the patients have macroscopic hematuria, the onset of which is often associated with upper respiratory infections. Approximately one-third of the patients are asymptomatic and the disease is discovered during routine urinalysis because of the associated hematuria and/or proteinuria. Exceptions to the usually benign course of this disease have been reported and in the series we presented, three of nine children with mesangial IgA nephropathy progressed to renal insufficiency (66). We noted at that time that each of the cases with progression had glomerulosclerosis in contrast to the patients with a benign course, most of whom had either diffuse mesangial proliferative findings, focal and segmental proliferation, or normal histology. Similarly, in the group of children followed by Levy, et al., such lesions were not associated with decreased renal function over periods of observation ranging up to approximately 10 years (67). In the rare instances in which renal insufficiency is progressive, renal transplantation has been generally successful; however, recurrence of the disease in the transplanted kidney has been reported (68). IgA nephropathy was initially described in France by Berger (68) but is now recognized to have a world wide distribution. The incidence in France where it constitutes approximately 25% of primary glomerulonephropathies is similar to the incidence in Spain and Australia, although in England and the United States IgA nephropathy constitutes approximately 5% of primary glomerulonephropathies (69,70,71,72,73). It has been our experience that with the decreased incidence of acute post streptococcal glomerulonephritis there has been a relative increase in mesangial IgA nephropathy. It is entirely possible that if incidence surveys in the United States were more current than the ones cited above, that IgA nephropathy would constitute a higher proportion of the cases of primary glomerulonephritis.

The pathogenesis of IgA nephropathy is not known and although most studies have shown elevated serum IgA levels (72) there is no clinical or histologic findings. Some authors have indicated that elevated serum levels of IgA are associated with a more benign course in this disease (62). Apparently the IgA in addition to being elevated is also abnormal in many instances and some authors have reported the presence of high serum levels of Polymeric IgA, including the secretory component, in some but not all patients with IgA nephropathy (74). It is interesting that although IgA is capable of activating the complement cascade via the alternative pathway, serum complement levels have consistantly been found to be normal in IgA nephropathy.

The association of IgA nephropathy with various HLA antigens has been reported. Probably the strongest association is with HLA-Bw35 antigen in which the disease risk ahs been reported to be four times higher than in the general population (75). In addition, IgA nephropathy has been described in two pairs of HLA identical siblings who shared the HLA-Bw35 antigen (76). Close association f the DRw4 antigen in patients with IgA nephropathy has been described by several groups (77). Several other groups, however, have failed to find association between specific HLA antigens and IgA nephropathy (78,79,80).

Over the past few years there has been an emphasis on a possible relationship between IgA nephropathy and anaphylactoid purpura (Henoch-Schönlein) nephritis. Histologically these two entities may be indistinguishable. Serum IgA has been found to be elevated in both diseases, recurrence of nephritis in a transplanted kidney has been documented in both as well as similar HLA antigen associations and high serum levels of Polymeric IgA, some of which are present as immune complexes. These have been reviewed by Egido et al., who have suggested that there may be a common pathogenic mechanism between the two diseases with a basic defect consisting of an abnormal increase in IgA polymerization (81). Alcoholic liver disease is another circumstance in which a predominance of glomerular IgA deposits may be found. Berger et al., found that the majority of 100 autopsy samples and 11 biopsy samples had prominent IgA deposits (82). The renal histology, however, was quite varied in this series and not all of the patients had alcoholic cirrhosis. The pathogenesis of these IgA nephropathies and their potential pathogenic interrelationships are unknown. At this point, whether or not the mere prominence of IgA deposition justifies linkage in etiopathogenesis remains speculative.

PATHOGENIC MECHANISMS IN ANS

It is generally assumed that the deposition of immunoglobulins found in virtually all forms of the ANS represent immune complex induced glomerular injury. This concept is best supported by experimental and human nephropathies in which a specific antigen has been identified in both the circulation and the glomerular basement membrane, and the well described pathogenic mechanisms involving the complement cascade which are associated with alterations in serum complement levels (83).

As will be seen later, there are similarities and differences in the patterns of immunoglobulin involvement among the various nephropathies of the ANS. The mediators of immunologically induced renal injury are varied and complex. In the most widely applicable mechanism, antibodies react with their antigen either in tissues (as occurs in anti-glomerular basement membrane antibody nephritis) or in the circulation and the complement cascade is activated (84). These mechanisms are extensively reviewed by Schreiber and Müller-Eberhard (85) will be briefly summarized below.

Activation of the complement system can occur by the classical or alternative pathways and many of the nephropathies associated with the acute nephritic syndrome involve both (85). The classic pathway is activated by immune complexes (IgG and IgM) which bind, via the F_c region, the Cl_q subunit of the Cl complex (Clq, Cl_r, Cl_s) of the complement system. Cl_r acquires the capacity to activate Cls which is then converted to its natural substrates, C2 and C4. C4 is divided into a and b fragments with the larger $C4_b$ fragment binding to the immune complex. C2 is also cleaved into a and b fragments with $C2_a$ forming classical pathway C3 convertase and exposing a binding site through which $C3_b$ can bind the immune complex.

The C5-C9 "membrane attack" complex, possessing factors for opsonization, anaphylaxis and cytolysis is initiated by $C4_b$, $C2_a$, $C3_b$ complex induced cleavage of C5 into $C5_a$ and $C5_b$. The interaction of cells with the $C5_b$-C9 complex overcomes the charge barrier of cell membranes and alters the hydrophobic barrier resulting in formation of tiny membrane channels and allowing cellular damage to occur (85). In addition, several of the activated components of the complement system can be shown to acquire specific biological properties such as immune adherence and opsonization ($C3_b$), and chemotaxis for polymorphonuclear leukocytes and anaphylotoxins ($C3_a$).

The alternative complement pathway includes properdin, factor B, C3 and factor D and does not require antibody or early classical components (Cl, C4, C2) for activation. It can be activated by lipopolysaccharides (bacterial components, insulin, zymosan) and IgA (49). The reaction between factor B and $C3_b$ (which may be produced by activation of the classical pathway or earlier components of the alternative pathway which are not well understood) generates C3 convertase called $C3_{bB}$, an enzyme, which is a weak complex with its B molecule possessing C3 activating capacity (85). In the presence of activated D, $C3_{bBb}$, a more active component than $C3_{bB}$ is formed. Nephritic factor, or C3NeF, is an IgG autoantibody found in patients with hypocomplementemic progressive glomerulonephritis (49) which increases the initial production of $C3_b$ and increases the duration of biologic activity of $C3_{bBb}$ (49) resulting in potent activation of C3.

Despite the apparent role of the complement cascade and immune complex deposition in human glomerulonephritis, attention has recently been drawn to the hypothetical nature of this association (86). For example, in membranoproliferative glomerulonephritis with subendothelial deposits, it appears that the pathogenic process is not directly affected by the complement abnormalities, since the prognosis is similar whether the process is normo or hypo-complementemic (87). Furthermore, Berger et al. have recently published the case of an 11 year old girl who had circulating immune complexes and glomerulonephritis with congenital absence of the third component of complement. Her kidney showed heavy accumulations of IgG, IgM and Cl_q while deposits of C3 were absent (88). In addition, removal of complement by cobra venom factor (an analogue of human $C3_b$ that activates the alternative pathway and depletes the complement system from C3 to C9 (89), does not prevent the development of lesions in rabbit kidney with Masugi nephritis induced by injection of heteroantibodies to the glomerular basement membrane (90). Hence other mediators of glomerular inflammation need to be explored.

REFERENCES

1. Rothfield, NF: DM Disease a Month: 29:46,1982 (Oct.).

2. Pohl, MA, Krakauer, R, Gephardt, G, Hunsicker, L, Roberts, JL, Schwartz, MM, & Lewis, EJ: Modified Criteria for the Diagnosis of Systemic Lupus Erythematosus in the Presence of Diffuse Proliferative Nephritis. Kid. Internat. 23:131,1983.

3. Leehey, DJ, Katz, AI, Azaran, AH, Aronson, AJ, & Spargo, BH: Silent diffuse lupus nephritis: Long-term follow-up. Am. J. Kidney Dis. Vol. 11, No. 1 Suppl. 1, July 1982.

4. Ackroyd, JF: Allergic purpura including purpura due to foods, drugs, and infections. Am. J. Med. 14:605,1953.

5. Greifer, I, Bernstein, J, Kikkawa, Y, & Edelmann, CM, Jr: Histologic evidence of nephritis in patients with Henoch-Schönlein syndrome without clinical evidence of renal disease. Proc. Am. Soc. Nephrol. 1966.

6. Meadow, SR, Glasgow, EF, White, RHR, Moncrieff, MW, Cameron, JS, & Ogg, CS: Schönlein-Henoch nephritis. Q. J. Med. 41:241,1972.

7. Urizar, RE, Singh, JK, Muhammad, T, & Hines, O : Henoch-Schönlein anaphalactoid purpura nephropathy: electron microscopic lesions mimicking acute poststreptoccal nephritis. Human Pathol. 9:223,1978.

8. Hurley, RM, & Drummond, KN : Anaphalactoid purpura nephritis: Clinicopathological correlations. J. Pediat. 81:904,1972.

9. Lieberman, E: Hemolytic-uremic syndrome. J. Pediat. 80:1,1972.

10. Sanchez Avalos, J, Vitacco, M, Molinas, F, Penalver, J, & Gianantonio, CA: Coagulation studies in the hemolytic-uremic syndrome. J. Pediatrics 76:538,1970.

11. Kim, Y, Miller, K and Michael, AF: Breakdown products of C3 and Factor B in Hemolytic Uremic Syndrome. J. Lab. Clin. Med. 89:845, 1977.

12. Kaplan, BS.: Hemolytic-uremic syndrome with recurrent episodes: An important subset. Clin. Nephrol. 8:485,1977.

13. Seegal, D, Lyttle, JD, Loeb, EN, Jost, EL, & Davis, G: On the exacerbation in chronic glomerulonephritis. J. Clin. Invest. 19:569.1940.

14. Hyman, LR, Jenia, EH, Hill, GS, Zimmerman, SW, & Burkholder, PM : Alternate C3 pathway activation in pneumococcal glomerulonephritis. Am. J. Med. 58:810,1975.

15. Moncrief, MW, Glasgow, EF, Arthur, JH, & Hargraves, HM: Glomerulonephritis associated with Staphylococcus albus in a Spitz Holter valve. Arch. Dis. Child. 48:69,1973.

16. Treser, G , Acosta-McVicar, M, Semar, M, Lange, L : Localization of Autologous and Homologous 7-S Gamma-globulin on Kidney Biopsies of Patients with Early Acute Glomerulonephritis. Science, 163:676,1969.

17. Glassock,, RJ, Cohen, AH, Bennett, CM, & Martinez-Maldonado, M. Primary Glomerular Diseases. In B Brenner & F Rector, Jr (eds) The Kidney. Saunders,Toronto, 1981, Vol. II, p. 1384.

18. Schacht, RG, Gallo, GR, Gluck, MC, Iqbal, MS, & Baldwin, DS: Irreversible Disease Following Acute Poststreptococcal Glomerulonephritis in Children. J. Chron. Dis. 32:515,1979.

19. Lewy, JE, Salinas-Madrigal, L, Herdson, PB, Pirani, CL,& Metcoff, J: Clinicopathologic correlations in acute poststreptococcal glomerulonephritis. Medicine.50:453,1971.

20. Meadow, SR: Poststreptococcal nephritis - a rare disease? Arch. Dis. Child. 50:379,1975

21. Rammelkamp, CH, Jr, & Weaver, RS : Acute glomerulonephritis. The significance of variations in the incidence of disease. J. Clin. Invest. 32:345,1953.

22. Dillon, HC : Streptococcal infections of the skin and their complications: Impetigo and nephritis. In Wannamaker, LW, & Matsen, JM, (eds) Streptococci and Streptococcal Diseases. Academic Press, New York, 1972, p. 571.

23. Kaplan, EL, Anthony, BF, Chapman, SS, & Wannamaker, LW : Epidemic acute glomerulonephritis associated with type 49 streptococcal pyoderma. I. Clinical and laboratory findings. Am. J. Med. 48:9,1970.

24. Dodge, WF, Spargo, BF, & Travis, LB: Occurrence of acute glomerulonephritis in sibling contacts of children with sporadic acute glomerulonephritis. Pediat 40:1029, 1967.

25. Bengtsson, U, Ekedahl, C, & Holm, SE : Acute post-streptococcal glomerulonephritis. A retrospective study, Scand. J. Infect. Dis. 5: 111, 1973.

26. Hall, WD, Blumberg, RW, & Moody, MD : Studies in children with impetigo; bacteriology, serology, and incidence of glomerulonephritis. Am. J.Dis. Child. 125 :800, 1973.

27. Sagel, I, Treser, G, Ty, A, Yoshizarva, N, Kleinberger, H, Yuceoglu, AM, Wassermann, E & Lange, K : Occurrence and nature of glomerular lesions after group A strepto-cocci infections in children. Ann. Intern. Med. 79:492, 1973.

28. Anthony, BF, Kaplan, EL, Wannamaker, LW, Briese, FW, & Chapman, SS: Attack rates of acute nephritis after type 49 streptococcal infection of the skin and of the respiratory tract. J.Clin. Invest. 48:1697,1969.

29. Fleisher, DS, Voci, G, Garfunkel, J, Puragganan, H, Kirkpatrick, J, Jr, Wells, CR & McElfresh, AE : Hemodynamic findings in acute glomerulonephritis. J. Pediatr. 69:1054,1966.

30. Eisenberg, S : Blood volume in patients with acute glomerulonephritis as determined by radioactive chromium tagged red cells. Am. J. Med. 27:241, 1959.

31. Heymann, W, Rothenberg, MB, Gilkey, C, Lewis, M: Differences in color of hematuria in the nephrotic syndrome and glomerulonephritis. Pediat. 21:375,1958.

32. Potter, EV, Lipschultz, SA, Abidh, S, Poon-King, T, Earle, DP: Twelve to seventeen year follow-up of patients with poststreptococcal acute glomerulonephritis in Trinidad. N. Engl. J. Med. 307:725, 1982.

33. Repetto, HA, Lewy, JE, Brando, JL, & Metcoff, J : The renal functional response to furosemide in children with acute glomerulonephritis. J. Pediatr. 80:660, 1972.

34. Johansson, B, Strandgaard, S, & Lassen, NA : On the pathogenesis of hypertensive encephalopathy. Circ. Res. (Suppl. 1) 34-35:167,1974.

35. Schwartz, WB & Kassirer, JP : Clinical aspects of acute poststreptococcal glomerulonephritis. In Strauss, MB, & Welt, LG (eds): Diseases of the Kidney, Vol. 1. Little, Brown, & Co., Boston, 1971.

36. Kholy, AE, Hafez, K, Krause, R: Specificity and sensitivity of the streptozyme test for the detection of streptococcal antibodies. Appl. Microbiol. 27:748, 1974.

37. Lange, K, Graig, F, Oberman, J, Slobody, L, Ogur , G, & LoCasto, F: Changes in serum complement during the course and treatment of glomerulonephritis. Arch.Intern. Med. 88:433, 1951.

38. West, CD, McAdams, AJ, McConville, JM, Davis, NC, & Holland, NH : Hypocomplementemic and normocomplementemic persistent (chronic) glomerulonephritis: Clinical and pathologic characteristics. J. Pediatr. 67:1089,1965.

39. Strife, CF, McEnery, PT, McAdams, AJ, & West, CD: A third type of membranoproliferative glomerulonephritis. Clin. Nephrol. 7:65, 1977.

40. White, RHR : Membranoproliferative Glomerulonephritis. In Edelman, CM (ed) : Pediatric Kidney Disease, Vol. II. Little, Brown, & Co., Boston, 1978.

41. Strife, CF, McAdams, AJ, West, CD: Membranoproliferative glomerulonephritis characterized by focal, segmental proliferative lesions. Clin. Nephrol. 18:9, 1982.

42. Cameron, JS, Ogg, CS, White, RHR, & Glasgow, EF: The clinical features and prognosis of patients with normocomplementemic mesangiocapillary glomerulonephritis. Clin. Nephrol. 1:2,1973.

43. Habib, R, Kleinknecht, C, Gubler, M-C, & Levy, M: Idiopathic membranoproliferative glomerulonephritis in children. Report of 105 cases. Clinc. Nephrol. 4:194, 1973.

44. Alternate day steroid therapy in membranoproliferative glomerulonephritis: A randomized controlled clinical trial. A report of the ISKDC. Kid. Internat. 21:150, 1982.

45. Mandalenakis, N, Mendoza, N, Pirani, CL, & Pollak,VD: Lobular glomerulonephritis and membranoproliferative glomerulonepritis. Medicine 50:319, 1971.

46. Antoine, B, & Faye, C: The clinical course associated with dense deposits in the kidney basement membranes. Kidney Int. 1:420,1972.

47. Cameron, JS, Glasgow, EF, Ogg, CS, & White, RHR : Membranoproliferative glomerulonephritis and persistent hypocomplementaemia. Br. Med. J. 4:7, 1970.

48. Kim, Y, Vernier, RL, Fish, AJ, & Michael, AF : Immunofluorescence studies of dense deposit disease. The presence of railroad track and mesangial rings. Lab. Invest. 40:474, 1979.

49. Vallota, EH, Götze, O, Speigelberg, HL, Forristal, J. West, CD, & Müller-Eberhard, HJ : A serum factor in chronic hypocomplementemic nephritis distinct from immunoglobulins and activating the alternate pathway of complement. Journal of Experimental Medicine 139:1249,1974.

50. Ooi, YM, Vallota, EH, & West, CD : Classical complement pathway activation in membranoproliferative glomerulonephritis. Kidney International 9:46,1976.

51. Austen,KF : Homeostasis of effector systems which can also be recruited for immunologic reactions. Journal of Immunology 121:793, 1978.

52. Peters, DK, & Williams,DG : Complement and mesangiocapillary glomerulonephritis. Role of complement deficiency in the pathogenesis of nephritis. Nephron 13: 189, 1974.

53. West, CD, & McAdams, AJ : Serum Beta 1C globulin levels in persistent glomerulonephritis with low serum complement: Variability unrelated to clinical course. Nephron 7:193, 1970.

54. Herdman, RC, Pickering, RJ, Michael, AF, Vernier, RL, Fish, AJ, Gewurz, H, & Good, RA : Chronic glomerulonephritis associated with low serum complement activity (chronic hypocomplementemic glomerulonephritis). Medicine 49: 207, 1970.

55. Arroyave, CM, Vallota, E, & Müller-Eberhard, HJ : Lysis of human erythrocytes due to activation of the alternate complement pathway by nephritic factor (C3NEF). J. Immunol. 113:764,1974.

56. Davis, BK, & Cavallo, T: Membranoproliferative glomerulonephritis. Am. J. Pathol. 84:283, 1976.

57. Anders, D & Thoenes, W : Basement membrane changes in membranoproliferative glomerulonephritis. A light and electron microscopic study. Virchows Arch. (Pathol. Anat.) 369:87, 1975.

58. Case records of the Massachusetts General Hospital, N. Engl. J. Med.197:713, 1977.

59. Holland, NH, & Bennett, NM : Hypercomplementemic (membranoproliferative) glomerulonephritis. Immunosuppressive therapy. Am. J. Dis. Child. 123:439,1972.

60. Kincaid-Smith, P: The treatment of chronic mesangiocapillary (membranoproliferative) glomerulonephritis with impaired renal function. Med. J. Aust. 2:587, 1972.

61. West, CD : Membranoproliferative Glomerulonephritis: Classification and Treatment. In Grusin, AB & Norman, ME (eds). Pediatric Nephrology (Proceedings of the V International Congress of Pediatric Nephrology). Martinus Nijhoff, Boston,1981

62. Giordano, C: Protein restriction in chronic renal failure. Kidney International Vol. 22: 401, 1982.

63. Chandra, M, Susin, M, Teichberg, S, McVicar, M : Experimental Focal Segmental Glomerulosclerosis: Correlation with Protein Excretion, Glomerular Filtration Rate and Renal Plasma Flow. Pediat. Res., (In press.)

64. Alternate day steroid therapy in membranoproliferative glomerulonephritis: A randomized controlled clinical trial. A report of the ISKDC. Kid. Internat. 21:150, 1982.

65. Neugarten, J, Feiner, H, Schacht, RG, Gallo, GR and Baldwin, DS: Aggravation of experimental glomerulonephritis by superimposed clip hypertension. Kidney Internat. 22:257,1982.

66. McVicar, M, Gauthier, B, Nicastri, AD: Mesangial IgA:IgG nephropathy in children. Proceedings 14th International Congress of Pediatrics. p 169, 1974.

67. Levy, MH, Beaufils, Gubler, MC, Habib, R: Idiopathic recurrent macroscopic hematuria and mesangial IgA-IgG deposits in children (Berger's Disease). Clinical Nephrology, 1:63, 1973.

68. Berger, J: IgA glomerular deposits disease. Transplantation Proceedings. 1:939, 1969.

69. Clarkson, AR, Seymour, AE, Thompson, AJ: IgA nephropathy: A syndrome of uniform morphology, diverse clinical features and uncertain prognosis. Clin. Nephrol. 8:459, 1977.

70. Droz, D : Natural history of primary glomerulonephritis with mesangial deposits of IgA. Contrib. Nephrol. 2:150, 1976.

71. Davies, DR, Tighe, JR, Jones, NF: Isolated glomerulonephritis with mesangial IgA deposition. Br. Med. J. 4:103, 1975.

72. Egido, J, Rivera, F, Sancho, J, et al: Estudio del sistema HLA. Factores de riesgo para la insuficiencia renal en la glomerulonefritis mesangial IgA. Nefrologia 1:21, 1981.

73. Hyman, LR, Wagnild, JP, Beirne, GJ, et al: Immunoglobulin A distribution in glomerular disease. Analysis of immunofluorescence localization and pathogenic significance. Kidney Internat. 3:397, 1973.

74. Lopez Trascasa, M, Egido, J, Sancho, J, et al: IgA glomerulonephritis (Berger's Disease). Evidence of high serum levels of polymeric IgA. Clinic. Exp. Immunol. 42:247, 1980.

75. Gagne, A, Sabatier, JC, et al: HLA-Bw35 and mesangial IgA glomerulonephritis. N. Engl. J. Med. 298:1034, 1978.

76. Sabatier, JC, Genin, C, Assenot, H, et al: Mesangial IgA glomerulonephritis in HLA identical brothers. Clin. Nephrol. 11:35, 1979.

77. Guegren, M, Genetet, B, et al: HLA-DR antigen and IgA nephropathy (Berger's Disease). N. Engl. J. Med. 302:1033, 1980.

78. Silvestri, MG, et al: HLA antigens and HLA mesangial glomerulonephritis. Clin. Nephrol. 12:45, 1979.

79. Nagy, J, Hamori, A, Ambrus, M, et al: More on IgA glomerulonephritis and HLA antigens. N. Engl. J. Med. 300:92, 1979.

80. Mouzon-Cambron, A, Ohaydon, E, Bouissou, F, et al: HLA-DR typing in children with glomerular diseases. Lancet 11:868, 1980.

81. Egido, J, Sancho, J, Mampaso, F, et al: A possible common pathogenesis of the mesangial IgA glomerulonephritis in patients with Berger's disease and Schönlein-Henoch syndrome. Proc. Eur. Dial. Transplant Assoc. 17:660, 1980.

82. Berger,J, Yaneva, H, Nabarra, B: Glomerular changes in patients with cirrhosis of the liver, in Hamburger, J, Crosnier, J, Grunfeld, JP, et al. (eds.): Advances in Nephrology. Chicago, Year Book Medical Publishers, 7:3, 1977.

83. Hunsicker, LG, Ruddy, S, Carpenter, CB, Schur, PH, Merrill, JP, Muller-Eberhard, HJ, Austen, KF: Metabolism of third component of complement (C3) in nephritis. N. Engl. J. Med., 287:835, 1972.

84. Müller-Eberhard, HJ: Complement: Molecular mechanisms, regulations and biologic function. In: Molecular Basis of Biological Degradative Processes, R. Berlin, H. Hermann, I. Lepow, and J. Tanzer, Editors. Academic Press, New York, 1978,p. 65.

85. Schreiber, RD, Müller-Eberhard, HJ: Complement and renal disease. In:Immunologic Mechanisms of Renal Disease. Ed. C.B. Wilson, Churchill Livingstone, N.Y., 1979, p. 67.

86. Couser, WG: What are immune complexes doing in glomerulonephritis? N. Engl. J. Med. 304:1230, 1981.

87. West, CD: Pathogenesis and approaches to therapy of membranoproliferative glomerulonephritis. Kid. Internat. 9:1, 1976.

88. Berger, M, Balow, JE, Wilson, CB, Frank, MM: Circulating immune complexes and glomerulonephritis in a patient with congenital absence of the third component of complement. N. Engl. J. Med. 308:1009, 1983.

89. Cochran, CG, Müller-Eberhard, HJ, Aikin, BS: Depletion of plasma complement in vivo by a protein of cobra venom: Its effect on various immunologic reactions. J. Immunol. 105:55, 1970.

90. Thomson, NM, Naish, PF, Simpson, IJ, Peters, DK: The role of C3 in the autologous phase of nephrotoxic nephritis. Clin. Exp. Immunol. 24:464, 1976.

CIRCULATING IMMUNE-COMPLEXES IN GLOMERULAR DISEASE

Guido O. Perez, M.D.

The formation of immune complexes is a crucial component in the normal defense of the organism against pathogens and other foreign substances. Unfortunately, in certain cases immune complexes may become pathogenic, causing injury to the host. Typical examples of diseases associated with increased levels of circulating immune complexes (CIC) are systemic lupus erythematosus, rheumatoid arthritis, various forms of glomerulonephritis, chronic inflammatory bowel disease, malignancy and many chronic infections.

Immune complexes are formed when antibodies from the host react with endogenous or exogenous antigens in tissues or in the systemic circulation. A number of factors are known to contribute to the pathogenicity of CIC. They include the nature of the antigen and antibody, the quantitative relationship between antigen and antibody and the function of the reticuloendothelial system. Complexes which are formed when the levels of antigen and antibody are similar or at a slight antigen excess, fix complement, are not completely phagocytized by the reticulo system, and tend to lodge in the wall of blood vessels causing tissue damage by their interaction with complement, polymorphs, macrophages, and other effector cells.

MEASUREMENT OF CIRCULATING IMMUNE COMPLEXES

In the last ten years numerous methods have been described to measure CIC. These methods are based on 1) the physicochemical properties of the complexes or 2) their interaction with humoral or cellular receptors (Table 1). Among the most useful tests currently available are the Clq binding assay or one of its modifications, the conglutinin binding assay, and the Raji cell radioimmunoassay (Fig. 1A,B,C).

These tests, however, suffer from several limitations, and a positive test cannot be taken as absolute proof that CIC are present. In fact, none of the tests available differentiates antigen-antibody complexes from nonspecifically aggregated immunoglobulins. An additional constraint is that as of this moment there are no generally available reference preparations in the form of stable immunoglobulin aggregates of different size or stabilized antigen-antibody complexes which can be used by various laboratories around the world.

Positive tests for CIC may be found in approximately 3-4% of normal subjects and there is evidence that IgA immune complexes may be found in healthy individuals after eating food. On the other hand, these tests may be negative in diseases associated with tissue deposition of complexes. In these cases it has been suggested that the tests may not be sensitive

Table 1. Methods Used for the Determination of Immune Complexes

1. Physicochemical methods

   - Cryoprecipitation
   - Precipitation with polyethylene glycol
   - Analytic ultracentrifugation

2. Methods that utilize protein or cellular receptors

   A. Humoral Receptors

      - Rheumatoid factors
      - Conglutinin
      - Clq and complement

   B. Cellular Receptors

      - Platelets, WBC, RBC
      - Macrophages
      - Lymphocytes (Raji cells)

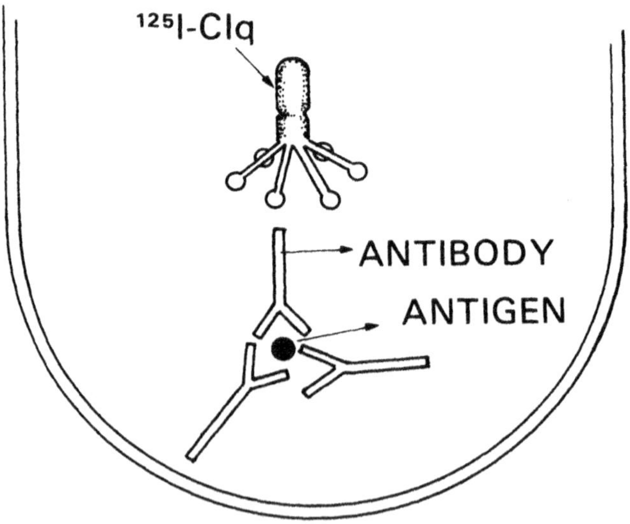

Figure 1-A. Clq binding assay (liquid phase). The test serum is incubated with ^{125}I-Clq and CIC are precipitated with polyethylene glycol. The precipitate is isolated by centrifugation and the precipitated radioactivity is counted.

Figure 1-B. Conglutinin assay (solid phase). In this test conglutinin, fixed to the walls of the test tube, reacts with a fragment of C3 that has been fixed in the immune complex. Labelled antibodies against human IgG alone or conjugated with alkaline phosphatase are then added. The complexes are then identified either by adding a reagent to develop the color with the alkaline phosphatase or by adding radiolabelled Protein A.

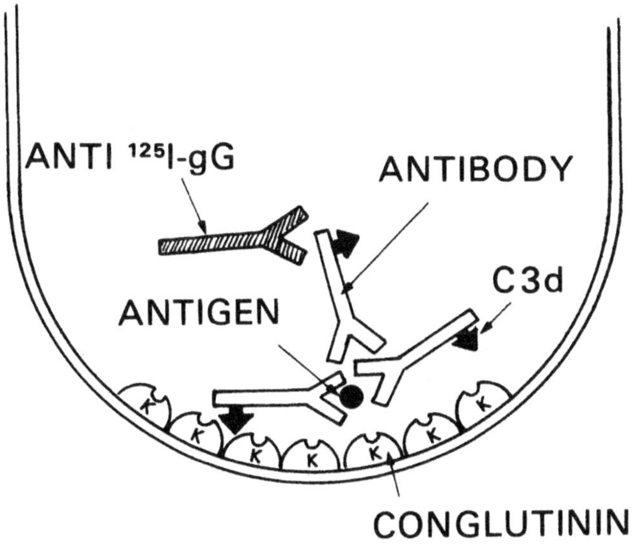

enough, that CIC appear intermittently or that the complexes are formed in situ.

Because of the idiosyncrasies and specificities of the different tests, certain CIC may react preferentially with one reagent and not with another. Since none of the tests currently available is capable of detecting complexes of all Ig classes, both complement fixing and non-complement fixing, and of all sizes, optimal screening for CIC requires that a panel rather than a single test be used.

It is important to emphasize that the detection of CIC in disease states does not necessarily implicate the complexes in the pathologic process. Thus, the ultimate criterion is the demonstration that CIC are concentrated in the main lesions associated with the disease. One additional important limitation found in many studies is that a single determination of CIC does not reflect the severity or frequency of the immunological insult during the course of the illness. In this regard, it has been shown in several diseases that changes in the activity of the illness may be associated with a switch of immunoglobulin class in the complex.

Despite the aforementioned diagnostic limitations, assays for CIC have been used to follow the clinical activity of the disease and to gauge the response to treatment. In addition, it is hoped that modification of these tests may provide the tools for immune complex isolation and characterization of their components.

Figure 1-C. Raji cell assay. Raji cells have complement receptors but no surface-bound IgG. After incubation of the test serum with Raji cells the immune complexes bound to cells are detected by adding labelled antibodies against human IgG.

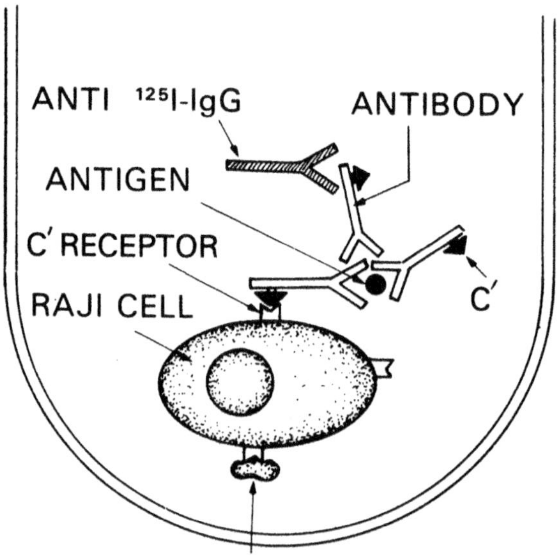

IMMUNE COMPLEXES IN PATIENTS WITH GLOMERULAR DISEASES

Positive CIC are frequently found in patients with glomerulonephritis associated with systemic diseases. In patients with systemic lupus erythematosus, various high and low molecular weight substances reacting in CIC assays have been identified. A high prevalence of immune complex-like substances has been found in sera of patients with systemic vasculitis, bacterial endocarditis and Wegener's granulomatosis. In some instances the levels of CIC in these diseases correlate with the activity of the illness, its prognosis or both.

Qualitative differences between CIC have been found which may prove useful in terms of diagnosis. For example, a low molecular weight serum Clq reactant appears to be a marker for the syndrome of hypocomplementemic cutaneous vasculitis which may be associated with mild proliferative glomerulonephritis. IgA immune complexes are found preferentially in certain diseases such as Henoch-Schönlein purpura, IgA nephropathy and Behcet's syndrome.

Numerous studies have evaluated the prevalence of CIC in patients with primary glomerular diseases. In general, the prevalence of CIC in these patients is lower than in those with systemic illnesses. In patients with the nephrotic syndrome the detection of CIC varies considerably depending on the nature of the disease and the timing and type of assays used (Table 2).

Table 2. Immune Complexes in Patients with Minimal Change Disease and Membranous Glomerulopathy.

First Author/Year	Test	No.	Prevalence (%)
	MINIMAL CHANGE DISEASE		
Stuhlinger (1976)	Macrophage inhibition	12	83
Sobel (1976)	Clq deviation	19	42
Smith (1975)	Rosette inhibition	14	100
Levinsky (1978)	Inhibition of agglutination of latex particles	18	94
Abrass (1980)	Clq and Raji tests	14	79
	MEMBRANOUS GLOMERULOPATHY		
Adam (1973)	Cryoimmunoglobulins	12	11
Nydegger (1974)	Cryoimmunoglobulins	10	40
Stuhlinger (1976)	Macrophage inhibition	7	86
Gluckman (1976)	Rosette inhibition	26	31
Rossen (1979)	Clq binding assay	10	10
Sobel (1976)	Clq deviation	26	69
Woodroffe (1977)	Clq and Raji tests	2	0
Tung (1978)	Clq binding assay	8	13
Zayer (1978)	Raji cell assay	26	6
Abrass (1980)	Clq binding assay	52	42

Minimal change disease, a condition in which IC are not found in the renal lesions, is associated with CIC in a high proportion of the cases. These complexes contain IgG and do not bind Clq. The prevalence of CIC in membranous glomerulonephritis is highly variable. It appears that assays utilizing the Raji cells have lower sensitivity than the Clq binding assay. In other studies, the prevalence of CIC in patients with focal sclerosing and membranoproliferative glomerulonephritis has also been found to be increased.

The results of the collaborative study of the adult idiopathic nephritic syndrome are of great interest. CIC, as determined by reactivity in one or more assay techniques, were more prevalent in patients with minimal change (11/14), focal glomerular disease (13/27), and membranous glomerulopathy (26/55) as compared to control sera. Unfortunately, the presence of CIC was not specific for a particular disease category. In addition, their presence did not correlate with the clinical activity of the disease.

Recently Cairns, London, and Mallick measured levels of CIC with four different assays in a large group of adults with idiopathic glomerulonephritis and attempted to correlate the levels of CIC with the renal biopsy changes. Three groups were evaluated: 1) twenty-four patients with minimal change disease, 2) thirty-six patients with membranous glomerulopathy, and 3) sixty-two patients with mesangial hypercellularity without antecedent history of acute glomerulonephritis. Thirty patients exhibited mesangial IgM deposition, thirteen had IgA deposits and in nineteen patients no immune deposits were detected. In addition, twelve patients with Henoch-Schönlein syndrome were evaluated.

In minimal change disease, in at least one assay, 63% of the sera were positive and CIC could be found at sometime in 62.5% of patients. In the group as a whole CIC levels did not correlate with time from onset, the most recent relapse or the severity of proteinuria. Similar findings were observed in the other two groups. Only in minimal change disease did a specific pattern of CIC emerge. These patients exhibited non-Clq binding IgG complexes, an observation first made in children by Levinsky and co-workers.

Although in this study no correlation was found between the type of CIC detected and the immunoglobulin deposited in the kidney, not all CIC assays were performed in sera taken at the time of the biopsy. The authors failed to demonstrate a predominant size of CIC in five of six sera examined. They concluded that the pattern of distribution of different types of CIC does not allow different forms of glomerulonephritis to be distinguished, with the possible exception of minimal change disease, and that the overall levels of CIC do not provide useful information about the clinical activity of the disease.

Serial measurements of CIC have been used to estimate the efficacy of newly developed forms of therapy such as plasmapheresis and immunosuppression. These studies have been performed particularly in catastrophic illnesses such as idiopathic rapidly progressive glomerulonephritis and systemic lupus erythematosus associated with proliferative nephritis.

Some investigators have reported a relationship between acute transplant rejection and CIC levels; however, these results have not been confirmed in recent studies. Our own studies have documented a high incidence of CIC (45%) in patients with non-immunologic renal diseases undergoing regular hemodialysis. Thus, it appears that the level of CIC prior to transplantation and the presence of systemic infections are the most common causes of CIC positivity in renal transplant patients.

A great deal of progress has been made to establish the nature of the antigen in CIC. The immune complexes have been isolated from pathologic sera utilizing Raji cells or columns coated with Clq or conglutinin. The constituents of the complex can then be eluted and separated by electrophoretic techniques. Unfortunately, in many studies, the antigen in the immune complex has not been recognized. It is possible that extrinsic antigens may cross-react with self-proteins so that the continuing presence of the antigen in the circulation is no longer necessary to maintain disease activity. An alternative possibility is that many of the immune complexes measured are non-specific, being induced by an antigen which causes polyclonal activation of B lymphocytes with the result that rheumatoid factors and other autoantibodies are formed.

In conclusion, the diagnostic usefulness of CIC assays at the present time appears to be limited. The tests may be of value in following the activity of certain diseases and in gauging the efficacy of new treatment modalities. It is hoped that the future design of large scale clinical studies and the introduction of improved technology will lead to a better understanding of immune complex-associated diseases.

REFERENCES

Border, W.A.: Immune complex detection in glomerular diseases. Nephron 24:105-113, 1979.

Wilson, C.B., Neale, T.J., Holdsworth, S.R.: Nephritogenic immune reactions involving immune complex forms in the circulation and in situ within the kidney. Aust. NA J. Med.; 11(SUPPL 1): 88-93, 1981.

Theofilopoulos, A.N., Dixon, F.J.: Immune complexes in human diseases: A review. Am. J. Pathol. 100. a:529-94, 1980.

Couser, W.G.: What are circulating immune complexes doing in glomerulonephritis? (Editorial). N. Eng. J. Med. 304:1230-1232, 1981.

Agnello, V.: Immune complex assays: The first ten years. Ann. Intern. Med. 94:266-267, 1981.

Levinsky, R.J.: The measurement of immune complexes. Is it clinically useful? Immunology Today, May, 1981, pp. 94-97.

Theofilopoulos, A.N., Dixon, F.J.: The biology and detection of immune complexes. Adv. Immunol. 28:89, 1979.

WHO Scientific Group: The role of immune complexes in disease. Technical Series 606. WHO, Geneva, 1977.

Cairns, S.A., London, R.A., Mallick, N.P.: Circulating immune complexes in idiopathic glomerular disease. Kidney Int. 21:507-512, 1982.

Levinsky, R.J., Malleson, P.N., Barratt, T.M., et al: Circulating immune complexes in steroid responsive nephrotic syndrome. N. Engl. J. Med. 298:126-129, 1978.

Abrass, C.K., Hall, C.A., Border, W.A., et al: Circulating immune complexes in adults with idiopathic nephrotic syndrome. Kidney Int. 17:545-553, 1980.

Woodroffe, A.J., Border, W.A., Theofilopoulos, A.N., et al: Detection of circulating immune complexes in patients with glomerulonephritis. Kidney Int. 12:268-278, 1977.

ACUTE MANIFESTATIONS OF SYSTEMIC LUPUS ERYTHEMATOSUS

Melinda McVicar, M.D.

The diagnosis of systemic lupus erythematosus (SLE) rests on clinical criteria prosposed by the American Rheumatism Association. These have recently been revised to incorporate several serologic criteria and the revision (Table 1) is currently in press (1). Any four of the cited 11 manifestations in any sequence of time constitutes the diagnosis of SLE.

The majority of patients with SLE have renal involvement and approximately 30-50% have the more severe form called diffuse proliferative lupus nephritis (DPLN). It is not unusual, therefore, for the nephrologist to be entrusted with the care of patients with this multisystem disease. The acute manifestations of SLE are many and ideally there is a multidisciplinary approach to the care of these patients. Table 2 lists the acute manifestations of SLE and it can readily be appreciated that many of these manifestations are also complications of the immunosuppressive, especially steroid, therapy so frequently administered in this condition. The distinction between acute manifestations of SLE activity and complications of immunosuppressive therapy may be difficult to assess. This assessment must be made with great skill and speed since the decision to initiate or intensify immunosuppressive therapy versus discontinuation of therapy is critical. An incorrect evaluation can have devastating consequences. Baseline physical examination must be carefully performed and recorded for serial evaluation at the time of an acute manifestation. For example, moderate elevation of blood pressure is not as likely to result in an acute encephalopathy as a more rapid and severe elevation of BP. Home monitoring of BP can be an invaluable asset in distinguishing hypertensive from other encephalopathies. A superimposed intracranial bleeding episode, perhaps associated with thrombocytopenia, may result in encephalopathic findings similar to those which occur secondary to hypertension in a patient with only modest elevation of BP.

In addition, baseline and serial lab evaluation of indicators of lupus activity are very helpful in the assessment of acute manifestations. Some of these are listed in Table 3.

Table 1. Proposed revised criteria for the diagnosis of SLE

Malar rash
Photosensitive rash
Discoid lupus
Oral mucosal ulcerations
Proteinuria >.5 g/day or cellular casts
Nonerosive arthritis
Pleuritis or pericarditis
Hematologic manifestations:
hemolytic anemia
leukopenia
lymphopenia
thrombocytopenia
Seizures or psychosis
Positive FANA
Antibody to DNA or Sm antigen or LE cells or false positive STS

In this chapter, we will present a synopsis of those acute manifestations of SLE which are more commonly encountered in children. Major emphasis will be placed on the acute renal manifestations of SLE.

ACUTE RENAL MANIFESTATIONS

The acute nephritic syndrome is by far the most frequently encountered acute renal manifestation of SLE. Occasionally acute renal failure occurs. Hypertensive crises are almost invariably associated with the acute nephritic syndrome but may be a manifestation of systemic activity or steroid toxicity. Renal vein thrombosis is a rare complication which will not be discussed here.

The diagnosis of SLE should be considered in any patient who presents with the acute nephritic syndrome. The major

Table 2. Acute manifestations of systemic lupus erythematous in children and adolescents

Renal
Acute nephritic syndrome
Acute renal failure
Hypertensive crisis
Renal vein thrombosis
Cardiac
Pericarditis ± Effusion
Pericardial tamponade
Neuropsychiatric
Seizure
Organic brain syndrome
Stroke
Gastrointestinal
Intestinal perforation
Acute pancreatitis
Hematologic
Severe anemia
Severe leukopenia
Severe thrombocytopenia
Skeletal
Aseptic necrosis
Severe Infection
Acute Fulminant SLE with Multisystem Involvement

diagnostic considerations in primary and secondary forms of the acute nephritic syndrome have already been discussed in the chapter entitled Glomerulonephropathies Causing the Acute Nephritic Syndrome: Similarities and Differences, which appears elsewhere in this text. Although approximately 70% of children have renal involvement at the time of diagnosis of SLE (2), only about 5% have either acute nephritic syndrome or a rapidly progressive form of renal failure, with the majority having a more indolent course (3). Although unusual, renal disease may be the initial manifestation of SLE and antedate other clinical manifestations (4). Some patients present with or

Table 3. Baseline and serial tests for evaluation of acute manifestations of SLE.

Fluorescent Antinuclear Antibody
Anti-DNA Antibody
Complete Blood Count and Differential
Platelet Count
Serum Complement
Urinalysis
Serum Creatinine
C-Reactive Protein
Sedimentation Rate

develop a rapidly progressive glomerulonephritis, sometimes followed or accompanied by fulminant manifestations of SLE. This clinical syndrome is usually associated with a crescentic form of glomerulonephritis and intracapillary glomerular thrombi may be prominent (5).

The diffuse proliferative form of lupus nephritis is the most serious renal manifestation, though it does not always present as an acute manifestation. Prompt and aggressive therapy appears to be beneficial in this form of nephritis. Although knowledge of the pathogenesis, histology, natural history and therapy of systemic lupus erythematosus has increased significantly over the past decade, it seems that it is nevertheless difficult to find consensus about what constitutes optimum therapy. Similarly, the classification of renal involvement in SLE has undergone revisions. No sooner has the World Health Organization established a histologic classification of renal involvement in SLE than two distinguished groups offer modifications of that classification (Table 4). It becomes immediately clear that variation in classification will affect data concerning outcome of therapy, particularly for the more severe lesion which has been termed diffuse proliferative lupus nephritis.
is extremely variable and it may mimic other renal diseases. The pattern varies between patients and, not infrequently, the lesion varies from one glomerulus to another in the same patient. In addition, it is now well recognized that the lesion is not static and that there is evolution from one classification to another in approximately 20% of patients (6). It has

Table 4. Histology of lupus nephritis. Modified WHO classifications

A. Light microscopy[1]

I. Normal or minimal
II. Pure mesangial alteration
III. Focal segmental glomerulonephritis
IV. Diffuse glomerulonephritis
V. Diffuse membranous glomerulonephritis
VI. Advanced sclerosing glomerulonephritis
Difficult to classify by light microscopy

B. Light microscopy, immunofluorescence and electron microscopy[2]

		LM		IF		EM		
	Patterns +‡	Mes.	PCW	Mes.	PCW	Mes.	SEn	SEp
I.	Normal	0	0	0	0	0	0	0
IIA.	Mes. Deps.	0	0	+	0	+	0	0
IIB.	Mes. Glom.	+	0	+	0	+	0	0
III.	Focal-Segm. GN	+	+ (< 50%)	++	+	++	+	±
IV.	Diffuse GN	++	++ (> 50%)	++	++	++	++	±
V.	Membr. GN	+	++	+	++	+	±	++

* Modified from Finlander, P., Koss, M., Kitridou, R. and Border, W.A.: Glomerulonephritis in systemic lupus erythematosus. Amer. J. Nephrology 1:53-67, 1981.

\+ For patterns III and IV, qualify if active or inactive.

‡ In mixed forms, indicate which patterns are present.

1. Grishman, E., Gerber, M.A., Churg, J.: Patterns of renal injury in systemic lupus erythematosus: Light and immunofluorescence microscopic observations. Am. J. Kid. Dis. 11:135, 1982 (Suppl).

2. Pirani, C.L., Olesnicky, L.: Role of electronmicroscopy in the classification of lupus nephritis. Am. J. Kid. Dis. 11:150, 1982 (Suppl).

recently been emphasized that intraglomerular thrombi are an important histologic finding which is predictive of further glomerulosclerosis on subsequent renal biopsies (7). Similarly, subendothelial deposits, long known to be associated with progressive renal insufficiency, are also predictive of further glomerulosclerosis (7). Immunofluorescent findings of several immunoglobulins and complement components in lupus nephropathy are typical. The most characteristic of these is the finding of IgA as a prominent feature. Electronmicroscopic findings include the presence of discrete electron dense subendothelial deposits which in DPLN are quite numerous and often confluent forming "wire loop" lesions.

A recent modification of the criteria for diagnosis of SLE in patients with DPLN has been proposed by Lewis and his group (8). The modification allowed a diagnosis of all patients with DPLN thought to have lupus in which the overall clinical criteria were incomplete. They followed a series of 26 out of 38 patients in which the traditional criteria did not allow the diagnosis of SLE. By utilizing the modification which added to the criteria the presence of a low C_4 and a positive band test in the skin, 37 of the 38 patients (97%) met at least 4 criteria and all of the patients did so within 6 months of biopsy. They suggested that the traditional criteria have not dealt adequately with SLE as a renal disease and appear inadequate for patients with DPLN.

Ever since the early 1960's when Pollack and his associates (9) reported the marked differences in outcome between patients with DPLN treated with high versus low steroids, treatment with large doses of adrenocortico-steroids has become the main stay of therapy in this form of nephropathy. Since then, there have been many uncontrolled studies and a few controlled suggesting that the addition of azathioprine, cyclophosphamide, or other immunosuppressive agents to steroids, induced remission of active lesions either more rapidly or more completely than with steroids alone (10,11,12,13). However, there have been an almost equal number of reports suggesting that the addition of these cytotoxic agents to steroids was of little or no value (14,15,16). In the search for better modes of treatment for this devastating disease it has become popular to treat DPLN with high dose intravenous methylprednisolone and favorable outcomes have been reported by several authors. Among these, probably the most impressive is that of Kimberly et al. (17). In this series, an improvement of renal function was obtained in twelve patients given pulse therapy with methylprednisolone. However, there was virtually no improvement in an additional 22 patients treated in the same fashion. In what is probably the largest pediatric group treated with pulse therapy to date, Barron et al. (18) treated 22 children with DPLN. Fifteen were treated with prednisone p.o. 2 mg/kg/day and seven patients with similar renal pathology were treated with daily pulses of methylprednisolone 30 mg/kg/day not exceeding 1 gm/day and followed by prednisone orally at 2 mg/kg/day. The two groups had comparable side effects and there were no deaths in either group. Although there was a more rapid improvement in GFR in the pulse therapy group, the long term effects were no different between the two groups over a mean follow-up period of 59 months.

There have been many reports of the results of plasma exchange on the course of DPLN. Several authors have suggested impressive improvement in clinical outcome (19,20,21). In what is probably the only randomized trial of plasma exchange for systemic lupus erythematosus there was no difference between 9 patients treated by plasma exchange and 9 other patients treated by a sham procedure with respect to the frequency and degree of clinical improvement. All the patients had mildly active systemic lupus erythematosus with GFR's greater than 20 cc per minute and were not segregated according to the diagnosis of DPLN (22). Although one cannot extrapolate from this study to patients with DPLN, it appears that there is still no clear evidence that any mode of therapy thus far evaluated, with the possible exception of high dose adreno-corticosteroids, is definitely beneficial for patients with DPLN. Hence, the outlook for these patients continues to be dismal with a poor long and short-term prognosis. In a recent publication by the Lupus Nephritis Collaborative Study Group (23), data were collected from 12 participating centers on the outcome of patients with severe DPLN treated with various pharmacologic regimens during one calendar year following biopsy. Among 44 patients with a mean serum creatinine of 2.4 mg/dl and urinary protein of 3.9 gm/day, 7 died and 4 went into end stage kidney disease within the initial year, and 12 increased their serum creatinine by more than 40%. Crude mortality rates for those with creatinine less than 1.2 mg/dl was 21.5%, for those with creatinine 1.3 mg/dl,21%,and for creatinine greater than 2 mg/dl,36%. The authors concluded that the renal biopsy finding of DPLN in SLE continues to identify a group with poor prognosis irrespective of the serum creatinine at the time of biopsy. The highest mortality or end stage renal disease rate was among those with initial serum creatinine greater than 2 mg/dl.

Hence, it seems clear that this lesion continues to identify patients with the potential for a grave prognosis. It also continues to be difficult to evaluate and identify therapeutic maneuvers which are beneficial. In marked contrast to the experience cited above, Platt et al. (2) followed patients in the first 2 decades of life during the years 1974 through 1981 and reported a five year survival in patients with DPLN (21 patients) which was similar to that of the total group. However, the prognosis was poor at the end of seven years, indicating that analysis of outcome will probably require long term follow-up. Some authors have made an argument for renal biopsy in SLE even in the absence of clinical renal manifestations (23A).

ACUTE RENAL FAILURE

Sometimes patients with SLE present with acute renal failure and are assumed to have DPLN warranting aggressive immunosuppressive therapy. A biopsy may in some instances be omitted because frequently these patients are acutely ill and it is presumed that the acute renal failure is secondary to a diffuse proliferative lesion. However, we have seen a 13 year old girl who presented with acute renal failure and virtual anuria over a period of three weeks. Our presumptive diagnosis had been DPLN. When a biopsy was performed, however, the child had membranous nephropathy associated with some areas of necrosis and tubular regeneration. Hence, her renal failure was caused by an acute tubular necrosis and not by the membranous lesion. Recently, Cohen et al (24) have reported six similar adult patients who presented with acute renal failure. Five of the patients received pulse methylprednisolone and/or cyclophosphamide and/or plasma exhange before other causes of acute renal failure were considered. A subsequent renal biopsy showed that the patients actually had mesangial lupus nephritis associated with acute tubular necrosis, rather than DPLN. These authors pointed out that a biopsy must be done prior to therapy for a presumed DPLN in order to avoid unnecessary aggressive therapy. One of their patients in fact died of opportunistic infection probably related to the aggressive treatment. Also of interest was the fact that the acute renal failure in four of the patients was related to non-steroidal anti-inflammatory drugs. Two had been treated with Ibuprofen and two had been treated with Naprosyn. This serves as a reminder that pre-existing renal disease is one of the predisposing factors in acute renal failure, and may potentiate the effects of drugs which may cause acute renal failure, such as the non-steroidal anti-inflammatory drugs. Awareness of these possibilities is helpful in treating the arthritis which so often is present in patients with SLE.

INFECTIONS

Infections associated with SLE and also as complications of intensive immunosuppressive therapy are an ever present threat to the patient. Fever may be a particularly difficult sign to interpret. As many as 80% of the patients who are initially diagnosed with SLE present with fever, and fever is frequently associated with exacerbations in the course of the disease (25). Recurrent infections are also quite common in SLE and have been the major cause of death in this disease. Wallace et al (26) reported 10 bacterial or fungal infections in 45 children with SLE. Platt et al (2) noted 55 episodes of infection in 70 children with SLE. Infections were the cause of death in 9 of 11 children in this study of SLE in the first two decades of life.

Proper diagnosis and management of such infections are among the most challenging circumstances in medical practice. A recent finding which may be helpful to the clinician is the confirmation by Honig et al (27) of the observation initially made by Hill in 1951 (28) that in 4 patients with active SLE there was no detectable increase in C-reactive protein (CRP). Others (29), however, did not find very good correlation of infection with CRP elevations. A simple semi-qualitative precipitant capillary tube test for CRP was used by Bravo, et al (30) who found that all but three of 50 sera which were taken at the time of infections were positive for CRP, whereas 80 of 115 sera taken at the time of SLE activity without infection were negative for CRP. They suggested that the high correlation of positive CRP with infection in their study and the discrepancy with other studies may be because of the use of more sensitive radioimmunodiffusion methods by other authors. They also point out that others (31) have shown that rheumatoid factor can interfere with the detection of CRP. At the present time, it is uncertain whether the test is as reliable with viral and fungal infections as it appears to be with bacterial infections. Becker et al (32) have found significant differences using statistical analysis of CRP levels derived by electroimmunoassay which demonstrate higher levels in patients with proven infections, thus confirming this finding even with a more sensitive measurement of CRP. These authors found that none of the patients in the active SLE group exceeded CRP of 16 mg/l. They found that the severity of infection tended to correlate with the level of CRP.

It seems that the greatest value of CRP determination would be in serial determinations in an individual patient. It appears than an elevation above baseline levels may provide early warning of occult infection and may facilitate interpretation of findings when patients become acutely ill with fever and the differential diagnosis between active SLE and infection is difficult. The non-specific nature of the CRP response must always be borne in mind when utilizing it as an aide to diagnosis of infection. Extensive tissue necrosis which may be a result of SLE activity and drug reactions, particularly those in which fever and rash occur, are two important examples of situations in which CRP may be elevated without infection.

Treatment of infections in SLE must be prompt with careful choice of antibiotics and consideration of whether it is appropriate to reduce immunosuppressive therapy. Adrenocorticosteroids are needed in "stress" doses if adrenal suppression is present. It is our custom to utilize infectious disease consultation in all but the simplest problems because it sometimes becomes necessary to utilize the extensive armamentarium of newly developed and experimental drugs.

ACUTE CARDIAC MANIFESTATIONS

Pericarditis is the most common cardiac manifestation of SLE. The incidence in various series ranges from about 20-30% of all patients at some time during their disease. A typical presentation is with substernal pain, usually aggravated with motion and sometimes respirations. Pericardial friction rub may be heard, although it does not necessarily correlate with the symptoms of pericarditis (33). Electrocardiograms are usually abnormal, showing ST-segment and T-wave abnormalities. The most sensitive and simple method for confirming the presence of pericardial fluid is by echocardiography. Studies performed in patients whether or not they were symptomatic have shown that up to two-thirds of patients with active SLE have evidence of pericardial effusions by echocardiography (34).

Pericardial tamponade, an acute emergency, has been reported with SLE, but fortunately is rare. Among 159 cases of lupus pericarditis reported by DuBois (33) there were no cases of tamponade.

There is no standardization of therapy for lupus pericarditis. Non-steroidal anti-inflammatory drugs as well as prednisone in varying doses have been used but not adequately evaluated. DuBois (33) has suggested parenteral hydrocortisone in doses of 1 gram or more.

ACUTE PULMONARY MANIFESTATIONS

Among the various pulmonary manifestations of SLE, acute pneumonitis and pulmonary hemorrhage are the most serious. Matthay (35) found 12 cases of acute pneumonitis among 102 hospitalized patients with SLE after exclusion of those with infections or chronic pulmonary manifestations. Dyspnea was the major complaint in almost all of these patients. About half had pleuritic chest pain. Fever and pulmonary crepitations were found in all. In six of the patients the pneumonitis was the presenting finding for SLE. Aggressive therapy was utilized with a mortality of 50%.

Pulmonary Hemorrhage

The nephrologist who encounters the association of massive pulmonary hemorrhage and glomerulonephritis will think immediately of Goodpasture's Syndrome. Patients with SLE may have a very similar presentation (36). Aggressive immunosuppressive therapy is indicated for both conditions. The diagnosis of pulmonary hemorrhage may be difficult to make, but sputum which is filled with macrophages containing iron may be very helpful. It has been speculated that the pulmonary hemorrhage occurs secondary to damage to the pulmonary capillaries by immune complexes which have been demonstrated in autopsy studies along with electron dense deposits in the alveolar septae and vessel walls. It is likely, however, that other mechanisms are involved. In antiglomerular basement membrane antibody nephritis, intercurrent infection has been shown to precipitate episodes of pulmonary hemorrhage despite stable levels of antiglomerular basement membrane antibodies (37). There are no clear guidelines for treatment of pulmonary hemorrhage. Symptomatic relief with administration of oxygen and blood transfusions is helpful. It is not clear whether dialysis can relieve the pulmonary edema, and the role of aggressive immunosuppressive therapy is unknown.

Acute Pneumonitis

Most patients with acute pneumonitis present with dyspnea, fever and basal rales which is frequently accompanied by pleuritic chest pain. Radiologic chest findings are generally diffuse and associated with pleural effusions. Mortality and residual pulmonary defects are common despite aggressive therapy. The characteristic histologic finding is lymphocytic and plasma cell infiltration. In one series, acute pneumonitis was the presenting complaint in 6 of 102 patients hospitalized with SLE (35).

ACUTE CENTRAL NERVOUS SYSTEM MANIFESTATIONS OF SLE

In one of the largest studies of SLE in the first two decades of life, Platt et al. (2) reported 21 out of 70 patients (30%) with evidence of central nervous system involvement after exclusion of those patients who merely had headaches, uncomplicated depression, amenorrhea due to hypothalamic insufficiency, or abnormal EEG's (all of which might be classified as having CNS manifestations of SLE). In their series, the most common manifestation of CNS lupus was psychosis or depression, followed by chorea, cranial nerve involvement, and seizures. Among the 45 patients with childhood lupus, studies by Wallace, et al (26), 49% were found to have neurological manifestations. The neurologic manifestations generally did not differ from those found in adults. Seizures, psychosis, cerebral dysfunction, strokes, chorea and neuropathies are relatively common CNS manifestations in adults. Electroencephalograms are frequently abnormal and may be abnormal when clinical neurologic manifestations are absent.

The psychiatric manifestations in SLE are difficult to evaluate particularly in adolescents who are emotionally labile and may be thought to have reactive symptoms associated with chronic illness. Most reports in the literature do not distinguish between functional and organic psychiatric disorders. In addition, the potential of corticosteroids for producing psychosis adds further to the difficulty in making this diagnosis in patients who are treated with high doses. It seems that the psychiatric manifestations appear more commonly than organic neurologic features which might be confused with psychosis. A reasonable classification of psychiatric disorders in SLE has been proposed by Bresnihan and associates (38). These authors separated out an acute brain syndrome either with or without psychosis, a chronic brain syndrome, and an organic depressive disorder. We will consider here only the acute brain syndrome since it is the one most commonly encountered. It has arbitrarily been defined as a cognitive impairment which is characterized by memory and attention deficit without disorientation and which persists for less than a month. When they co-exist with psychosis, there are delusions or hallucinations.

The contribution of corticosteroids to psychiatric manifestations is difficult to assess. In one series, 9 of 28 patients on high dose corticosteroids developed psychosis with reversal when the dose was reduced in six of the patients (39).

On the other hand, Gurland and associates and Baker and colleagues (40,41) concluded that the onset of psychiatric manifestations was rare after an increase in corticosteroid dose. It has been our practice to increase the dose of steroids in acute psychosis to maximum therapeutic levels, on occasion using pulse methylprednisolone therapy. If the manifestations do not subside or improve over several days in a patient who has received high enough doses of steroids to make steroid induced CNS toxicity a possibility, the dose is then diminished. Hypertensive encephalopathy, CNS infection or hemorrhage and extreme uremia are other causes of CNS manifestations in SLE which must be seriously considered. Cerebral spinal fluid findings in acute brain syndrome are usually non-specific and CSF pressures are usually normal (42). In one study (43), elevation of the CSF cell count was found in six of eight specimens in which organic neurologic disease was present. In contrast, all 11 specimens obtained during psychiatric disease alone were negative. In a few cases neurologic and psychiatric disease may co-exist. These authors were further able to distinguish psychiatric disorders from neurologic disease because of elevated CSF cyclic GMP in the patients with neurologic manifestations. Elevated CSF protein values have been an inconstant finding, as has been the finding of immune complexes in CSF during CNS disease. Several authors have reported lowering of the CSF C_4 levels in association with active CNS lupus (44,45). More recently, however, doubt has been cast on the value of this finding (46).

The results of computed cranial tomography were shown in at least one series to correlate well with central nervous system disease. This finding corresponds well with our experience. The most common finding in CNS lupus was cortical atrophy with or without ventricular enlargement, while infarction and hemorrhage were found less frequently (47). Figure 1A demonstrates an area of intracranial hemorrhage in the left frontal lobe in one of our patients with SLE who developed an acute organic brain syndrome. In another section (Fig. 1B) cortical atrophy which had been noted in previous studies was obscured because of brain edema. In the following study, one month later, cortical atrophy is apparent with dilated ventricles and prominence of the sulci, particularly the Sylvian fissures. As seen in this case, cortical atrophy may be masked by edema during an acute CNS problem.

The treatment of CNS lupus is difficult, and rests principally on symptomatic measures. In addition to anti-convulsive medication for seizures, increased doses of corticosteroid therapy and appropriate sedation and anti-depressive therapy are used for the milder psychological or depressive disturbances. We attempt to have a psychiatrist and psychiatric social worker follow each of these patients during periods of remission as well as during acute exacerbations. The less stressful contact during more stable periods enhances their effectiveness in crisis intervention. As mentioned earlier, high doses of steroids, sometimes given as intravenous pulse therapy, are the mainstay of therapy for severe neurologic manifestations or acute organic psychosis with or without

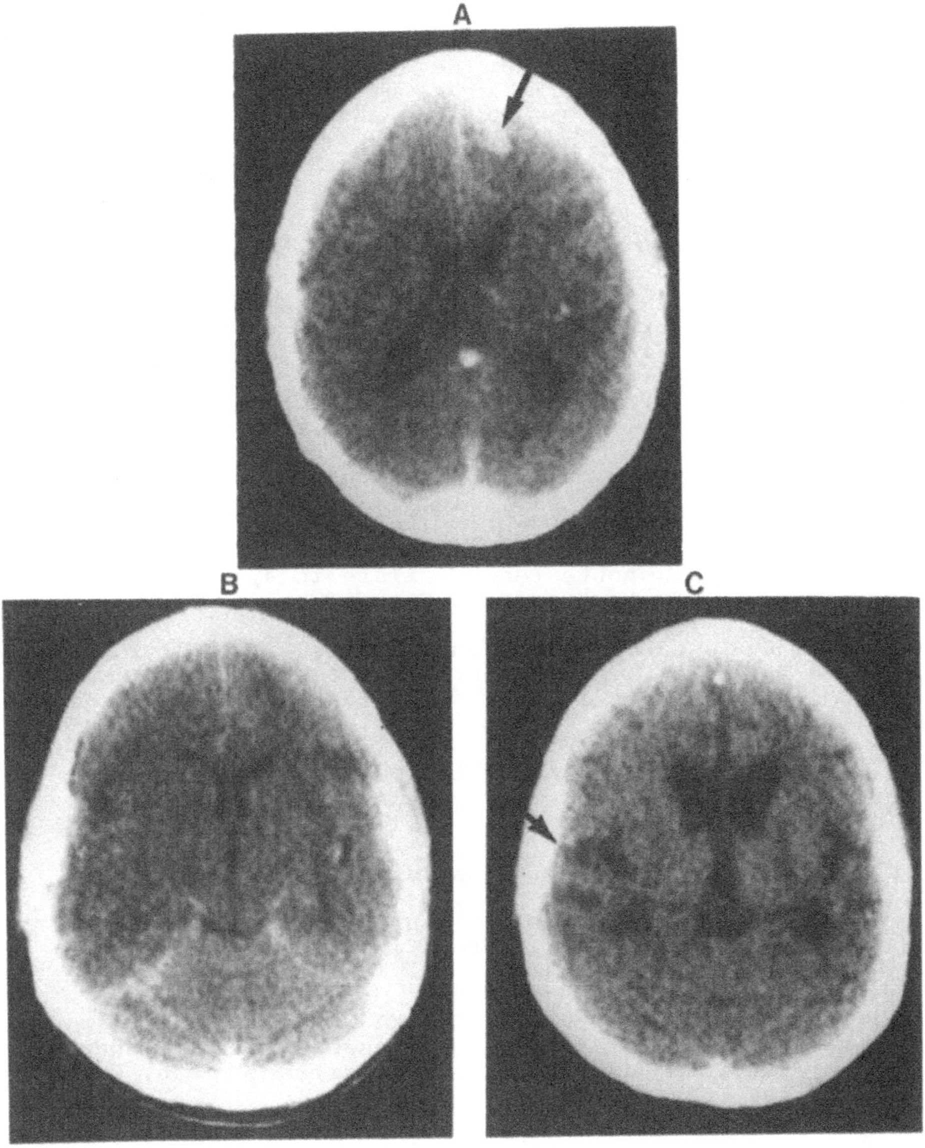

Figure 1

A Area of intracranial hemorrhage in the left frontal lobe.

B Cortical atrophy obscured by brain edema.

C Same view as 1B one month later showing cortical atrophy. The ventricles are dilated and the sulci are prominent, especially the Sylvian fissures (arrow).

convulsions. Other conditions which usually require high doses of steroids are stroke, transverse myelitis, or deteriorating consciousness which is not related to infection. Every effort must be made to rule out the presence of infection prior to initiating high dose steroid therapy.

REFERENCES

1. Rothfield, N.F.:DM Disease a Month: 29:46,1982 (Oct).

2. Platt, J.L., Burke, B.A., Fish, A.J., Kim, Y., & Michael, A.F.:Systemic Lupus Erythematosus in the First Two Decades of Life. Am. J. of Kid. Dis. Suppl.11:212,1982.

3. Estes, D. & Christian, C.: The natural history of SLE by prospective analysis. Medicine 50:85,1971.

4. Adu, D., and Cameron, J.S.: Lupus Nephritis. Clinics in Rheumatic Diseases 8:153,1982 (April).

5. Ponticelli, C., Imbasciati, E., Brancaccio, D., Tarantino, A., & Rivolta, E.: Acute renal failure in systemic lupus erythematosus. British Medical Journal iii:716,1974.

6. Baldwin, D.S., Gluck, M.C., Lowenstein, J., & Gallo, G.R.: Lupus nephritis. Clinical course as related to morphologic forms and their transitions. American Journal of Medicine 62:12,1977.

7. Pollak, V.E., & Dosekun,A.K.: Evaluation of treatment in Lupus Nephritis: Effects of Prednisone. Am. J. of Kid. Dis. Suppl. 11:170,1982.

8. Pohl, M.A., Krakauer, R., Gephardt, G., Hunsicker, L., Roberts, J.L., Schwartz, M.M., & Lewis, E.J.: Modified Criteria for the Diagnosis of Systemic Lupus Erythematosus in the Presence of Diffuse Proliferative Nephritis. Kid. Internat. 23:131,1983.

9. Pollak, V.E., Pirani, C.L., & Kark, R.M.: Effect of Large Doses of Prednisone on the Renal Lesions and Life Span of Patients with Lupus Glomerulonephritis. J. Lab. Clin. Med. 57:495,1961.

10. Hayslett, J.P., Kashgarian, M., & Cook, C.D., et al: The effect of azathioprine on lupus glomerulonephritis. Medicine 51:393,1972.

11. Shelp, W.D., Bloodworth, J.M.B., Jr., & Rieselbach, R.E.: Effect of azathioprine on renal histology and function in lupus nephritis. Arch. Intern. Med. 128:566,1971.

12. Decker, J.L., Steinberg, A.D., & Reinertsen, J.L., et al: Systemic lupus erythematosus: Evolving concepts. Ann. Intern. Med. 91:587,1979.

13. Donadio, J.V., Jr., Holley, K.E. & Ferguson, R.H., et al: Treatment of diffuse proliferative lupus nephritis with prednisone and combined prednisone and cyclophosphamide. N. Engl. J. Med. 299:1151,1978.

14. Donadio, J.V., Jr., Holley, K.E., & Wagoner, R.D., et al: Treatment of lupus nephritis with prednisone and combined prednisone and azathioprine. Ann. Intern. Med. 77:829, 1972.

15. Hahn, B.H., Kantor, O.S., & Osterland, C.K.: Azathioprine plus prednisone compared with prednisone alone in the treatment of systemic lupus erythematosus: Report of a prospective controlled trial in 24 patients. Ann. Intern. Med. 83:597, 1975.

16. Donadio, J.V., Jr., Holley, K.E., & Ilstrup, D.M.: Adrenocorticoid and cytotoxic drug treatment of lupus nephropathy. Proceedings of the 8th International Congress of Nephrology, Athens,Greece, pp. 643, 1981.

17. Kimberly, R.P., Lockshin, M.D., & Sherman, R.L., et al: High-dose intravenous methylprednisolone pulse therapy in systemic lupus erythematosus. Am. J. Med. 70:817, 1981.

18. Barron, KS, Person, DA, Brewer, EJ,Jr., Beale, MG, Robson, AM: Pulse methylprednisolone therapy in diffuse proliferative lupus nephritis. J. Pediatr. 101:137, 1982.

19. Jones, J.V., Cumming, R.H., & Bacon, P.A., et al: Evidence for a therapeutic effect of plasmapheresis in patients with systemic lupus erythematosus. Q.J. Med. 48:555, 1979.

20. Lockwood, C.M., Worlledge, S. & Nicholas, A., et al: Reversal of impaired splenic functions in patients with nephritis or vasculitis (or both) by plasma exchange. N.Engl. J. Med. 300:524, 1979.

21. Jones, J.V., Robinson, M.F. & Parciany, R.K., et al: Therapeutic plasmapheresis in systemic lupus erythematosus: Effect on immune complexes and antibodies to DNA. Arth. Rheum. 24:1113, 1981.

22. Wei,N, Huston, DP, Lawley, PJ, Steinberg, AD, Klippel, JH, Hall, RP, Balow, JE, Decker, JL: Randomized trial of plasma exchange in mild systemic lupus erythematosus. Lancet 1:17, 1983.

23. The Lupus Nephritis Study Group. Short-term Prognosis in Severe Lupus Nephritis. Kidney Internat. 23:129, 1983.

23A. Leehey, D.J., Katz, A.I., Azaran, A.H., Aronson, A.J. & Spargo, B.H.: Silent diffuse lupus nephritis: Long-term follow-up. Am. J. Kidney Dis. Vol. 11, No. 1 Suppl. 1, July 1982.

24. Cohen, A.H., Wang, H., Border, W.A., & Glassock, R.J.: Acute renal failure due to acute tubular necrosis in lupus nephritis. Kidney Internat. 23:119, 1983.

25. Dubois, E.L., & Tuffanelli, D.L.: Clinical Manifestations of Systemic Lupus Erythematosus. JAMA 190:104,1964.

26. Wallace, C., Schaller, J.G., Emery, H.M., & Wedgwood, R.: Prospective Study of Childhood Systemic Lupus Erythematosus (SLE). Arth. and Rheum. 21:599,1978.

27. Honig, S., Gorevic, P. & Weissman, G.: C-reactive protein in systemic lupus erythematosus. Arth. and Rheum. 20:1065,1977.

28. Hill, A.G.S.: C-reactive protein in chronic rheumatic diseases. Lancet 1:807,1951.

29. Zein, N., Ganuza, C. & Koshner, I.: Significance of serum C-reactive protein elevation in patients with systemic lupus erythematosus. Arthritis and Rheum. 22:7,1979.

30. Bravo, M.G., & Alarcon-Segovia, D.: C-reactive protein in the differential diagnosis between infection and disease reactivation in SLE. J. Rheum. 8:291,1981.

31. Deyo, R.A., Pope, R.M., & Persellin, R.H.: Interference by rheumatoid factor with the detection of C-reactive protein by the latex agglutination method. J. Rheum. 7:279,1980.

32. Becker, G.J., Waldburger, M., Hughes, G.R.V., & Pepys, M.B.: Value of serum C-reactive protein measurement in the investigation of fever in systemic lupus erythematosus. Ann. of Rheum. Dis. 39:50,1980.

33. Dubois, E.L.: The clinical picture of systemic lupus erythematosus. In Lupus Erythematosus: A Review of of the Current Status of Discoid and Systemic Lupus Erythematosus and Their Variants (Ed.) Dubois, E.L. Los Angeles: U. California Press, 1974, pp. 265,402.

34. Davis, P., Atkins, B., Josse, R.G., & Hughes, G.R.V.: Criteria for classification of SLE. British Medical Journal. iii,88,1973.

35. Matthay, R.A., Schwarz, M.I., Petty, T.L., Stanford, R.E., Gupta, R.C., Sahn, S.A., & Steigerwald, J.C.: Pulmonary manifestations of systemic lupus erythematosus: a reveiw of 12 cases of acute pneumonitis. Medicine. 54:397, 1975.

36. Rajani, K.B., Ashbacher, L.V., & Kinney, T.R.: Pulmonary haemorrhage in systemic lupus erythematosus. Journal of Paediatrics. 98:810,1978.

37. Rees, A.J., Lockwood, C.M., & Peters, D.K.: Enhanced allergic tissue injury in Goodpasture's syndrome by intercurrent bacterial infection. British Medical Journal, ii,723,1977.

38. Bresnihan, B., Hohmeister, R., Cutting, J., Travers, R.L., Waldburger, M., Black, C., Jones, T., & Hughes, G.R.V.: The neuropsychiatric disorder in systemic lupus erythematosus: evidence for both vascular and immune mechanisms. Annals of the Rheumatic Diseases. 38:301,1979a.

39. Cade, R., Spooner, G., Schlein, E., Pickering, M., deQuisada, A., Holcomb, A., Juncos, L., Richard, G., Shires, D., Levin, D., Hackett, R., Free, J., Hunt, R., & Fregly, M.: Comparison of azathioprine,prednisone, and heparin alone or combined in treating lupus nephritis. Nephron. 16:37,1973.

40. Gurland, B.J., Ganz, V.H., Fleiss, J.L., & Zubin J.: The study of the psychiatric symptoms of systemic lupus erythematosus. Psychosomatic Medicine. 34:199,1972.

41. Baker, M., Hadler, N., Whitaker, J.N., Dunner, D.L., Gerwin, R.D., & Decker, J.L.: Psychopathology in systemic lupus erythematosus: II Relation to clinical observations, corticosteroid administration and cerebrospinal fluid C4. Seminars in Arthritis and Rheumatism. 3:111,1973.

42. Abel, T., Gladman, D.D., & Urowitz, M.B.: Neuropsychiatric lupus. Journal of Rheumatology. 7:325,1980.

43. Kassan, S.S. & Kagen, L.J.: Central nervous system lupus erythematosus. Measurement of cerebrospinal fluid cyclic GMP and other clinical markers of disease activity. Arthritis and Rheumatism. 22:449,1979.

44. Hadler, N.M., Gerwin, R.D., Frank, M.M., Whitaker, J.N. Baker, M., & Decker, J.: Fourth component of complement in the cerebrospinal fluid in systemic lupus erythematosus. Arhtritis and Rheumatism. 16:507,1973.

45. Petz, L.D., Sharp, G.C., Cooper, N.R., & Irwin, W.S.: Serum and cerebrospinal fluid complement and serum autoantibodies in systemic lupus erythematosus. Medicine. 50:259,1971.

46. Lockshin, M.: Personal communication.

47. Gonzalez-Scarano, F., Lisak, R.P., Bilaniuk, L.T., Zimmerman, R.A., Atkins, P.C., & Zweiman, B.: Cranial computed tomography in the diagnosis of systemic lupus erythematosus. Annals of Neurology. 15:158,1979.

RENAL IMAGING IN ACUTE RENAL DISORDERS - RENAL EMERGENCIES

G. N. Sfakianakis, M.D.

OVERVIEW

Under this topic one can classify a great variety of renal disorders which have as a common characteristic their acute onset. History, patient examination and laboratory data usually establish or indicate the diagnosis and imaging is applied to rule out correctable pathology and probably help in the specific diagnosis. A functional imaging study may also serve as a baseline for future reference.

The procedures to visualize kidneys are First Line examinations (non-invasive) and Second Line (invasive).

The first group includes Urography (IVP), Ultrasonography (US), Scintigraphy (Radioisotope or Radionuclide studies) and Computerized Tomography (CT). Arteriography, Venography, Retrograde Pyelography and Percutaneous Antegrade Pyelography are invasive procedures and they carry varying degress of morbidity.

Excretory Urography (IVP) may identify obstruction, trauma or other cause of renal disease. The quality of the study depends on the degree of renal insufficiency present. Urographic assessment of the kidney in renal failure has limited use and it has been replaced by US, scintigraphy or CT. Furthermore, in many disorders the results are nonspecific. Immaturity of the kidney in the neonate poses another limitation. There is risk from the contrast media and significant radiation exposure (1).

Ultransonography is independent of renal function and assesses renal size, provides information about renal parenchyma and detects hydronephrosis and cysts, even in the presence of severe renal insufficiency. It does not obtain physiologic information and it is not specific for parenchymal and collecting system disorders. It is well tolerated and carries no risks.

Scintigraphy provides structural and functional information. It is successful with advanced renal insufficiency (BUN above 100 mg/dl), easily identifies location and size of kidneys, hydronephrosis and, usually level of obstruction; it can separate cysts from hydronephrosis, acute from chronic disease. It can detect trauma and, nonspecifically, space occupying lesions. It provides images of the cortex and of the collecting system (Tc-99m-Glucoheptonate and Tc-99m-

DMSA). With the different radiopharmaceuticals available for renal scintigraphy and the dynamic approach, Blood Flow, GFR, ERPF and Filtration Fraction can be studied. The information can be quantitated for GFR (Tc-99m-DTPA) and ERPF (I-131 Hippurate) and semiquantitated for Blood Flow. It can, reportedly, separate ATN from cortical necrosis, hepatorenal syndrome, renal vein thrombosis and renal artery stenosis and occlusion. There is no evidence, however, that scintigraphy can make the specific diagnosis of the nephrotic or the nephritic syndromes, although it may help with the diagnostic work-up and assess effect of treatment. Infection and interstitial nephritis give focal and diffused patterns of hyperactivity, respectively, on Gallium-67 scintigraphy. Scintigraphy is well tolerated and delivers less radiation to the patient than Urography and CT.

Computed tomography (CT) provides the structural information of US and the functional of IVP but it carries the risks of the latter method. Availability and cost, and lack of specificity for many disorders, limit the application of CT. Lack of retroperitoneal fat limits the resolution in many children.

Comparative studies, in general, favor scintigraphy over urography and underline the complementary role of scintigraphy and ultrasonography (23). Further experience with specific radiopharmaceuticals and the application of scintigraphic tomography may increase the usefulness of this approach. Tissue characterization with US or CT, Digital Subtraction Radiography and Nuclear Magnetic Resonance are under current investigation.

It is the experience at our institution that scintigraphy is very successful as the first approach in patients with acute renal disorders or renal emergencies, when structural and functional information is needed to complement the clinical and laboratory investigation.

IMAGING PROCEDURES IN ACUTE RENAL DISORDERS

Excretory Urography (IVP)

The help we may expect from the different imaging procedures in the evaluation of patients who have acute renal disease is weighed against the risks. IVP may identify obstruction, may show if there is a trauma or other cause of renal disease, but lacks the specificity for many parenchymal diseases and the quality of the study depends upon the degree of renal insufficiency. If renal insufficiency is present, IVP should not be performed because the expected usefulness is not worth the radiation exposure nor the danger of damage from contrast media reaction. In case, however, an IVP is done, nephrotomography may be required and may be helpful. The patient need not be dehydrated but bowel cleansing is needed if possible. Also delayed films after 24 hours are useful and should be performed. In renal insufficiency, IVP has been replaced by scintigraphy and ultrasonography because of lack of success, radiation and contrast media reactions (4). In the neonate and the young infant, immaturity ofthe kidney is another limitation for IVP, particularly when renal insufficiency has been superimposed.

Ultrasonography (US)

Since US is independent of function and is entirely non-invasive it is useful in the study of acute renal disease. It does not provide, however, functional information; this is a limitation of the method. It can assess renal size, but has difficulty in finding an ectopic kidney. It separates the renal parenchyma from the collecting system and may be diagnostic of cystic disease. It detects hydronephrosis but is not useful in differentiating obstruction from hydronephrosis of other etiology or residual hydronephrosis after obstruction has been corrected surgically. It is not always possible for US to indicate the level of obstruction; it can detect and characterize cysts (multicystic kidney, polycystic kidney disease - adult and infantile type , and other cystic diseases). In cases of advanced hydronephrosis in ureteropelvic junction obstruction or even in distal ureteric obstruction, ultrasonography separates a multicystic kidney from obstructive uropathy. Finally, US is not helpful in renal trauma (because it does not detect extravasations) or in renal vascular diseases. Despite its limitations, ultrasonography is a non-invasive procedure easily performed and readily available and many times provides valuable information if applied when indicated.

Nuclear Scintigraphy (Radionuclide studies)

Nuclear scintigraphy in acute renal disease has no risks except for the radiation exposure, which is in the range of the IVP or lower. It provides structural and functional information (5). It is successful with advanced renal insufficiency (BUN > 100 mg/dl and serum creatinine > 10 mg/dl). It provides information about the existence, location, function, anatomy of the kidneys, and is helpful in separating acute from chronic renal insufficiency. Scintigraphy can diagnose hydronephrosis but also shows obstruction and it can detect the level of the obstruction. It may diagnose cystic disease and differentiate it from advanced hydronephrosis. It can be helpful in the diagnosis of renal parenchymal disease if there is a thorough and careful use of the information derived from flow studies, GFR (DTPA), effective renal plasma flow (ERPF, Hippuran), image and quantitation. The individual function of each kidney separately can easily be determined using any renal radiopharmaceutical.Scintigraphy detects space occupying lesions but cannot separate solid tumors from cysts. It is at this point that complementary use of ultrasonography may provide the definitive diagnosis. Scintigraphy is very sensitive for the diagnosis of trauma of the kidney and may also reveal trauma to the adrenals, useful information at any age but especially in the neonate. Renal scintigraphy provides information about renovascular disease and with the help of Gallium scintigraphy,may detect focal or diffuse renal infection. With improving instrumentation which increased the resolution of scintigraphy and with availability of the emission computed tomography (ECT), scintigraphy may become more useful.

Computed Tomography (CT)

This diagnostic modality provides combined information provided by US and IVP. Even though CT has the disadvantages of the IVP (radiation exposure and reaction to contrast media),it may be diagnostic in trauma, cyst, obstruction, tumors, renovascular disease (by showing clots within vessels) and abscesses. In children, however, because of lack of sufficient retroperitoneal fat, CT has limited resolution ability and it cannot be applied as much as in adults. In children ultrasonography plays part of the role which CT plays in adults. In addition to the risks of radiation exposure and reaction to contrast media, CT is the most costly test and there are problems with availability of the equipment.

DIAGNOSTIC INFORMATION FROM IMAGING PROCEDURES IN INDIVIDUAL ACUTE RENAL DISORDERS

Urinary Tract Obstruction

In urinary tract infection associated with obstructive uropathy, the IVP may be diagnostic if sufficient function is retained,while ultrasonography would show the dilated collecting system but not the obstruction. Advanced hydronephrosis may be confused with cystic disease on the ultrasonogram; this modality seldom demonstrates the cause of the hydronephrosis. Ultrasonography is very useful for the insertion of a nephrostomy tube and certainly to locate the kidney for percutaneous biopsy. In urinary tract obstruction, the radionuclide study shows enlarged kidneys with thin parenchyma, dilated collecting system and delayed drainage. Cysts do not visualize; instead, they remain as photopenic areas on the scintigram. Delayed imaging (3-4 hours after injection) can show the level of obstruction. The CT usually shows a dilated collecting system and may show the level of obstruction but, for reasons mentioned before, it is not widely applied in children. The specific diagnosis may be made with a retrograde study.

Acute Tubular Necrosis (ATN), Glomerulonephritis, Nephrotic Syndrome

The IVP may show a dense nephrogram throughout the procedure, or no visualization. Neither IVP nor US are sensitive or specific because they reveal a similar renal image in ATN, acute suppurative pyelonephritis, acute glomerulonephritis and other diseases. Scintigraphy provides a specific diagnosis (see below).

Renal Vein Thrombosis (RVT)

In RVT the IVP may be useful if there remains sufficient function of the involved kidney; it shows increased size, persistent nephrogram with increasing density with time, and underfilling of the collecting system. The ultrasound is again non-specific, although some parenchymal changes may be apparent. In the acute phase of RVT, the radionuclide studies may show increased size, decreased perfusion and function, and a persistent nephrogram without obstruction; in the subacute or compensated RVT, the flow, GFR and ERPF imaging studies may be diagnostic.

The CT in RVT is non-specific although some parenchymal changes have been described in the literature but they are not commonly found; however, CT may show the clot in the renal vein, thus establishing the diagnosis. Venography makes the specific diagnosis of RVT.

Renal Artery Occlusion

Renal artery obstruction, embolism, aortic aneurysm and aortic dissection are not common in children. The IVP is non-specific, usually resulting in non-visualization of the kidney involved. In renal scintigraphy the flow study may be diagnostic and focal defects may be found in the parenchymal phase of the scintigram if there is branch embolism. The ultrasound is non-specific for the kidney but may show clots in vessels. The CT shows a non-functioning kidney and may show clots in vessels. Arteriography makes the specific diagnosis.

Trauma to the Kidneys

Trauma cases are usually diagnosed with IVP. This is a good approach because usually the kidney had nearly normal function before trauma and, unless there is total obliteration of the flow or absence of the kidney, the information is diagnostic. Ultrasound has questionable value. Scintigraphy is very sensitive and usually diagnostic even in cases where IVP provides a false negative result or is non-specific. The CT is equally sensitive and diagnostic; in addition, it provides information about the surrounding organs. Angiography may give a specific diagnosis but many times it is not more informative that CT and, of course, is an invasive procedure.

COMPARISONS AND COMPLEMENTARY STUDIES, SEQUENCES AND INDICATIONS

If there is sufficient clinical information, the radiologist can suggest the imaging modality best indicated for the patient. If the information is not sufficient, a general approach for imaging in acute renal disorders should be followed. There are comparative studies in the literature which favor scintigraphy over urography and they underline the complementary role of scintigraphy and ultrasonography. In general, ultrasonography should be used as the first study to attain structural information, while scintigraphy should be used first for functional and structural information. Both (one after the other) give the answer in most nephro-urologic problems in the pediatric age.

Many times in clinical practice the question has been raised, is there a single imaging modality, sensitive and specific enough which can be applied in every instance to obtain sufficient information in most clinical conditions to direct us to the specific diagnosis? It is the experience at our institution that nuclear scintigraphy is very successful as the first approach in patients with acute renal disorders or renal emergencies. Recently, we reviewed our data (3) and out of 140 studies there was one case in which non-contributory information was obtained when scintigraphy was performed; in fourteen instances information was partially diagnostic and in 114 cases scintigraphy was in complete agreement with the diagnosis; there was only one case where scintigraphy provided the wrong information. In this retrospective study, we found that in 98% of the cases renal scintigraphy was in agreement with the final diagnosis when performed or reviewed as a first study and without the information from other imaging studies. Renal ultrasonography was in agreement with the final diagnosis in 82% of the cases and excretory urography in only 55%.

We suggest the use of Tc-99m-Glucoheptonate as the choice for the first procedure. We inject 200 microcuries per kilogram of body weight intravenously and perform a flow study, sequential imaging for 20 minutes and delayed studies 3-4 hours later. Since ^{99m} Technetium Glucoheptonate is filtered by the glomeruli (90%), it provides GFR information; 10% of the injected dose is bound to the renal tubules and enables cortical imaging. This radiopharmaceutical has the unique ability to provide information about blood flow and GFR (semiquantitatively)and also to show the cortices on delayed imaging. The study can be performed at the bedside with a portable camera.

RENAL SCINTIGRAPHY IN ACUTE RENAL DISORDERS (5)

Normal Study

The normal scintigram is characterized by the appearance of uniform kidney bean shaped activity in the renal bed within one minute after injection. The collecting system may be visible or not; if visible it appears early (4-5 minutes) and later (10-15 minutes) shows less activity. The ureters may or may not be visible intermittently but they must empty eventually.

Congenital Anomalies

Agenesis can be easily diagnosed. There is no renal activity and the background is normal without photopenic defects (the characteristic of cystic lesions). The multicystic kidney is visualized in two forms, depending on residual function: if there is no residual function, there is a photopenic region; if there is some function left, there appears a central area of activity surrounded by a photopenic halo. Polycystic kidney disease is characterized by large kidneys, some ilets of perfusion in the flow and ilets of functioning tissue surrounding cysts on the delayed images; there is no obstruction. Ectopic, hypoplastic, hypertrophic and horse-shoe kidneys can be diagnosed easily with anterior or posterior early or delayed views. Hydronephrosis has the opposite image from multicystic kidney; there is a rim of activity surrounding a central photopenia and there is delayed and persistent activity in the collecting system. If there is proximal obstruction with hydronephrosis, there is persistent renal pelvic activity which increases continuously and the ureters are not visualized. If there is distal obstruction, at 1-4 min. the rim of hydronephrosis is evident, then persistent pelvic activity increases, sometimes plateaus, the ureter is visualized late (between 10 minutes and 4 hours) and occasionally there is photopenia at the beginning. In patients with duplication, the radionuclide study provides information about the function of each of the two components of each kidney. If there is acute renal vein thrombosis in the neonate, the diagnosis can be suggested as the findings include a large kidney, solid but decreased activity (decreased function without obstruction) and a renogram image which remains for a long period of time. In trauma during delivery, bilateral adrenal hemorrhage
kidneys.

Acquired Diseases

In acute renal obstruction of any etiology there is decreased blood flow and function, slight, if any, hydronephrosis and continuous accumulation of cortical activity. The collecting system is not visible if there is total obstruction; if there is late collecting system visualization, it signifies partial obstruction. The renogram curves show the typical image of continuously increasing activity. In chronic renal obstruction the kidney may not be visible or may show reduced blood flow and function depending on the degree and duration of obstruction. There is evident hydronephrosis, and a rim of cortex around the dilated collecting system. The kidney size depends on the duration of the obstruction; if it is enlarged, relative function is preserved and the obstruction is new or partial; if it is normal or small, the kidney is probably undergoing atrophy. In renal artery occlusion, if it is total and acute, there is total absence of flow and function and a photopenic area. In old renal artery occlusion there is no flow but average background activity in the renal bed. Detection of trauma is prompt by scintigraphy. Contusion appears as focal lack of function, hematoma (focal defect) compresses and displaces the kidney, extravasation appears as activity outside the kidney. Finally, tumor can be diagnosed by scintigraphy as a focal defect, which may displace and distort the kidney.

Functional Studies with Radioisotopes In Acute Renal Disorders (5,6)

Functional information can be acquired by applying two different radiopharmaceuticals in the study of GFR and ERPF, global or split. The information obtained with computer analysis and other calculations is specific (renography, clearances), and it helps in making a specific diagnosis in various clinical presentations.

The hypertensive patient can be studied to rule out a renovascular component. In renal artery stenosis, the flow is decreased and delayed; technetium complexes (imaging) show small kidney size and persistence of cortical activity; functional images of 131-I-Hippurate provide the specific pattern of continuously increasing activity in the kidney cortex. In the patient with ATN the diagnosis can be made when there is relative preservation of renal blood flow (although reduced down to one-third of normal), a decreased but present cortical retention of 99m-DTPA (or Glucoheptonate), and a prompt uptake and retention of 131-I-Hippurate. With these studies we can differentiate between rejection of a renal transplant and ATN. ATN can be separated from cortical necrosis, hepato-renal syndrome, and renal artery occlusion, because in all the other conditions there is absence of renal uptake of 131-I-Hippurate and absence of DTPA flow and function. RVT shows characteristics discussed above. In glomerular diseases, there is preservation of the Hippurate image but there is a disproportionate decrease in the DTPA flow and function. In acute pyelonephritis with renal insufficiency scintigraphy with 99m-Tc-Complexes may show cortical defects and decreased function; still, 67-Gallium scintigraphy is the best choice, because it will show focal accumulation or intense and diffuse accumulation.

There is recent information about Filtration Fraction (FF) determination using GFR and ERPF measurements with 99m Tc-DTPA and 131-I-Hippurate (6). It is increased in acute tubular necrosis (95% sensitivity), hypoproteinemia, pyelonephritis, and congestive heart failure; decreased in glomerulonephritis, cortical necrosis, and obstructive uropathy; and normal in most chronic situations.

Finally, with the use of furosemide diuresis renography we differentiate between the non-obstructed dilated collecting system and the obstructed dilated collecting system.

As our experience in functional radioisotopic studies increases, more information about the functional applications of the radionuclides in pediatric nephrology will become available.

REFERENCES

1. Lopez, S.A. and Kumar, R.: Medical Diseases of the Kidneys. In Ney, Charles and Friedenberg, Richard, Radiographic Atlas of the Genitourinary System, 2nd Edition. Philadelphia: Lippincott, 1981, pp 753-790.
2. G. N. Sfakianakis, E. Sfakianaki and F. Bowen: Radionuclide Renal Study in Neonatal Clinical Problems. J Nucl Med 19:698, 1978.
3. G. N. Sfakianakis, E. Sfakianaki, R. Lopez, G. Zilleruelo, M. Freundlich, H Gorman, J. Strauss and A. Serafini: Renal Scintigraphy in Neonatal and Infantile Clinical Problems. J Nucl Med 23 (5), p 98,1982.
4. R. A. Olden, M. Corobkin, D.M. Cleeve, et al: Contrast-Induced Acute Renal Failure: Persistent Nephrogram as Clue to Early Detection. AJR 134:339-342, 1980.
5. R.A. Sherman, K.J. Byun: Nuclear Medicine in Acute and Chronic Renal Failure. Semin Nucl Med 12 (3):265-279, 1982.
6. E.V. Dubovsky, C.D. Russell: Quantitation of Renal Function with Glomerular and Tubular Agents. Semin Nucl Med 12(4):308-329, 1982.

ANTIMICROBIAL AGENTS IN URINARY TRACT INFECTIONS

Heinz F. Eichenwald, M.D.

In order for an antimicrobial agent to be reasonably effective in the treatment of acute or chronic urinary tract infection, three requirements must be met. The drug must:

1) produce serum levels sufficiently high to inhibit or kill the bacterium causing the infection,
2) appear in the urine in adequate concentrations and in active form,
3) achieve proper tissue levels.

Failure to meet any one of these requirements usually means that the drug has no or only limited use in infections of the urinary tract. Examples include <u>nitrofurantoin</u> which produces neither adequate tissue nor serum levels and is useful only in the suppression of bacteruria; the polymyxins, whose use results in serum but usually not tissue or urine levels and thus are relatively ineffective in the treatment of infections of the kidney, and <u>chloramphenicol</u> which produces good serum and tissue levels but appears in the urine only in limited amounts as a microbiologically inactive metabolite, and whose efficacy in any type of urinary tract infection is relatively poor.

In addition to the so-called "true antibiotics", a number of synthetic chemicals are available for use in the treatment of urinary tract infections. These include:

1) Methenamine mandelate
2) Nalidixic acid, and its close relatives, oxolinic acid and cinoxacin
3) Nitrofurantoin
4) The sulfonamides
5) Trimethoprim, also offered in combination with sulfamethoxazole.

Several of these drugs can be dismissed out of hand: <u>methenamine</u> mandelate is, at best, a weak urinary antiseptic. It is claimed to be useful for the suppression of bacteruria but, in our experience, has proven difficult to administer and of low, if any, efficacy.

Nalidixic acid is approved for use in children, while oxolinic acid and cinoxacin are not. No situation exists where these agents might be useful in a child. All three drugs show relatively low efficacy, high toxicity, and the tendency to produce resistant organisms quite rapidly. In addition to causing a number of other serious side-effects, such as arthritis, nalidixic acid acts as a central nervous system stimulant; it may precipitate seizures in a child with a history of convulsions and it may produce considerable irritability and insomnia in children and adults.

Nitrofurantoin has been in use for many years and is available both in oral and intravenous form. The drug appears in the urine in high concentrations but serum and tissue levels are low. The major advantages of this drug are its broad activity against both gram-positive and gram-negative bacteria, excluding pseudomonas and most strains of proteus, and the fact that bacterial resistance develops slowly, indicating that its primary use is in the suppression of bacteruria. Administration in the fasting state often results in nausea, anorexia, and abdominal pain. These reactions can be reduced in frequency and severity by giving the drug only with meals. The use of the formulation "macrodantin" reduces the incidence of gastritis but does not eliminate the problem.

A more serious side effect consists of peripheral neuritis, which occurs primarily in patients with reduced renal function in whom elevated blood levels of this drug may appear; nitrofurantoin should be used with caution, if at all, in children with significant renal disease. The agent also produces hemolysis in children with congenital deficiencies of erythrocyte glucose-6-phosphate dehydrogenase. Patients on prolonged and/or repeated courses may develop an eosinophilic, probably allergic, pneumonia which may progress to pulmonary fibrosis. While the exact incidence of this potentially serious reaction remains unknown, it is believed to be quite rare, especially in children. More recently, use of the drug has been associated with the occasional appearance of chronic active hepatitis. These observations would indicate the need for careful follow-up of patients receiving nitrofurantoin repeatedly or for long periods of time.

The sulfonamides have a long history of efficacy in the treatment of acute urinary tract infection and in the suppression of bacteruria. The presently available preparations, especially sulfisoxazole and its relatives, and the preparation triple soluble sulfas U.S.P. are considerably safer to administer than the sulfonamides of the past. Toxic effects, while rare, may be serious and include the Stevens-Johnson syndrome, aplastic or hemolytic anemia, and chemical hepatitis. The newer preparations rarely produce crystalluria or hematuria even in highly acid urine. Sulfonamides still represent excellent therapy for acute uncomplicated urinary tract infections by combining high efficacy, considerable safety, and low cost.

Sulfonamides have also been used in the suppression of bacteruria and in the prophylaxis of urinary tract infection following various surgical manipulations. They are effective but bacterial resistance develops fairly rapidly.

Trimethoprim is available for use in adults as a single agent but is marketed for children only as the trimethoprim-sulfamethoxazole combination (TMS-SMX) which is effective against most gram-negative organisms that cause urinary tract infection with the exception of some strains of proteus and most pseudomonas. It is approved for use in children two months or older and does represent a highly effective mode of therapy. The label, however, states that "it is recommended that initial episodes of uncomplicated urinary tract infections be treated with a single effective antibacterial agent rather than the combination". We believe this admonition to be entirely correct; our own studies have not shown a superiority of trimethoprim-sulfa over either sulfa or amoxicillin in the treatment of acute disease. This combination drug represents a good choice, however, if initial therapy has failed to clear the infection. In addition, it is widely prescribed for the suppression of bacteruria; such use is not an FDA approved indication although when employed for this purpose, TMS-SMX is effective and probably quite safe; furthermore, the emergence of resistant bacteria is likely to be delayed for longer than would be the case where a sulfonamide is used alone.

The toxicity rate of trimethoprim-sulfa is relatively low; whether the combination is more likely than the sulfonamides to cause reactions such as Stevens-Johnson syndrome or hepatitis remains unclear. A serious but rare problem is the occurrence of rapidly deteriorating renal function in children with some pre-existing renal disease. It would seem prudent to avoid the use of TMS-SMX in patients known to have kidney disease; more effective and less toxic drugs are available.

True antibiotics useful in the treatment of urinary tract infections may be divided into four groups:

1) "Miscellaneous" agents

2) Aminoglycosides

3) Penicillins

4) Cephalosporins

Among the miscellaneous group are the polymyxins (polymyxin B and colistin), tetracyclines, and chloramphenicol. Both polymyxins combine high toxicity with relatively low efficacy. The tetracyclines possess unacceptable toxicities for children, but equally important is the fact that most common gram-negative bacteria have become resistant. The observation that chloramphenicol represents a poor choice in the treatment of urinary tract infection has already been mentioned.

The aminoglycosides, on the other hand, have been extraordinarily useful. They possess high activity against most bacteria responsible for urinary tract infections, especially E. coli. and klebsiella-enterobacter, and produce high serum, tissue, and urine levels. Their action on bacteria is rapid and they are therefore especially useful in those children with acute renal infections associated with bacteremia. Antibacterial activity is greatly enhanced by an alkaline urine.

Aside from streptomycin, whose use is archaic, the various aminoglycosides possess approximately the same toxicity, although there are data to indicate that tobramycin produces less renal and eighth nerve damage in adults than does gentamicin. Since such toxic effects rarely occur in infants and young children when these drugs are administered appropriately, it is not possible to demonstrate such superiority of tobramycin in the pediatric age group. Much information exists about the use of gentamicin and kanamycin in children; with the newer drugs tobramycin and amikacin, data are less complete. Tobramycin possesses an essentially similar spectrum of activity as gentamicin, and may be used interchangeably with it. Amikacin is effective against most bacteria that have become gentamicin resistant and thus is used primarily in situations where resistance to the latter drug is known or can be inferred from the epidemiologic situation.

The third group of antibiotics useful in the treatment of urinary tract infections is the penicillins, specifically ampicillin and related drugs and the so-called "gram-negative" or "anti-pseudomonas" penicillins such as carbenicillin, ticarcillin, piperacillin, etc.

The "ampicillin-like penicillins" include ampicillin itself, amoxicillin, cyclacillin, and bacampicillin. The latter three are marketed for oral use only and, when administered by this route, are absorbed better than ampicillin, which is the only member of the group that is available for parenteral use. All of them are highly effective against most strains of E. coli, but generally inactive against klebsiella-enterobacter and pseudomonas. One important feature is that they are active against most strains of enterococci, bacteria that may often be highly resistant to other drugs, such as the cephalosporins.

In our experience, the preferred oral drug is amoxicillin which is relatively inexpensive, quite well tolerated, and produces high serum, tissue and urine levels. Cyclacillin and bacampicillin are more expensive and no more effective than the older drug. For those patients who routinely develop diarrhea on amoxicillin, bacampicillin may be useful since, in general, it produces fewer gastrointestinal disturbances.

A different group of penicillins, while possessing some activity against gram-positive bacteria, is useful primarily in the treatment of gram-negative infections. This group consists of carbenicillin, ticarcillin, mezlocillin, azlocillin, and piperacillin. All five are active against pseudomonas, although carbenicillin is less so than the others. Mezlocillin, piperacillin, and azlocillin are effective in the treatment of enterococcal infections while, in general, carbenicillin and ticarcillin are not. Mezlocillin, piperacillin and azlocillin have more activity against klebsiella-enterobacter than do the others; all of these agents are equally effective clinically against E. coli (Table 1).

Aside from some minor side effects such as rashes, each of these five drugs is inherently very safe; the limiting factor to dosage is related more to the amount of sodium they contain than to any intrinsic toxicity. As a result, they have been administered to adults in truly enormous dosages. One problem shared by all five is the relatively rapid appearance of resistant strains, often during the course of therapy. To minimize this problem, most experts recommend that these drugs not be used alone but only in combination with aminoglycosides such as gentamicin. As a group, these penicillins are more useful in adults and in children that are immunosuppressed than they are in the average child with acute or persistent urinary tract infection.

Table 1. "Anti-Pseudomonas" Penicillins

Characteristic	Carbenicillin	Ticarcillin	Mezlocillin	Piperacillin
Trade Names	Geopen, Pyopen	Ticar	Mezlin	Pipracil
Activity against:				
Ps. aeuruginosa	+	++	++	+++
Enterococcus	0	0	++	++
Serratia	+	+	++	++
Klebsiella-Enterobacter	+	+	++	++
B. fragilis	+	++	+++	+++
E. coli	++	++	++	++
Sodium content (mg/g)	110	120	42	45
Penetration into CSF	+	+	+++	+++

0 = None; + = Fair; ++ = Good; +++ = Excellent

The fourth group of antibiotics consists of the cephalosporins. While a sizable number of these drugs are available, discussion will be limited to those agents of particular interest in the treatment of urinary tract infection. Of the oral agents, *cefaclor*, *cephalexin* and *cefadroxil* share very similar microbiologic properties, although cefadroxil and cefaclor may be more active against klebsiella. Administration of each of these three agents results in high and predictable serum levels with most of the drug appearing in the urine in active form. In terms of efficacy, all three agents are about the same. Cefadroxil has a longer half-life and thus needs to be administered only twice a day; the other two drugs are given on a three times a day schedule.

Should they be employed in the usual case of acute urinary tract infection? In such patients, amoxicillin and the sulfonamides are as effective as the cephalosporins and much less costly, but the latter drugs are useful in children in whom other medications have failed to eradicate the infection; they possess an advantage over trimethoprim-sulfa by being virtually free of nephrotoxicity.

A number of the cephalosporins available for parenteral administration have proven useful in the treatment of severe urinary tract infections.

Of the so-called "first and second generation" drugs intended for parenteral use, cefamandole and cefuroxime are most useful. They are highly active against klebsiella and E. coli but possess relatively little activity against pseudomonas. Their use in recommended dosage produces high serum, tissue and urine levels; they are exceedingly safe drugs, even in circumstances where kidney function is limited. The major problem associated with their use is the fact that they are painful on intramuscular injection and may produce thrombophlebitis when given intravenously. Cefoxitin possesses very similar activity against gram-negative enterobacteria as the other two but is generally more effective in anaerobic infections (Table 2).

Table 2. Antimicrobial Activity of Parenteral Cephalosporins

	Cephalothin	Cefamandole	Cefoxitin*
Gram positive cocci	++++	++++	+
B. fragilis	0	+	+++
H. influenzae	+	+++	++
Enterobacter	0	+++	+
Indole pos. Proteus	0	0	+++

*Actually a cephamycin

Three "third generation" cephalosporins are available: cefotaxime, cefoperazone, and moxolactam. Each of these three drugs possesses enormous activity against E. coli and other gram-negative enterobacteria, including pseudomonas. Enterococci, however,are usually resistant. Cefoperazone is metabolized in the liver, rather than being excreted in the urine; the other two drugs therefore represent better choices in the treatment of urinary tract infection (Table 3). Few toxic effects have been reported in children but in adults a bleeding diathesis occasionally occurs with their use.

While their greater activity suggests that moxolactam and cefotaxime should prove superior to cefamandol or cefoxitin in the treatment of urinary tract infection, few data exist to support this view.

In summary then, the physician can choose from many different drugs to treat a child with urinary tract infection. In normal children, acute uncomplicated infection responds satisfactorily to sulfonamides and the

Table 3. Comparison of "Third Generation" Cephalosporin Derivatives*

Characteristic	Cefotaxime	Moxalactam	Cefoperazone
Trade Name	Claforan	Moxam	Cefobid
Activity against:			
Ps. aeruginosa	++	++	+++
Coliform bacilli	+++	+++	++
Aminoglycoside-Resistant Coliforms	+++	+++	++
Non-fermenters	++	++	++
Haemophilus	+++	+++	+++
Neisseria	+++	+++	+++
Pneumococci	+++	+	+++
Group B streptococci	+++	+	+++
Staphylococci	++	+	++
Enterococci	0	0	0
Listeria	0	0	0
Concentration in:			
Urine	++	+++	+
Bile	+	++	+++
CSF	++	+++	++
Activity of Metabolites	+	+++	N/A
Dosage Adjustment in Renal Failure	Moderate	Moderate	None
Dosage Interval	6-8 hr	6-12 hr	6-8 hr

*Adapted from Nelson, J.D., Ped. Inf. Disease 1 (Supplement) 58, 1982

ampicillin-like agents; it is only in the more complex patients with diminished renal function, malformations of the urinary tract, mixed infections, and the occasional highly resistant organism that the use of other antibiotics needs to be considered. In such cases, the selection should be based on the organisms involved, the safety of the drug, its reliability, and ease of administration.

REFERENCES

1. Assael, B.M. et al: Ototoxicity of aminoglycoside antibiotics in infants and children, Ped. Inf.Disease, 1, 357, 1982

2. Eichenwald, H.F. and McCracken, G.H., Jr.: Antimicrobial therapy in infants and children, J. Ped. 93, 37, 1978

3. Hellerstein, S.: Recurrent urinary tract infection in children, Ped. Inf. Disease 1, 271, 1982

4. Lafierre, C.I. and Marks, M.I.: Chloramphenicol: properties and clinical use, Ped. Inf. Disease 1, 257, 1982

5. McCracken, G.H., Jr. and Nelson, J.D.: Third generation cephalosporins, Ped. Inf. Disease 1, 123, 1982

6. Nelson, J.D. and McCracken, G.H., Jr.: Mexlocillin and related antibiotics, Ped. Inf. Disease 1, 42, 1982

PANEL DISCUSSION: ACUTE RENAL DISEASES

Moderator: José Strauss, M.D.

QUESTION: I have two questions. First, did you screen the urine of these children, and if so, what did you find in terms of dip sticks?

RESPONSE: Unfortunately, we did not screen the urine, a question that Dr. Strauss immediately asked during that luncheon when we first talked about the study. It would have been simple enough to do but we were doing a great many other things, including photography, and we were limited to getting a certain amount of information. It certainly would have been useful and it would have been interesting to do several weeks after that visit as well, since we were getting the patients back in three weeks.

QUESTION: The second question I have is, what is your current recommendation in terms of the use of topical drugs to treat impetigo vs oral drugs?

RESPONSE: I think as a rule the topical drugs are most ineffective for cutaneous pyoderma. Now, I will use topical antibiotics for other disorders, acne for example. But not for cutaneous pyoderma, and I don't like a topical antibiotic in a disease that may have a sequella such as streptococcal disease; perhaps staphylococcal disease as well because of the spread to other family members, etc. who may be more vulnerable for a serious sequella. I don't use topical antibiotics for pyoderma.

QUESTION: I have two questions. First, did you make any attempt to see if the streptococcal infections were really nephritogenic or just simply strep infections? Second, was there any nephritis following staph infections?

RESPONSE: The second question was another one that Dr. Strauss had posed. We had no incidence of nephritis with staph infections. We had this patient population locked into a system and we had no incidence of post-staphylococcal renal disease in these patients. Again, when I was writing this protocol, conducting it, it was very early in my stay in Miami and I had little in hand. I was looking for research funds, looking for what I could get for what I most wanted. I certainly would have loved and would still like to repeat the study, looking for a number of things such as what you mentioned. It took us a long time; we had to lyophilize the staph before we had the funding to even phage type them. We found some very interesting things about the phage typing, too. It wasn't only group 2, type 71, for example, it was across the board groups 1, 2, and 3 in our own population. It would have been a very significant adjunct to the study as done and I would love to have had the funding to do them at the time.

QUESTION: As a point of interest, I've been in practice for six years, and from the day I walked into practice probably 90% of our skin infections have looked like staph and we've been treating them with anti-staphylococcal drugs. I just sat here amused that it took so long to change down here, though classically in the pediatric literature there have always been reports of nephritis in the warmer areas being skin and in the colder areas being throat. We've always had staph in our skin infections, for many, many years (in Long Island).

RESPONSE: We've always had staph in our skin infections for many years, too. I did my pediatric training in the same neighborhood. I was at Montefiore Hospital and at Albert Einstein. I was convinced in those years that we were seeing increased staph as well. But I defy you to find that in the pediatric literature.

RESPONSE: It's probably present at Einstein also. There I don't recall but I know that in our area it has clearly been staph for many years.

COMMENT: I felt the same when I was in New York, that we were seeing increased incidence, though not predominance of staphylococcal disease, not only in infants but also in the adolescent and young adult population. At Montefiore we had an adolescent program that went to 21-22 years of age. But, if you take a look at the reviews of pyodermas or the reviews of streptococcal disease, the last one being in the New England Journal around 1979-1980, they will tell you that streptococcal disease predominates as the pyoderma across the country, and mixed infections will be penicillin responsive. Find a reference elsewhere in the literature if you can; I would appreciate it. We wrote the one that will be in the Clinics of North America.

MODERATOR: I wonder whether I could impose upon our friend who knows so much about so many things and ask him to comment on the shifting patterns of infections or diseases that may or may not be related to infections.

COMMENT: First, it has been our impression that post-streptococcal glomerulonephritis is less frequently seen than we used to see it. Second, with rare exceptions, the disease is much less severe. I have seen two severe cases in the last few years, and one of those two was a Vietnamese boat refugee who required dialysis but then recovered completely. She had a very interesting finding. She had very severe tubulointerstitial involvement. If you look at the literature in the last 10 or 20 years, you hardly ever see tubulointerstitial involvement mentioned in post-streptococcal GN. But if you go back to the forties, to the early days of the association between streptococcal infection and renal disease, you will see that it is mentioned much more often. Now, in France there has been a reduction in the incidence of membrano-proliferative GN. There was an abstract in Kidney International last year pointing this out. We have had the feeling that we are not seeing MPGN either. I'm not talking about Type II, but Type I, and I'm not saying that this is related to streptococcal infection. I'm just mentioning that there has been a change in the disease. In the northern United States and Canada there seems to be no impetiginous streptococcal glomerulonephritis but in the Artic among the Eskimo, it does occur.

In South Africa, there was a big series of patients with streptococcal infections resulting in nephrotic syndrome with epimembranous deposits, a membranous type of nephrotic syndrome which I found to be quite astonishing. At the time I didn't agree with the lady doctor who reported the series but the more I think about it, the more I think she had good evidence to say that there was epimembranous GN secondary to streptococcal infection. I was also struck by the fact that there was such a high incidence of membranous GN in black children in that country, but not in white children. Nephrotic syndrome is completely different in that country in whites and blacks. In whites it is predominantly minimal lesion and this is true for Asian children as well; in black children it's predominantly membranous - a very high association of membranous GN with hepatitis B infection, I think it is. I don't know what the experience is in that regard in the United States. Certainly in Japan and East Asia there is some suggestion that hepatitis B can cause glomerulonephritis. My last comment about post-infectious GN is about the report of a case of mycoplasma pneumoniae complicated by glomerulonephritis several years ago. We thought that we had demonstrated the mycoplasma antigen in the glomeruli of this patient. Subsequent to that report, there have been a number of case reports, and we have seen a few cases either of hematuria or glomerulonephritis and one case of classical Berger's disease associated with mycoplasma pneumoniae. I'm sure that I have said much more than you expected me to, probably not what you hoped me to.

MODERATOR: You said just the right amount of very valuable information. We have not talked about the other possible infections like the one suggested in Argentina for the hemolytic uremic syndrome, but I guess we have said enough. Now, we shall go to other questions. What is the criterion to diagnose systemic disease with a glomerulopathy? In other words, if you take post-infectious glomerulonephritis and say that that is not a systemic disease - what we in general tend to say - we need to think of work like that of Guiseppe Andres in Buffalo who had a patient with post-infectious glomerulonephritis. This patient, an adolescent, recovered and did very well, had a motorcycle accident, his spleen was removed and it was loaded with immune complexes. In situations like that, how can we refine our diagnosis of systemic involvement?

RESPONSE: That's a very difficult question. I think all these diseases have the potential of being systemic. Unless you have an in situ formation of immune complexes, or you have a disease like Goodpasture's Syndrome, for instance, where you have the cross reactivity between the basement membrane of the kidney and the lung, you have the potential of having systemic disease. The reasons why immune complexes are localized in specific vascular beds are not known. Nobody has any idea why in polyarteritis nodosa, the immune complexes go into certain types of vessels and why in nephritis they go into other types, why in lupus sometimes you get cerebritis or why you don't. I think that's a mystery. As I mentioned before, immune complex formation is probably a normal event. Probably we all form immune complexes during the day.

MODERATOR: What about during the night?

RESPONSE: Yes, during the night, too, if you take a glass of milk before going to bed!

QUESTION: I just wanted to verify...did you say that the urticaria hypocomplementemic nephritis syndrome had increased C1Q complexes?

RESPONSE: Right, they have a low molecular weight, C1Q precipitants.

QUESTION: You then mentioned another disease after that?

RESPONSE: Yes, lymearthritis.

QUESTION: Lymearthritis. Does it have C1Q? It doesn't have renal disease, does it?

RESPONSE: It does have C1Q of a specific type. As far as I know, it does not have renal disease but the tests are helpful in predicting - I believe that the rheumatologists used to predict involvement in the CNS and other extra-renal involvement. They used the test to gauge the prognosis of the patients with that. But you are right. This is not related to renal involvement.

QUESTION: What role does histopathology play in the history of the urticaria - hypocomplementic syndrome?

RESPONSE: It's a mild form of proliferative, mostly mesangial glomerulonephritis.

QUESTION: I would like for you to pinpoint a little better if you could tell us, from the practical point of view in the daily clinical practice, how can we and how should we, what should we do about circulating immune complexes? On top of everything, with logistic problems, we are, for example, faced with a patient with rapidly progressive glomerulonephritis who needs, let's say, plasmapheresis. We want to gauge what we are doing but it takes us eight, ten, twelve days, two weeks until we get the results back. How do we work that out in our mental scheme of daily clinical applications?

RESPONSE: Of course, remember the immune complexes are helpful in other areas of medicine. It's not only in nephrology. For instance, in cancer. There are all kinds of immune complex diseases. I think that now in nephrology, these tests are generally available. Most of the big labs do it. Bio-Science now does everything, Raji cells, everything. The whole group in La Jolla has commercialized all these products and there are several labs that do the conglutinin and the C1Q binding assay and the Raji cells. These are the three most commonly used tests. Now you do have a logistics problem if you have to mail the tests. In Miami our Division of Immunology has all these tests available and you should get these tests within 24 hours; the results are available right away. Now, as far as using them, the tests are helpful if you are looking for a presumptive marker of immunologic diseases or immune complex disease.

For instance, if you suspect a systemic immune complex disease, you can use them the same way you use complement and other tests like ANA as a screening. For immune complex disease that may be helpful, especially if the titers are very high. That's one usefulness of the tests. The other usefulness, of course, is what I outlined. You can use them for assessing the activity of the disease and the efficacy of your therapy, whether you are giving corticosteroids or immune suppression or whether you are using plasmapheresis.

MODERATOR: On the practical level, continuing, sometimes we get opposite results with one of these three tests. I think we are not using the conglutinins yet on a routine basis. I didn't realize it was available commercially. I thought that you were setting that up as a special test. We do routinely now send to the La Jolla laboratory, Scripps laboratory, the ClQ and Raji cells tests. Sometime, one is normal, the other is abnormal. Can you tell us what our approach should be, which one is more liable to give false results?

RESPONSE: You always have to do more than one because you cannot do too much with one since each test is specific for certain types of complexes. For instance, the ClQ doesn't detect low molecular weight complexes. So, if the patient that you are looking at is forming low complexes, you won't detect them. As I mentioned, they interfere more often. If you have endotoxin in the blood, that will give you a false positive, or a DNA in the blood,that will give you a false positive test. I think that certain other tests are specific for immunoglobulin components. Certain immunoglobulins do not react in certain types of assay. So, if you are forming complexes with IgM, you may not detect them with certain tests. Also, it depends on the complexes,whether they fix complement or not. The combination of conglutinin and ClQ is fairly good because conglutinin detects different size complexes, the whole spectrum of complexes, and detects complexes that are complement bound while the other one doesn't require complement bound complexes. So, you really have to use several tests, preferably three tests: the Raji cells, the ClQ binding and the conglutinin are a good combination. Also, the rheumatoid factor-precipitation with monoclonal rheumatoid factor-is a pretty good test, too. And of course, you can use also screening tests. There's nothing wrong with doing cryoglobulins - there are a few tests that are used for screening.

MODERATOR: We have one last question, please.

QUESTION: In a very simplistic way, immune complexes of certain sizes, it seems like they would come out into the urine. When I was at Tulane we were able to follow a couple of children with lupus who did have immune complexes in a qualitative manner and when we had the patients in remission, there were none. I'm aware that Rawle McIntosh had demonstrated at least cryoglobulins in the urine. Has anybody systematically looked at urinary immune complexes?

RESPONSE: I am not aware of any systematic study. Probably the problem there is that all depends on the filtration characteristics of the glomerulus. It depends on the specific disease but basically on the severity of the disease. It may be like determining certain plasma inactivating factors in the urine; those tests used to be very popular. But, basically, they don't tell you much about what's going on in the patient. What they tell you is how much permeability, how much damage you have in the glomerulus. These are big macromolecules, by the way. Unless you have a generalized inflammation, they really shouldn't be in the urine. They are of use to follow the activity of the glomerular damage, not so much the activity of the immunological disease. The kidney will determine that.

MODERATOR: I would like to make a suggestion. Since we keep running out of time for a very exciting subject like this, I would like to request that you give me your written questions now before you leave and I will be sure that each speaker replies to those questions and they will be answered in the volume made from the Seminar. Now, we must stop. Many thanks to all the participants.

IV

ACUTE RENAL FAILURE

ETIOPATHOGENESIS AND DIFFERENTIAL DIAGNOSIS OF ACUTE RENAL FAILURE

Melinda McVicar, M.D.

Attention was first focused on acute renal failure in 1941 when Bywaters and Beall (1) noted that severe crush injuries which did not involve the abdominal cavity were frequently associated with decreased urine output and decreased renal function. Patients studied at autopsy had intratubular casts containing tubular epithelium and tubular necrosis as prominent findings. The terms lower nephron nephrosis and acute tubular necrosis were applied to this kind of injury. Since then active research in this area, particularly in experimental models, has led some clarification of the mechanisms involved in acute renal failure.

Clinical studies of acute renal failure have been limited by a number of factors which include varied diagnostic criteria, heterogeneous patient groups and inconsistencies in treatment and management. It is not surprising, therefore, that experimental models of acute renal failure have been utilized in attempts to elucidate its pathogenesis The following discussion will first consider the results of recent studies in the pathogenesis of acute renal failure. Since two of the most common clinical settings resulting in acute renal failure for adults and children are related to ischemia and aminoglycoside toxicity, experimental and clinical information relating to these forms will be discussed. This will be followed by a discussion of various etiologic factors which induce clinical acute renal failure in children and adults, and studies which are helpful in differential diagnosis.

PATHOGENESIS

Experimental Models

The experimental models may be divided into two general categories, those in which acute renal failure (ARF) is induced through use of nephrotoxins, and those in which decreased renal blood flow results in acute failure. The nephrotoxic models which have been well studied include the mercuric chloride model, the uranyl nitrate model, the myohemoglobinuric (glycerol) model, the aminoglycoside model, and the radio contrast model (Table 1). Ischemic ARF is most often induced by renal vasoconstriction by either clamping of the renal artery (complete or incomplete) or intravenous infusions of norepinephrine. In the nephrotoxic and ischemic forms of ARF, vascular and tubular effects have both been described.

There are 3 basic mechanisms which have been proposed for the pathogenesis of ARF. These are: altered hemodynamics, tubular backleak and tubular obstruction. The mechanisms frequently overlap and several experimental models develop ARF by the predominance of a particular

Table 1. Acute Renal Failure

Major Animal Models	Proposed Human Counterparts
Hemodynamic	
Norepinephine infusion renal artery	Decreased RBF
Clamping of renal artery (partial or complete)	Decreased RBF
Glycerol (intense vasoconstriction + Myo-hemoglobinuria)	Rhabdomyolysis Transfusion reactions
Toxic	
Aminoglycoside (gentamicin)	Aminoglycoside
Uranyl nitrate	ATN
Mercuric chloride (necrosis of proximal tubule)	ATN
Radiocontrast materials	Contrast Nephropathy

mechanism. The search for a critical pathogenic factor representing a final common pathway or unified pathogenic event has exercised many investigators for the past decade. It seems likely, however, that the varying ways in which ARF is induced have differing pathogenic mechanisms.

Maintenance of Acute Renal Failure

The factors which maintain ARF when the insult has been discontinued and when renal blood flow has been restored are not well understood and are the subject of much current research. The renin-angiotensin system has been suspect ever since an increase in the prominence of the juxtaglomerular apparatus was noted in patients with ARF following crush injury (2). Plasma renin has been shown to be increased in both clinical and experimental ARF and a diet high in sodium (which also suppresses plasma renin) has been shown to attenuate ARF. Although a pathogenic mechanism involving the renin-angiotensin system has been proposed, it is not well established. It has been shown, for example, that plasma renin activity may return to control levels while ARF is maintained (3). Nevertheless, some recent studies using inhibitors of angiotension II (A II) activity and which will be discussed below, suggest an important role for A II in the maintenance of ARF.

More recently, investigators have proposed that renal tubular cell injury and associated transport defects, particularly those associated with increases of intracellular calcium, are the final common pathway for the maintenance of renal insufficiency (4). Mitochondrial state 3 respiration and calcium levels of renal cortical homogenates have been used as parameters of biochemical renal tubular cell injury and are thought to be more sensitive than anatomic changes. In a recent study, the degree of gentamicin induced ARF has been shown to correlate directly with the decline in mitochondrial state 3 respiration and the rise in renal cortical calcium content (5). On the other hand, it is possible that changes in state 3 respiration and intracellular calcium content may merely reflect the early stages of cellular death.

There is some documentation that renal tubular transport function and microstructure may recover at different rates in ARF (6). Measurements of proximal renal tubular transport showed decreased absorption of sodium and glucose during the first hour after ischemic ARF and were associated with loss of proximal tubule brush border. However, even after the brush border regenerated (4 hours after release of 35 minutes of ischemia) these transport defects persisted. It seems likely that the application of methods which dissociate anatomic defects such as necrosis and loss of brush border from cellular functions, which more closely reflect cellular integrity, will offer better insights into the maintenance phase of ARF. Furthermore, continued study of maneuvers which are capable of protecting against ARF such as diets high in sodium or in calcium (7,8), administration of the calcium channel blocker, Verapamil (9), increased renal solute load (9,10), the diabetic condition in rats which may be independent of increased solute load (11), interference with the action of A II (12), administration of the Kallikrein antagonist, aprotinin (13,14), and inhibition of thromboxane with imidazole (14) should be valuable assets in future studies of the maintenance phase of ARF.

Hemodynamic and Toxic Models of Acute Renal Failure

Both complete and partial clamping of the renal artery are associated with a prompt decrease in renal blood flow which is accompanied by an increase in intrarenal vascular resistance. Following one hour of total renal artery occlusion, Arendeshorst (15) found that between 1 and 1½ hours after the release of the occlusion, renal blood flow was still reduced by approximately 40 percent and this was associated with increased renal resistance. Partial clamping of the renal artery was also found to result in approximately 40 percent decrease in superficial glomerular plasma flow after one hour (16).

The norepinephrine method of inducing experimental renal ischemia was first established by Fung (17) who demonstrated that prolonged intrarenal infusion of large doses of norepinephrine would cause unilateral oliguric ARF associated with blood flows and urine flows near zero. When the infusion is discontinued, there is slow restoration of blood flow which after 3 hours is still generally less than 50 percent of preinfusion values (18). Two factors which have been shown to influence the course of post-ischemic ARF are the duration of the ischemia and whether or not a normally functioning contralateral kidney is in place. In general, ischemia lasting for 3 minutes or less results in modest injury and is easily reversed. Progressive damage occurs the longer the ischemia persists. If ischemia is prolonged over a period of more than 2 hours, the injury is generally irreversible (19). It is of interest that when the contralateral kidney is removed in ischemic ARF, there is enhanced recovery of GFR compared to animals in which a normally functioning contralateral kidney is left in place (20).

Decreased renal blood flow does not seem to play a major role in maintaining renal functional impairment after the initial 24 to 48 hours of ARF. It has been shown in both the renal artery clamping and norepinephrine models that loading with Ringer solution has restored renal blood flow within 24 to 48 hours after the initial insult without significant improvement in GFR (15,19). Hence, although renal ischemia seems to be a common denominator in the initiation of the hemodynamic model, other factors must be responsible for the maintenance of ARF. There is evidence which strongly suggests that both tubular obstruction and tubular backleak play a role in the renal artery clamping model (15,21). But, both tubular obstruction and backleak vary with duration of ischemia and recovery, and backleak appears to be most prominent in the proximal straight tubules of juxtamedullary nephrons.

Several studies have focused on changes in the ultrafiltration coefficient (K_f) in ARF. In the norepinephrine model, a decrease in K_f has been noted by Cox et al. (19). Although structural findings may partially explain decreases in GRF their significance is uncertain. In the circumstances where vasoconstriction is present, K_f may fall in association with a decrease in surface of the glomerular capillaries, since it has been demonstrated that A II can cause a marked constriction of these capillaries (22). It has been demonstrated that there are specific A II receptors in the glomeruli (23). Studies have indicated that responses to A II were altered in ARF, suggesting that there may be an abnormal receptor response (24). However, studies performed at our institution to assess whether A II receptors were affected in ARF failed to show alteration (25). The binding of 1^{125} A II to isolated glomeruli was measured in rats with mercuric chloride induced renal failure. A high affinity binding site for A II in the rat glomerulus was found to be unaltered. Hence, the defect of glomerular response to A II does not appear to involve an abnormal receptor response.

GENTAMICIN NEPHROTOXICITY

Aminoglycoside nephrotoxicity is most commonly encountered secondary to administration of gentamicin and has become a relatively common cause of ARF in children and adults. The presentation is that of a gradual onset of non-oliguric renal failure which is frequently preceded by polyuria and decreased urine osmolality. The incidence is increased with serum gentamicin levels which exceed 10 ug/ml but it has also been reported in patients with therapeutic levels, and appears not to be directly related to total dose (26). Determinants of gentamicin nephrotoxicity include age, the balance between necrosis and regenerating cells, method of administration and duration of therapy (27, 28, 29). As in all categories of ARF sodium depletion, reduced renal mass and concomitant administration of other potentially nephrotoxic agents contribute to the incidence of ARF. Complete recovery after withdrawal of the drug is usual and all the aminoglycosides are readily dialyzed. Gentamicin therapy associated with other nephrotoxic drugs has been demonstrated to increase the nephrotoxic effects and in a controlled "double-blind" trial, Wade and colleagues (30) studied 90 patients treated for sepsis and demonstrated that aminoglycoside therapy associated with methacillin therapy resulted in renal toxicity in 7% of cases, whereas aminoglycoside and cephalothin therapy resulted in nephrotoxicity in 25% of patients. The recovery which occurs after withdrawal of the aminoglycosides may be delayed as much as 2 weeks and may be related to the half-life of the various aminoglycoside drugs. The half-life of gentamicin in human studies as well as in rat studies has been shown to be somewhere between 4 to 7 days (31).

The mechanism of gentamicin nephrotoxicity is still uncertain. The earliest anatomic correlate is an increase in the number and size of the secondary lysosomes followed by a decrease in the height and number of microvilli and swelling of mitochondria with cytoplasmic vacuolization (32). Formation of myloid bodies is prominent and reflects the intralysosomal accumulation of complex lipids. Studies of fibroblasts in tissue cultures shows uptake of gentamicin into lysosomes where it induces phospholipidosis with a decrease in lysosomal sphingomyelinase resulting in an increase in phospholipid content (33).

It is not understood precisely how these changes result in a persisting decrease in GFR in gentamicin nephrotoxicity. Despite the well proven functional and anatomic tubular effects of gentamicin, it has been difficult to demonstrate either tubular backleak or tubular obstruction. Baylis (34) has shown by micropuncture technique that at 10 days,40 mg/kg/day of gentamicin resulted in a 20 percent decrease of renal blood flow due to an increased resistance of the afferent and efferent arteries. But, at 4 mg/kg/day for 10 days the glomerular blood flow was not significantly reduced. Nevertheless, the GFR and single nephron GFR were reduced, and at all dose levels the GFR was proportionately more reduced than the renal blood flow. This relatively greater decrease in GFR than in renal blood flow was shown to be due to decreased permeability of the glomerulus (decrease K_f) and was the sole factor at lower doses of gentamicin. It was not possible to find a morphologic explanation for the decrease in K_f. Electron microscopic studies performed by Avasthi et al. (35,36), however, have shown anatomic changes in the glomeruli with gentamicin, or, more recently, with glycerol induced ARF. The fenestrae in the glomerular capillary were found to be decreased in area in comparison with controls. An effect of A II could explain the vascular effects which have been described. Angiotensin II converting enzyme inhibitor (Captopril) was given before and during gentamicin by Schor and his colleagues (12) to rats studied by micropuncture techniques. Whole kidney GFR and single nephron GFR were protected and did not decrease despite similar tubular damage in both the Captopril and control groups. Thus, the effects of gentamicin on glomerular microcirculation seem, at least in part, mediated by A II. Similar effects were shown by Ishikawa and Hollenberg (37) who demonstrated increased renal blood flow in glycerol induced ARF with both Captopril and an analogue of A II.

DIFFERENTIAL DIAGNOSIS OF ACUTE RENAL FAILURE IN CHILDREN

The conditions which are most commonly associated with ARF in children are listed in Table 2. Those related to volume contraction appear to be the most common, particularly secondary to gastrointestinal losses. Intrarenal causes secondary to a variety of severe glomerular nephropathies and toxic agents such as aminoglycosides are also common causes of ARF in children. Although post-renal (obstructive ARF) is uncommon, it is imperative to promptly rule out this possibility since surgical repair is usually curative, as in the case of congenital posterior urethral valves. Recent awareness, however, indicates that these children must be carefully followed since many have associated renal dysplasia and develop chronic renal insufficiency (38,39). Sonography performed at the bedside on admission is adequate to rule out obstructive causes of ARF. Examination of urine sediment and fractional excretion of sodium are most helpful in distinguishing renal parenchymal disorders when the history does not clarify the cause. Urine loaded with RBC, WBC, casts and containing excessive protein is typical of glomerular nephropathies. Interstitial nephropathies are characterized by predominately WBC excretion. Eosinophils in the urine sediment and sometimes associated with peripheral eosinophilia may be seen in hypersensitivity (allergic) nephritis. Fractional excretion of sodium (U sodium/P sodium $\div$ U creatinine/ P creatinine x 100) is less than 1 percent in children and less than 2 percent in young infants with a prerenal cause of ARF.

Table 2. Causes of ARF in infants and children*

Pre-renal: secondary to decreased effective renal blood flow or shock
- Dehydration
- Sepsis
- Heart failure
- Trauma
- Bilateral renal stenosis

Fulminant nephritis, especially
- Diffuse proliferative
- Interstitial allergic, toxic
- Rapidly progressive
- Necrotizing
- Possibly pyelonephritis

Congenital renal dysfunction
- Dysplasia
- Hypoplasia
- Agenesis
- Cystic kidney disease

Vascular and Thrombotic
- Hemolytic-uremic syndrome
- Renal vein thrombosis
- Acute cortical necrosis
- Malignant hypertension (especially with decreased GFR)
- Collagen-Vascular disease
- Post traumatic thrombosis

Post renal: secondary to outflow obstruction
- Posterior urethral valves
- Bilateral uretero-pelvic junction obstruction
- Inflammation
- Calculi
- Blood clots
- Tumors

*In approximate order of frequency

A number of substances have been used as intravenous provocative tests for pre-renal ARF. The objective is to increase the urine output to at least 2 cc/kg/hr within 30 minutes by the infusion of a test solution. Solutions which have been used are: normal or half-normal saline given in a dose of 40 cc/kg over 15-20 minutes; mannitol .5 g/kg of a 20% solution; and furosemide 2 mg/kg given over 10 to 15 minutes. If adequate urine flow, as defined above, is established the patient is then cautiously hydrated on the basis of the diagnosis of pre-renal ARF. If there is no adequate urine output after the provocative test, fluid is restricted to insensible water loss plus volume commensurate with urine output in order to avoid vascular volume overload. The distinction between ARF secondary to decreased intravascular volume and other mechanisms should be made decisively at the first opportunity since selection of opposite therapies (hydrate vs fluid restriction) depends on the outcome. Any urine obtained must be treasured as a golden elixir which upon examination will help to define the cause of ARF. The treatment of an established ARF is discussed in another section of this text and will not be dealt with here.

Table 3. Risk factors which predispose to ARF

Dehydration
Prior renal insufficiency
Hypertension
Diabetes mellitus (especially contrast ARF)
Hyperuricemia
Multiple nephrotoxic agents (e.g.: cephalothin plus aminoglycoside)
Advanced age

The most common cause of pre-renal failure is dehydration. This type of "failure" has been referred to as acute renal success because the renal response to decreased renal blood flow results in conservation of water and is appropriate. Nevertheless, with persistence, true acute renal failure ensues with decrease in GFR and urine flow even after adequate hydration is established. Children, and especially neonates who are acutely ill with sepsis, shock, acutely diminished plasma volume, heart failure and hypoxia,are at risk for developing ARF. Renal failure, secondary to renal vascular or parenchymal diseases is most frequently encountered in children in the setting of toxic nephropathies, renal vein thrombosis and hemolytic uremic syndrome, although virtually any rapidly progressive or severe proliferative nephritis can result in ARF. The two most commonly encountered causes of post-renal failure in children are posterior urethral valves and bilateral ureteropelvic or ureterovesical obstruction. These are readily identified by skilled sonography and relieved by prompt surgical intervention.

Factors which have been found to be important prognostic indicators in ARF are the age of the patient, amount of urine output, severity and reversibility of the cause, the clinical setting in which the ARF occurred and the associated biochemical and clinical abnormalities. Cowan and associates (40) confirmed the clinical observation which suggested that infants may be more resistant to gentamicin nephrotoxicity than older individuals. In a study of young puppies, they found that the relative resistance correlated with the lower GFR and lower cortical renal blood flow in the very young animals, hence although older age is a factor for increased risk, very young age provides the potential for a relative resistance to gentamicin nephrotoxicity.

Acute renal failure is a true emergency in which prompt and appropriate intervention will save patients' lives. The incidence of clinically significant ARF has fortunately diminished considerably over the past decade, probably because of increased awareness of predisposing factors and maneuvers in the early stages which may help reverse the process. For example, gentamicin nephrotoxicity is now recognized and monitored. At the first hint of decreasing renal function the drug is discontinued resulting in prompt restoration of function. Beneficial effects of the addition of .5 g/kg body weight of mannitol to the pump prime of cardiopulmonary bypass procedures has been shown to decrease the incidence of ARF in children in a randomized prospective study (41). In addition, risk factors predisposing to ARF are well recognized and averted (Table 3). With further understanding of the pathogenic mechanisms it can be expected that the incidence of ARF may decline even further in the future.

REFERENCES

1. Bywaters, EGL., and Beall, D.: Crush injuries with impairment of renal function. Brit. Med. 1:427, 1941.
2. Goormaghtigh, H.: Vascular and circulatory changes in renal cortex in the anuric crush-syndrome. Proc. Soc. Exptl. Biol. Med. 59:303, 1945.
3. Hayes, J.M., O'Connell, S.M.B., Siegel, L., Pryce, F.H., and Schreiner, G.E.: Renal renin and renin release in acute renal failure in the rat. Federation Proc. 27:629, 1968.
4. Humes, H.D.: Cellular pathophysiology of acute renal failure, Introductory Lecture. Am. Soc. of Nephrol., 15th Annual Meeting.
5. Sastrasinh, M., Weinberg, J.M., and Humes, H.D.: The degree of gentamicin (G)-induced acute renal failure in various states of Na balance is due to structural rather than functional renal abnormalities. Kidney Int. 23:207, 1983.
6. Johnston, P.A., Rennke, H., and Levinsky, N.G.: Effect of ischemia on proximal tubule fluid and glucose reabsorption. Kidney Int. 23:205, 1983.
7. Weinberg, J.M., Harding, P.G. and Humes, H.D.: Saline (NS) loading protects against tubular cell injury in H_gCL_2 (Hg) nephrotoxicity. Kidney Int. 21:226, 1982.
8. Elliott, W.C., Gilbert, D.N., DeFehr, J., Bennett, W.M., and McCarron, D.A.: Protection from experimental gentamicin (G) toxicity by dietary calcium (ca) loading. Kidney Int. 21:216, 1982.
9. Burke, T.J., Arnold, P.E., and Schrier, R.W.: Impairment of Mitochondrial (Mito) respiration (MR) and calcium (Ca) kinetics in ischemic acute renal failure (ARF): Prevention by impermeant solute (IS) and Ca membrane blocker. Kidney Int. 21:215, 1982.
10. Teschan, P.E. and Lawson, N.L.: Studies in acute renal failure. Prevention by osmotic diuresis and observations on the effect of plasma and extracellular volume expansion. Nephron 3:1, 1966.
11. Gouvea, W., Kelley, J., Alpert, H., Pardo, V., and Vaamonde, C.A.: Enhanced solute excretion fails to protect against gentamicin acute renal failure (G-ARF) in the phlorizin treated rat. Kidney Int. 21:217, 1982.
12. Shor, N., Ichiawa, I., Rennke, H.G., Troy, J.L., and Brenner, B.M.: Role of angiotensin II (A II) in gentamicin (G) nephrotoxicity. Clin. Res. 28:461, 1980.

13. Sinsteden, T.D., O'Neil, T.J., and Stein, J.H.: Studies on the protective effect of bradykinin (BR), mannitol (M) and furosemide (F) in norepinephrine (NE) induced acute renal failure (ARF) in the dog. Kidney Int. 21:224, 1982.
14. Klotman, P.E., Boatman, J., Baker, J.D., and Yarger, W.E.: Captopril stimulates thromboxane production and exacerbates nephrotoxic acute renal failure. Kidney Int. 23:205, 1983.
15. Arendhorst, W.J., Finn, W.F., and Gottschalk, C.W.: Pathogenesis of acute renal failure following renal ischemia in the rat. Circulation Res. 37:558, 1975.
16. Daugharty, T.M., Ueki, I.F., Mercer, T.F., and Brenner, B.M.: Dynamics of glomerular ultrafiltration in the rat. Response to ischemic injury. J. Clin. Invest. 53:105, 1974.
17. Fung, H.M.: Norepinephrine-induced unilateral acute renal failure. (Ph.D. Thesis). 1972. Winnepeg, Canada: University of Manitoba.
18. Mauk, R.H., Patak, R.V., Fadem, S.Z., Lifschitz, M.D., and Stein, J.H.: Effect of prostaglandin E administration in a nephrotic and a vasoconstrictor model of acute renal failure. Kidney Int. 12:122, 1977.
19. Cox, J.W., Baehler, R.W., Sharma, H., O'Dorisio, T., Osgood, R.W., Stein, J.H., and Ferris, T.F.: Studies on the mechanisms of oliguria in a model of unilateral acute renal failure. J. Clin. Invest. 53:1546, 1974.
20. Fried, T., Hishida, A., and Stein, J.H.: Studies on the protective effect of chronic uninephrectomy in renal ischemia in the rat. Kidney Int. 23:203, 1983.
21. Tanner, G.A., and Sophasan, S.: Kidney pressures after temporary renal artery occlusion in the rat. Am. J. Physiol. 230:1173, 1976.
22. Hornych, H., and Richet, G.: Dissociated effect of sodium intake on glomerular and pressure responses to angiotensin. Kidney Int. 11:28, 1977.
23. Sraer, J.D., Ardaillou, R., and Mimoune, O.: Evidence for renal glomerular receptors for angiotensin II. Kidney Int. 6:241, 1974.
24. Wilkes, B.M., Caldicott, J.H., Schulman, G., and Hollenberg, N.K.: Loss of the glomerular contractile response to angiotensin in rats following myohemoglobinuric acute renal failure. Circ. Res. 49:1190, 1981.
25. Bellucci, A. and Wilkes, B.M.: Glomerular angiotensin (A II) receptors are normal in acute renal failure. Kidney Int. 21:214, 1982.
26. Smith, C.R., Maxwell, R.R., Edwards, C.Q., Rogers, J.F., Leitman, P.S.: Nephrotoxicity induced by gentamicin and amikacin. Johns Hopkins Med. J. 142:85, 1978.
27. Houghton, D.C., Campbell-Boswell, M.V., Bennett, W.M., Portor, A.J. and Brooks, R.E.: Myeloid bodies in the renal tubules of humans: Relationship to gentamicin therapy. Clin. Nephrol. 10:140, 1978.
28. Kosek J.D., Mazze, R.I. and Cousins, M.J.: Nephrotoxicity of gentamicin. Lab. Invest. 30:48, 1974.
29. Fabre, J., Rudhart, M., Blanchard, P. and Regamey, C.: Persistence of sisomicin and gentamicin in renal cortex and medulla compared with other organs and serum of rats. Kidney Int. 10:444, 1976.
30. Wade, J.C., Petty, B.G., Conrad, G., Smith, C.R., Lipsky, J.J., and Ellner, J.: Cephalothin plus an aminoglycoside is more nephrotoxic than methicillin plus an aminoglycoside. Lancet II 604:1978.
31. Luft, F.C. and Kleit, S.A.: Renal parenchymal accumulation of aminoglycoside antibiotics in rats. J. Infect. Dis. 130:656, 1974.

32. Alfthan, O., Renkonen, O.V. and Sivonen, A. Concentration of gentamicin in serum, urine and urogenital tissue in man. Acta Pathol. Microbiol. Scand. (B) (suppl. 241):92, 1973.
33. Aubert-Tulkens, G., Van Hoof, F., Tulkens, P.: Gentamicin-induced lysosomal phospholipidoses in cultured rat fibroblasts. Lab. Invest. 40:481, 1979.
34. Baylis, C.: The mechanisms of the decline in glomerular filtration rate in gentamicin induced acute renal failure in the rat. J. of Antimicrobial Chemotherapy. 6(3):381, 1980.
35. Avasthi, P.S., Huser, J., and Evan, A.P.: Glomerular endothelial cells in gentamicin-induced acute renal failure in rats. Kidney Int. 16:771, 1979.
36. Avasthi, P., Evan, A.P., and Hay, D.: Glomerular endothelial cells in uranyl nitrate-induced acute renal failure in rats. J. of Clin. Invest. 65:121, 1980.
37. Ishikawa, I. and Hollenberg, N.K.: Pharmacologic interruption of the renin-angiotensin system in myohemoglobinuric acute renal failure. Kidney Int., (suppl. 183), Oct. 1976.
38. Warshaw, B.L., Edelbrook, H.H., Ettenger, R.B., Malekzadeh, M.H., Pennis, A.J., Vittenbogaart, C.H., and Fine, R.N.: Progression to end-stage renal disease in children with obstructive uropathy. J. of Pediat. 100:183, 1982.
39. Atwell, J.D.: Posterior urethral valves in the British Isles: a multicenter B.A.P.S. review. J. Pediat. Surg. 18:70, 1983.
40. Cowan, R.H., Jakkola, A.F. and Arant, B.S.: Pathophysiologic evidence of gentamicin nephrotoxicity in neonatal puppies. Ped. Research 11:1204, 1980.
41. Barratt, T.M. and Rigden, S.P.A.: In: Alan B. Gruskin and Michael E. Norman, eds. Pediatric Nephrology-Proceedings of the Fifth International Pediatric Nephrology Symposium, 1980. Boston: Martinus Nijhoff Publishers 1980, pp. 278-96.

MINERAL METABOLISM IN ACUTE RENAL FAILURE

Michael Freundlich, M.D., Gaston Zilleruelo, M.D.
and José Strauss, M.D.

Disturbances in divalent ion metabolism are well known consequences of chronic renal failure (CRF). An in-depth review of the recent extensive literature about these disturbances is beyond the scope and goals of this chapter. However, in brief, hyperparathyroidism secondary to CRF apparently develops through two major mechanisms (both with lowered serum ionized calcium): hyperphosphatemia and acquired vitamin D resistance. It has been suggested (1) that hyperphosphatemia resulting from decreased glomerular filtration rate is one of the main causes of the hypocalcemia and secondary hyperparathyroidism of CRF. The second mechanism, vitamin D resistance (truly a reduced generation of active vitamin D due to a diminished functional renal mass), decreases intestinal absorption of calcium resulting in hypocalcemia, secondary hyperparathyroidism, and delayed mineralization of osteoid (2). Furthermore, skeletal resistance to the calcemic action of both exogenous and endogenous parathyroid hormone (PTH) has been demonstrated in patients with CRF (3), partly due to deficiency of 1,25-dihydroxyvitamin D ($1,25(OH)_2D$) (4). Studies dealing with alterations of mineral metabolism in acute renal failure (ARF) are rather scanty, and limited almost exclusively to patients in the adult age group. Pertinent information from these studies follows.

Acute renal failure is defined as the sudden suppression of the kidney's ability to regulate urine volume and composition according to the body needs (5). It should not be surprising, then, that an abrupt cessation of renal functional capabilities could lead to disturbances in divalent ion metabolism. Indeed, hyperphosphatemia, hypermagnesemia and hypocalcemia have been noted during the oliguric phase of ARF (6,7). The elevated serum concentration of both inorganic phosphorus and magnesium is due to their retention secondary to the inability of the failing kidney to excrete them.

A systematic evaluation of several aspects of divalent ion metabolism in 10 adult patients with ARF was reported (6). Those patients were studied during the oliguric and diuretic phases of the illness and following recovery of their renal function. Hyperphosphatemia occurred in all patients during the oliguric phase, and the maximum elevation in serum inorganic phosphorus ranged from mild to severe (5.2 to 11.0 mg/dl). The levels fell to normal or lower during the diuretic phase, and normalized upon recovery from renal failure. Hypermagnesemia was an almost universal finding during the oliguric phase; serum magnesium fell to a normal or slightly subnormal level during the diuretic phase, and was normal after recovery of renal function.

Hypocalcemia was invariably noted during the oliguric phase and occurred as early as two days after the onset of renal failure. The lowest values of serum calcium observed in the various patients ranged from 5.3 to 7.5 mg/dl. Hypocalcemia usually persisted during the diuretic phase and normalized after recovery of renal function. Transient hypercalcemia developed during the diuretic phase in one of the patients studied. The levels of immunoreactive PTH were persistently elevated in almost all patients during the oliguric phase and remained elevated during the diuretic period in all except one patient who had normal values during the oliguric phase.

Several factors may contribute to the hypocalcemia of ARF, including hyperphosphatemia, hypomagnesemia and magnesium depletion, hypoalbuminemia or alterations in calcium binding by serum protein, failure of parathyroid gland function and skeletal resistance to the actions of PTH.

No relationship was found between the concentration of serum calcium and phosphorus during the oliguric and diuretic phases of ARF (6) (Figs. 1 and 2). Hypocalcemia was observed with low, normal or elevated serum phosphorus, suggesting that hyperphosphatemia is not the only cause of the hypocalcemia. Since hypocalcemia occurred with elevated serum magnesium concentration, hypomagnesemia could not be incriminated in the genesis of hypocalcemia (8). Inasmuch as serum albumin was normal in those patients, hypoalbuminemia was not the cause of the hypocalcemia.

The finding of elevated levels of PTH in patients with ARF (6,9) clearly demonstrates that hyperactivity of the parathyroid gland occurs early in the course of ARF; this was also present within hours after the onset of ARF in rats (10). Furthermore, the inverse relationship between serum calcium and PTH concentrations indicates that the parathyroid gland responds appropriately to the hypocalcemia (6) (Fig. 3).

The infusion of PTH extract did not cause a significant increase in serum calcium concentration during the oliguric and diuretic phases, in contrast to the normocalcemic response (1.4 ± 0.14 Δ mg/dl) after recovery of renal function (6). Based on this information, it may be concluded that patients with ARF rapidly develop (within days) skeletal resistance to the calcemic action of PTH, and that this may be the primary cause of the hypocalcemia (6,11).

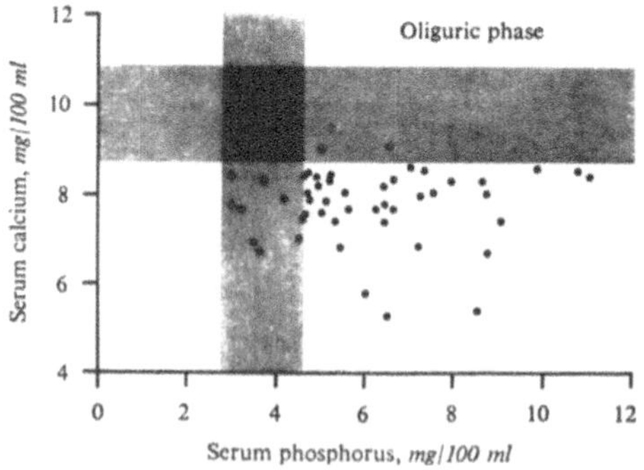

Figure 1. Relationship between the concentrations of serum calcium and phosphorus in adults during the oliguric phase of acute renal failure. Shaded areas represent the normal range. (Reproduced from p. 439 of Massry SG, Arieff AI, Coburn JW et al.: Divalent metabolism in patients with acute renal failure: Studies on the mechanism of hypocalcemia. Kidney Int 5:437-445, 1974 with permission.)

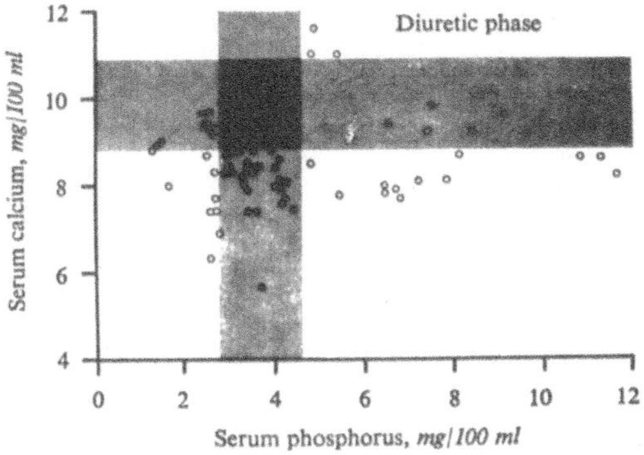

Figure 2. Relationship between the concentrations of serum calcium and phosphorus in adults during the diuretic phase of acute renal failure. (Reproduced from p. 441 of Massry SG, Arieff AI, Coburn JW et al.: Divalent metabolism in patients with acute renal failure: Studies on the mechanism of hypocalcemia. Kidney Int 5:437-445, 1974 with permission.)

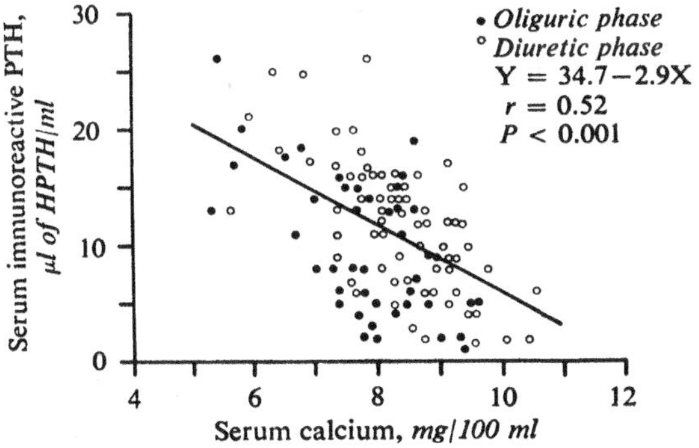

Figure 3. Relation between PTH and serum calcium in a group of adults with acute renal failure. (Reproduced from p 441 of Massry SG, Arieff AI, Coburn JW et al.: Divalent metabolism in patients with acute renal failure: Studies on the mechanism of hypocalcemia. Kidney Int 5:437-445, 1974 with permission.)

The precise mechanisms for the skeletal resistance are not entirely understood, but recently acquired data demonstrated low levels of 25-hydroxycholecalciferol (about 50% of normal) (12) and 1,25 $(OH)_2D$ (13) in the sera of patients with ARF. The low levels of 1,25 $(OH)_2D$, by decreasing intestinal calcium absorption, may further contribute to the persistence of hypocalcemia.

Various clinical circumstances, when associated with ARF, may accentuate disturbances of serum calcium and phosphorus.

1. Patients with rhabdomyolysis-induced ARF display a more prominent hyperphosphatemia and hypocalcemia than patients with ARF due to other causes (13,14), presumably due to the exaggerated phosphorus generation by the damaged tissues. The excess phosphorus, once in the extracellular space, should enhance deposition of calcium from the extracellular space into the injured muscle, thus leading to more severe hypocalcemia. Calcification of damaged muscles has been documented in those patients (11).
2. Hyperphosphatemia and hypocalcemia have been noted to occur in children with acute lymphoblastic leukemia hours after the initiation of chemotherapy, presumably by the high phosphorus load resulting from destruction of lymphoblasts, in a manner similar to the hyperuricemia which results from purine release (15,16).
3. The administration of fleet phospho-soda enemas has been associated with hypocalcemia and hyperphosphatemia in children with normal renal function (17) or with ARF (18); even tetany has been described in patients with chronic renal disease (19). The absorption of phosphate from the enemas leads to marked elevation of serum phosphate and concomitant lowering of serum calcium.
4. Newborn infants, in particular prematures, are prone to develop hypocalcemia shortly after birth (20); vitamin D deficiency or its altered metabolism, insufficient intake of vitamin D and calcium, exaggerated phosphate load from cow's milk, and hypercalciuria, seem to contribute to the hypocalcemia (21,22). It is conceivable that ARF in newborn infants is associated with more prominent changes in divalent ion metabolism; however, detailed studies are lacking.

Hypercalcemia also may occur with ARF, (mainly that associated with rhabdomyolysis) during the diuretic phase (11). The hypercalcemia observed in the recovery phase may be related to high levels of 1,25 $(OH)_2$ D, increased calcium mobilization from bone and soft tissue due to secondary hyperparathyroidism, and recovery of renal function (13). Finally, the type of renal disease leading to ARF may determine the alterations in mineral metabolism, since 1,25 $(OH)_2$ D is produced in the mitochondria of the tubular cells of the renal cortex (23). Children with CRF due to predominantly renal-tubular disease were shown to have lower levels of serum vitamin D than those with glomerulopathies (24). Similar data are lacking for patients with ARF.

The management of divalent ion disturbances in ARF includes utilization of phosphate-binding agents, appropriate nutritional support (to prevent excessive catabolism), and dialysis when clinically indicated. Hypocalcemia generally does not require treatment unless tetany or other symptoms occur. Attempts to correct hypocalcemia by the administration of supplemental calcium, without a lowering of the elevated serum phosphorus, can lead to widespread calcium deposition in soft tissues, involving vital organs such as the lungs and heart, and can cause severe cardiopulmonary insufficiency (11).

In summary, alterations in the serum concentration of divalent ions are frequently associated with the establishment of ARF. Those alterations, namely hyperphosphatemia, hypocalcemia and hypermagnesemia, can be accompanied by decreased circulating vitamin D and elevated serum PTH levels. The low levels of vitamin D seem to be an important contributing (or possibly initiating) factor to the hypocalcemia. The latter may lead occasionally to overt symptomatology (tetany, seizures), and only then is the parenteral administration of supplemental calcium indicated.

REFERENCES

1. Slatopolsky E, Caglar S, Pennell JP et al.: On the pathogenesis of hyperparathyroidism in chronic experimental renal insufficiency in the dog. J Clin Invest 50:492-499, 1971.
2. Massry SG, Ritz E, Verbeckmoes R: Role of phosphate in the genesis of secondary hyperparathyroidism. Nephron 18:77-81, 1977.
3. Massry SG, Coburn JW, Lee DBN et al.: Skeletal resistance to parathyroid hormone in renal failure: Studies in 105 human subjects. Ann Intern Med 78:357-364, 1973.
4. Massry SG, Stein R, Garty J et al.: Skeletal resistance to the calcemic action of parathyroid hormone in uremia: Role of $1,25\ (OH)_2\ D_3$. Kidney Int 9:467-474, 1976.
5. Williams GS, Klemk EL, Winters RW: Acute renal failure in pediatrics. In *The Body Fluids in Pediatrics*. Winters RW (ed). Boston: Little, Brown and Company, 1973, pp 523-557.
6. Massry SG, Arieff AI, Coburn JW et al.: Divalent ion metabolism in patients with acute renal failure: Studies on the mechanism of hypocalcemia. Kidney Int 5:437-445, 1974.
7. Grossman RA, Hamilton RW, Morse BM et al.: Non-traumatic rhabdomyolysis and acute renal failure. New Engl J Med 291:807-811, 1974.
8. Estep H, Shaw W, Waltington CO et al.: Hypocalcemia due to reversible hypomagnesemia and parathyroid hormone unresponsiveness. J Clin Endocrinol 29:842-848, 1969.
9. Kovithavongs T, Becker FO, Ing TS: Parathyroid hyperfunction in acute renal failure. Nephron 9:349-355, 1972.
10. Jastak JT, Morrison AB, Raisz LG: Effects of renal insufficiency on the parathyroid gland and calcium homeostasis. Am J Physiol 215:84-89, 1968.
11. Massry SG: Disturbances in divalent ions and vitamin D in acute renal failure. In *Acute Renal Failure*, Eliahov HE (ed). London: Libbeg, 1982, pp 277-282.

12. Pietrek J, Kokot F, Kuska J: Serum 25-hydroxyvitamin D and parathyroid hormone in patients with acute renal failure. Kidney Int 13:178-185, 1978.
13. Llach F, Felsenfeld AJ, Haussler MR: The pathophysiology of altered calcium metabolism in rhabdomyolysis-induced acute renal failure. New Engl J Med 305:117-123, 1981.
14. Koffler A, Friedler RM, Massry SG: Acute renal failure due to non-traumatic rhabdomyolysis. Ann Intern Med 85:23-28, 1978.
15. Zusman J, Brown DM, Nesbit ME: Hyperphosphatemia, hyperphosphaturia and hypocalcemia in acute lymphoblastic leukemia. New Engl J Med 289:1335-1340, 1973.
16. Jaffe N, Paed D, Kim BS et al.: Hypocalcemia-A complication of childhood leukemia. Cancer 29:392-398, 1972.
17. Davis RF, Eichner JM, Bleyer WA et al.: Hypocalcemia, hyperphosphatemia and dehydration following a single hypertonic phosphate enema. J Pediatr 90:484-485, 1977.
18. McConnell TH: Fatal hypocalcemia from phosphate reabsorption from a laxative preparation. JAMA 216:147-148, 1971.
19. Chesney RW, Haughton PB: Tetany following phosphate enemas in chronic renal disease. Am J Dis Chil 127:584-586, 1974.
20. Wald MK: Problems in chemical adaptation: Glucose, calcium and magnesium. In *Care of the High-Risk Neonate*, Klaus M and Fanaroff AA (eds). Philadelphia: WB Saunders Publishing Co., 1978, pp 224-242.
21. Freundlich M, Strauss J: Calcium, vitamin D and parathyroid hormone. Related aspects in the neonatal period. In *Neonatal Kidney and Fluid-Electrolytes*, Strauss J (ed.). Boston: Martinus Nijhoff, 1983, pp 127-135.
22. Arant BS: Renal handling of calcium and phosphorus in normal human neonates. Semin Nephrol 3:94-99, 1983.
23. Midgett RJ, Spielvogel AM, Coburn JW et al.: Studies on calciferol metabolism: VII. The renal production of the biologically active form of vitamin D, 1,25 dihydroxycholecalciferol: Species, tissue and subcellular distribution. J Clin Endocrinol 36:1153-1161, 1973.
24. Chesney RW, Hamstra AJ, Mazess RB et al.: Circulating vitamin D metabolite concentrations in childhood renal diseases. Kidney Int 21:65-69, 1982.

ANTIMICROBIAL THERAPY IN RENAL FAILURE

Heinz F. Eichenwald, M.D.

Whenever it is necessary to administer antimicrobial agents to a child with varying degrees of renal impairment, questions arise which have never been entirely satisfactorily resolved. Should dosage be decreased? Should the interval between doses be changed? How can the risk of drug toxicity be reduced? The situation is particularly difficult in infants and young children in whom renal function may be impaired by disease or immaturity while metabolic processes operate differently from those of older individuals. Because of the multiplicity of factors acting on the metabolism and/or excretion of an antimicrobial agent, these problems can only sometimes be solved by the use of tools such as a normogram which relates creatinine clearance and the proportion of an antibiotic excreted in the kidney to the amount and frequency with which a drug needs to be administered. Under some circumstances, such an approach may result in serious errors or over- or under-medication.

Furthermore, a related problem also requires solution: how does one treat a urinary tract infection in a child with depressed renal function? In addition, the problem of cumulative drug toxicity and interactions needs consideration or, to ask the question differently: how can synergistic toxicity of unrelated drugs on the kidney and other organs be avoided? Finally, a considerable body of data suggest that certain antimicrobial agents may damage the already damaged kidney further even when serum levels have been closely controlled. How can one deal with this situation?

Obviously, in the presence of decreased renal function, drugs that are excreted by the kidney need to be reduced in dosage, if accumulation of the agent in the blood is to be avoided. This is far simpler said than done; various schemes have been presented by which the physician can adjust dosage, either by increasing the interval or by using less drug in each dose. The use of these methods of calculation rarely, if ever, results in a dose-response curve identical to that found in normal children. The best that can be done is to attempt to approximate this; one is perpetually caught on the edge of producing drug levels too low to be optimally effective or so high as to be potentially toxic. Toxicity is, of course, a relative term and individual patients respond quite differently to what appear to be identical situations. Little harm is done, for example, if a drug depresses the upper frequency range of hearing to 18,000 hertz, an event probably not uncommon when aminoglycosides are administered to patients for significant periods of time. However, the severity of drug toxicity, like most biologic events, follows a bell-shaped distribution. There are recorded instances where infants received as much as 100 mg/kg/day of kanamycin for periods of two weeks or more: most of these babies escaped without permanent hearing loss, others were rendered totally deaf, with the majority demonstrating only hearing losses confined to the highest frequencies. Predictably also, some few children may experience major hearing losses following the use of aminoglycosides in entirely appropriate dosage. Thus, dosage that may be entirely safe in the great majority of patients may be harmful to individuals who cannot be identified to be at special risk prior to the start of treatment.

How does one adjust drug dosage in the presence of various degrees of renal failure? All the various schemes and mathematical formulations that have been proposed make certain assumptions which, in individual cases, may not be valid. These have been listed by Kauffman as follows:

1) The kinetics of the drug must be reasonably described as a one compartment, open model with first order elimination.
2) It is assumed that glomerular filtration and tubular function decrease to the same extent in renal failure, so that the elimination of a drug that undergoes tubular secretion and/or reabsorption is decreased proportionately to the decrease in glomerular filtration rate.
3) The distribution and nonrenal elimination of a drug are not altered in the presence of renal failure. There are instances where this assumption cannot be made.
4) There are no pharmacologically active metabolites that may

accumulate. Again, for a few drugs, this assumption is not valid.

5) The concentration-response relationship of the drug does not change in renal failure.

Nearly all methods that relate drug dosage to renal function utilize the creatinine clearance to determine the drug's elimination rate constant. Serum creatinine concentration has also been used but is so susceptible to large errors that it should not be employed for dosage calculations with drugs that have a narrow margin of safety. Creatinine clearance levels provide a better estimate but must be used cautiously in situations where there is changing renal function or the patient has certain metabolic derangements such as starvation, immobilization, acidemia, shock, myopathies and so forth. Kauffman and Habersang, basing their work on the methods of Dettli and Spring, developed a number of equations which provide reasonably accurate dosage information in a number of specified circumstances for drugs that are markedly, moderately, or slightly retained in patients with renal failure (Tables 1, 2, 3).

Table 1.

Antimicrobials <u>Markedly</u> Retained In Patients with Renal Failure	
Vancomycin	Polymyxins
Aminoglycosides	Tetracyclines

Table 2.

Antimicrobials <u>Moderately</u> Retained In Patients with Renal Failure	
All penicillins	Lincomycin
All cephalosporins	Clindamycin

Table 3.

Antimicrobials <u>Slightly</u> Retained In Patients with Renal Failure	
Erythromycin	Chloramphenicol
Nitrofurantoin	Isoniazid
Nalidixic acid	Amphotericin B

These schemes call for the administration of the usual loading dose; for drugs that are mostly excreted by the kidney, dosage adjustment is then made by increasing the interval of administration rather than by varying the individual doses. Obviously when a drug is being administered by a continuous intravenous infusion, no changes in interval are possible; in such a situation one simply multiplies the usual infusion rate by the patient's elimination rate of the drug as a fraction of normal which provides the proper infusion rate of the drug. Less obvious is the fact that dosage adjustment for drugs that are only partially excreted by the kidney cannot readily be made in increasing the interval but requires a reduction in the maintenance doses. This latter approach may result in instances where bactericidal levels are not reached because the calculated dosage tends to flatten the dose-response curve. Nevertheless, in children older than three or four years whose clinical problems relate primarily to the kidney, these various calculations do provide the physician with at least a dosage to start with. In younger children and especially infants with varying degrees of renal failure and/or other organ involvement, dosages based on creatinine clearance are often unsatisfactory, in some instances resulting in suboptimal levels of drug and, in other situations, potentially harmful ones. No amount of sophisticated calculation can provide the physician with entirely safe and reliable data in these young patients; only by direct measurement of drug levels at various intervals of time can appropriate adjustments in dosage be made (Table 4). This,

Table 4. Determination of Drug Dosages in Infants and Young Children with Renal Impairment

1) Administer usual loading dose
2) Obtain 4 - 6 serum specimens for drug assay at intervals over a 12 - 48 hour period (depending on degree of renal failure)
3) Plot measured antibiotic concentrations against time on semi-log paper
4) Estimate half-life from regression line
5) For moderate renal dysfunction, give 2/3 usual dose every 3 half-lives; for severe dysfunction, 1/2 usual dose every 2 half-lives

of course, produces a number of technical difficulties: many hospitals are unable to provide the physician with accurately measured antimicrobial blood levels. When these tests are available, they are generally performed by microbiologic methods requiring at least 24 hours for completion as well as sizable quantities of blood.

The use of high pressure liquid chromatography allows rapid and accurate determination of serial serum specimens using small amounts of blood. Most of our problems relating to dosage will be solved once this technique becomes generally available.

Failing the ability to measure antimicrobial concentrations directly, an approximation can be made using a scheme developed by my colleague John Nelson, which is shown in Table 5. While this approach provides reasonably accurate results, it does require certain assumptions. If these are not valid, the information obtained may be quite misleading. As a temporary "stopgap" measure, however, Dr. Nelson's method has much to recommend it, and in young children is clearly superior to those based on creatinine clearance.

Table 5. Determination of Drug Dosage in Infants and Young Children if Antibiotic Assay Cannot Be Done

1) Make 2-fold dilutions of patient's serum obtained 2, 4, and 8 hours after administration

2) Add 10^5 bacteria of strain isolated from patient

3) Incubate over-night, and read minimum inhibitory titer

4) Interpretation: for aminoglycosides, effective and non-toxic range is 1:2 - 1:8 against gram-negative bacteria. For penicillins and cephalosporins, effective and non-toxic range is 1:8 - 1:64 against Staphylococcus aureus.

The second problem relates to the use of antimicrobial agents to treat infections of the urinary tract in patients with reduced renal function. Under such circumstances, drugs excreted by the kidney to only a limited degree may not attain effective levels in the urine. For example, if only 5% of a drug is normally excreted by the kidney, the agent might prove ineffective when administered to an individual with considerable loss of renal function. It is often not possible to bypass the problem by increasing the dosage of medication to obtain higher serum levels, so that more drugs might appear in the urine, because the agent may then prove toxic to other organs. Even in those instances where a drug is normally completely cleared by the kidney, it may not be possible to achieve adequate urine levels; when high serum levels occur because of renal failure, the drug may be metabolized in other organs, leaving only inadequate quantities to be excreted in the urine. Nitrofurantoin represents an excellent example of such a drug; it is normally eliminated rapidly in the urine but if excretion of the agent is inhibited by renal failure, the amount of drug in circulation increases sufficiently to allow metabolism to an inactive form. Under such circumstances, effective urine levels cannot be achieved, no matter how high the serum levels might be.

A somewhat different situation applies to the aminoglycosides where the range between therapeutic and toxic level is small. Because of renal failure, little drug appears in the urine, often too little to treat an infection, and serum levels progressively rise. An increase in dosage in order to obtain therapeutic urine levels would carry with it unacceptable risks of toxicity.

How can this situation be circumvented? This has become quite easy because of the availabilty of relatively safe, highly effective, and reasonably nontoxic drugs such as the "gram-negative" penicillins, including ampicillin, amoxicillin, mezlocillin, azlocillin and piperacillin, as well as a number of cephalosporins. With these drugs, dosage may safely be increased to produce serum levels three to five times those of normal; under such circumstances, enough of the drug will appear in the urine to be effective.

A topic requiring only brief discussion relates to the occasional synergistic toxicity produced by interactions between unrelated drugs. Diuretics, such as ethacrynic acid, may potentiate the risk of auditory toxicity from gentamicin administration. Additionally, some data suggest that concurrent use of methicillin with an aminoglycoside enhances both the frequency of occurrence and the severity of renal toxicity. The first example can readily be avoided by using a penicillin or a cephalosporin (not cephaloridine) instead of an aminoglycoside while in the second instance, nafcillin can be used in older children instead of methicillin, or moxolactam instead of aminoglycosides in infants less than three months of age.

What can one do about the problem that certain antimicrobial agents may damage the already injured kidney further (Table 6)? There is only

Table 6. Antimicrobial Agents That May Further Injure Already Damaged Kidneys

Sulfonamides	Rifampin
TMP - SMX	Amphotericin B
Nitrofurantoin	Tetracyclines
Polymyxins	

one way to avoid this, and that consists of not using any of these drugs in patients with kidney disease. Little of therapeutic significance is lost if a physician has to avoid the use of polymyxins, sulfonamides, and tetracyclines, agents which rarely are drugs of first choice in the treatment of any infection. Amphotericin B may need to be used in certain systemic mycotic diseases, as does rifampin in tuberculosis or trimethoprim-sulfa in some unusual diseases; when these drugs are employed in patients with diminished renal function, careful monitoring of the kidney throughout the course of therapy is mandatory.

Taking into account all of these do's and don'ts, one might reasonably ask, "will there ever be an ideal antimicrobial drug for use in patients with renal disease?". Such an agent should possess sufficiently low toxicity that even five or tenfold increases in blood levels can be tolerated safely. The drug must have little or no nephrotoxicity, be excreted completely by the kidney in active form and be sufficiently active against bacteria causing urinary tract infections that even small amounts of drug in the urine would suffice. Finally, the agent should be stable in serum and not metabolized by the liver or other organs when high serum levels are achieved.

Drugs with all of these characteristics are already available to the physician among the cephalosporins and penicillins. Every one of the problems I have discussed can be avoided or at least greatly minimized by choosing a drug from among these two groups of antibiotics. Only for long term suppression of infection is an ideal agent not at hand because when these antibiotics are administered for a prolonged period, resistant strains of bacteria sooner or later appear.

REFERENCES

1. Dettli, L: Elimination kinetics and drug dosage in renal insufficiency, Triangle 14, 117, 1975.

2. Dettli, L: Drug dosage in renal disease, Clin. Pharmacokinet. 1, 126, 1976.

3. Jusko, W et al: Pharmacokinetics of gentamicin during peritoneal dialysis in children, Kidney Int. 9, 430, 1976.

4. Kauffman, RE and Habersang, R: Modification of dosage regimens in disease states of childhood, in "Clinical Pharmacology and Therapeutics: a Pediatric Perspective", BL Merkin (ed.) Year Book Publ. 1978.

5. Pagliaro, LA and Benet, LZ: Critical compilation of terminal half-lives, percent excreted unchanged and changes of half-life in renal and hepatic dysfunction for studies in humans with references. J. Pharmacokinet. Biopharm. 3, 333, 1975.

6. Sirinavin, S et al: Determining gentamicin dosage in infants and children with renal failure, J. Pediatr. 96, 331, 1980.

7. Spring, P: Calculation of drug dosage regimens in patients with renal disease: A new normographic method, Int. J. Clin. Pharmacol. Biopharm. 2, 76, 1975.

THERAPEUTIC APPROACH TO THE CHILD WITH ACUTE RENAL FAILURE

Alan B. Gruskin, H. Jorge Baluarte, Martin S. Polinsky, Bruce A. Kaiser, Sharon A. Perlman, Bruce Z. Morgenstern

General Overview

Acute renal failure (ARF) may be defined as a symptom complex that occurs when body fluid homeostasis is impaired by the rapid loss of kidney function. The diagnosis and pathophysiology of ARF are considered elsewhere in this volume. The past few decades have brought about major advances in the treatment of the biochemical derangements, hypertension, and fluid imbalance associated with acute renal failure. With widespread availability of dialysis, mortality has markedly decreased; those deaths that do occur are related more to the primary disorder and its complications than to renal failure. Therapy for acute renal failure depends upon the nature or the degree of renal impairment.

Two somewhat overlapping approaches are used to treat ARF. One is based primarily on identifying and treating the discrete biochemical and physiologic derangements associated with ARF, and the other is based on the consideration that the different disorders giving rise to ARF require different management priorities and perhaps specific treatment. Therapy for discrete complications of ARF as well as specific approaches to the management of children with pre-, intra-or post-renal ARF, will be considered. A number of reviews on various aspects of ARF in children are available (1-5) as are the details of treating neonates with ARF (6-8).

TRANSPORTATION TO SPECIALIZED PEDIATRIC NEPHROLOGY CENTERS

Depending upon the etiology and magnitude of renal impairment, children are often transferred to specialized pediatric centers for further care. A number of potential complications of acute renal failure should be considered when the acutely ill child is evaluated and stabilized prior to transfer. These problems include: hypervolemia with cardiac failure, acute pulmonary edema, acute hypertensive crisis, hypotension, encephalopathy, seizures, hyperkalemia, hyponatremia, and hypocalcemia. Whenever possible a physician should accompany the child during transport, because changes can occur rapidly. Appropriate supplies and medications should be available during transport.

SPECIFIC THERAPY FOR UNDERLYING DISORDERS

Acute renal failure may result from primary renal disorders as well as systemic and vascular disorders for which specific therapies are available.(9-13) Recognition of such disorders and prompt initiation of appropriate therapy may prevent the development of ARF. Stabilization of renal function and resolution of the underlying disease process may be achieved with specific and supportive therapy in such cases. These disorders and their current therapies are listed in Table I. Acute renal failure caused by nephrotoxins or drug-induced interstitial nephritis may be amenable to therapy and often requires nothing more than discontinuation or removal of the offending agent (Tables II & III).

Table I: SPECIFIC THERAPIES FOR DISORDERS ASSOCIATED WITH ARF

DISORDER	THERAPY
Hypovolemia: Acute Blood Loss	Blood Replacement
Acute Dehydration	Intra-vascular volume repletion
Hypoxemia	Oxygenation, Transfusion (if anemic)
Post Infectious Nephritis	
Streptococcus	Treatment of siblings
Ventriculo-Atrial Shunt	Removal of shunt, Antibiotics
SBE	Antibiotics, Cardiac surgery
Rapidly Progressive Glomerulonephritis (RPGN)	
Goodpasture Syndrome	Plasmapheresis
Idiopathic RPGN	Pulse methylprednisolone 30 mg/kg qod for 14 days Cyclophosphamide 2mg/kg day, or Azathioprine 2 mg/kg/day
Systemic Lupus Erythematosus	Pulse methylprednisolone, or Prednisone 2 mg/kg/day Cyclophosphamide 2mg/kg/day Plasmapheresis

Table I: (Continued)

Renal Artery Stenosis (bilateral)	Percutaneous transluminal angioplasty, Surgery
Vasculitis	
Hypersensitivity Angiitis	Prednisone 2 mg/kg/day, Cyclophosphamide 1-3 mg/kg/day
Polyarteritis	Prednisone 2 mg/kg/day Azathioprine 2 mg/kg/day, Cyclophosphamide 1-3 mg/kg/day
Wegener's Granulomatosis	Cyclophosphamide 2 mg/kg/day

Table II: AGENTS ASSOCIATED WITH NEPHROTOXIN INDUCED ARF

Acetaminophen	Fluorinated Anesthetic Agents
Antibiotics -	Heavy Metals- Mercury, arsenic, platinum,
Gentamicin	silver, copper, dichromate,
Cephalosporins	uranyl nitrate, lead, zinc
Polymyxins	
Sulfonamides	Mushroom toxins
Tetracycline	Organic solvents- carbon tetrachloride,
Amphetamine - abuse	chloroform,
Contrast media	tetrachlorethylene
Cholecystographic agents	Oxalate
D - Penicillamine	Paraquat
EDTA	Pigments: Hemoglobin, Myoglobin
	Uric Acid

Adapted from Porter, G.A., and Bennett, W.M.: Nephrotoxin induced acute renal failure. In: Brenner, B.M., and Stein, J.H., eds. Contemporary Issues in Nephrology 6. Acute Renal Failure, Churchill Livingstone, 1980, pp 123-162.

Table III: DRUGS ASSOCIATED WITH ACUTE INTERSTITIAL NEPHRITIS AND ARF

Beta-Lactam Antibiotics	Non Beta-Lactam Antibiotics
Amoxicillin	(?)Chloramphenicol
Ampicillin	Ethambutol
Carbenicillin	(?)Gentamicin
Cefataxime	(?)Isoniazid
Cephalexin	Polymyxin Sulfate
Cephalothin	Rifampin
Cephradine	Sulfonamides
Methicillin	Tetracyclines
Nafcillin	Trimethoprim-sulfamethoxazole
Oxacillin	Vancomycin
Penicillin G	
Nonsteroidal Anti-inflammatory Agents	**Others**
Diflunisal	Alpha methyldopa
Fenoprofen	Allopurinol
Ibuprofen	Aspirin
Indomethacin	Azathioprine
Mefanamic acid	Carbamazepine
Naproxen	Cimetidine
Phenazone	Clofibrate
Phenylbutazone	Glafenin
	Phenindione
Diuretics	Phenobarbital
Chlorthalidone	Phenylpropanolamine
Furosemide	Phenytoin
Thiazides	Sulfinpyrazone
Ticrynafen	

Adapted from Appel, G.B., and Kunin C.L.: Acute tubulo - interstitial nephritis. In: Brenner, B.M., and Stein, J.H., eds. Contemporary Issues in Nephrology 10. Tubulo-Interstitial Nephropathies, Churchill Livingstone, 1983, p 152.

COMPLICATIONS OF ACUTE RENAL FAILURE

EXTRACELLULAR FLUID (ECF) IMBALANCE

Alterations in ECF, either volume depletion or excess, commonly occur in children with ARF. Oliguria may result from actual volume depletion, or may reflect a lack of "effective" arterial filling. True ECF depletion may be due to the loss of whole blood, loss of ECF from body, loss of albumin, or internal rearrangement of solute and water. Reduction of such fluid losses may prevent the development of ARF due to circulatory insufficiency. Ineffective arterial filling may require specific therapy for the underlying disorder (e.g. cardiac dysfunction, sepsis) in order to stabilize or improve renal function. As the accompanying serum osmolality and serum sodium concentration may be normal, low or high, urinary indices are often helpful in making diagnostic and therapeutic decisions. (14-16) A high tubular reabsorption (> 97%) or low fractional excretion (< 3%) of sodium in the absence of gross urinary abnormalities usually indicates that extracellular volume depletion is present. One major exception is the child with acute post infectious nephritis who may have a high tubular reabsorption of sodium.

Rehydration in children who are oliguric and clinically acutely dehydrated should be initiated prior to considering any additional forms of therapy. The decision regarding insertion of intra-arterial, pulmonary artery, or central venous catheters should be individualized, but these devices are unnecessary in most children with pure volume depletion. Fluid resuscitation may be performed using 0.9% NaCl, lactated Ringers (if the small amount of potassium contained therein is not contraindicated), or an ECF-like solution made by adding 28 ml of 7.5% $NaHCO_3$ to 750 ml of 0.9% NaCl and 222ml of 5% dextrose in water, producing a solution with a total volume of 1000 ml and a chemical composition of 140 mEq/L of sodium, 115 MEq/L of chloride and 25 mM/L of bicarbonate. (17) As fluid therapy progresses, the state of hydration can be assessed by frequently checking vital signs and by noting the quality of the peripheral pulses, the return toward normal of skin turgor, the degree of moisture of the mucus membranes, urine output, etc. A predetermined rate of infusion of intravenous fluids and the total volume to be provided over a given period of time should be selected to avoid volume overload. A reasonable treatment scheme for the child in shock due to presumed ECF losses would be the administration of 10 ml/kg of solution as quickly as possible.

After reassessing the patient, two additional infusions of 5 ml/kg may be given, followed by subsequent infusions in increments of 3ml/kg, as needed. Urine output should increase within 1-2 hours of such therapy if dehydration alone is the cause of the oliguria.

Diuretic agents are reserved for those children whose urine output does not increase despite adequate rehydration. The two most commonly used agents are mannitol and furosemide. Mannitol may be given intravenously in a dose of 0.5 - 0.75 gm/kg over 60 minutes. This should be done with a bladder catheter in place. If the urine flow rate fails to increase to 1-1.5 ml/kg within 30 minutes, an intravenous infusion of furosemide, 2-3 mg/kg, may be given, followed by a second dose of 5-6 mg/kg two hours later if urine output has not returned. Furosemide alone can be used when attempting to induce a diuresis. Too rapid an infusion of furosemide may cause ototoxicity. In adults, it is recommended that furosemide not be given at a rate greater than 15 mg/min which corresponds to a weight related dose of 0.2 mg/kg/min. (18)

After the first 1-2 hours of rehydration, initial chemistries, BUN, and creatinine usually are available and the patient's status can be evaluated more thoroughly. If therapy has been successful in recovering urine output, the child will probably respond to additional volumes of fluid and perhaps further doses of mannitol or furosemide. Mannitol may be given either as another 1-hour infusion, or diluted five-fold and given as a continuous infusion in 0.2% NaCl at a rate equal to the urine output.

If the above measures do not lead to a significant diuresis despite adequate rehydration, the patient should be assumed to have developed acute intrinsic renal failure. The value of using mannitol in clinical intrinsic ARF remains unclear although experimental studies have shown that mannitol offers a protective effect if given prior to or at the time of development of ARF. In children whose acute renal failure is related to fluid loss i.e., intrinsic renal disorders such as the hemolytic uremic syndrome, extracellular volume is expanded and the primary therapeutic issues include the treatment of a volume overload syndrome and the consequences of hypertension. (19) The mechanism by which mannitol prevents the progression of ARF may involve a decrease in afferent arteriolar resistance, an increase in effective filtration pressure (20,21), or a reduction of edema in glomerular endothelial cells. (22) It is generally believed that mannitol does little, however, once

ARF has occurred. (23) The major disadvantage to using this osmotic agent is that, in the doses recommended, plasma volume is acutely expanded: one vial of 25% mannitol (50ml) will increase the plasma volume of an adult by 250 ml. (18)

Furosemide has been shown to prevent the progression of ARF in the cephaloridine (24) and methemoglobin (25) models of ARF. The protective effect probably is due to a generalized increase in renal blood flow and/or a redistribution of flow from inner to outer cortex. (26)

Because of the lack of clear-cut benefits associated with the use of mannitol we are conservative in our use of mannitol. We feel that the risks of mannitol in most situations outweigh its benefits and generally elect to use furosemide. Complications associated with the use of these agents include: worsening of dehydration, unless fluid intake is carefully monitored and losses replaced; proximal tubular epithelial swelling if too much mannitol is given; loss of the use of the urinary sodium concentration as an indicator of hydration or worsening intrarenal disease; and the false impression that as urine output increases, renal function is improving. (27).

The use of mannitol or furosemide may convert oliquric to non-oliguric (high output) ARF, (28) and such a conversion may make subsequent management easier. If the patient has become oligo-anuric, fluid management should be planned to provide an amount of water equal to that lost from kidneys and from insensible losses via the skin and lungs, minus that added to the extracellular compartment from the water of oxidation (10-15ml/100Cal/day), minus the addition of intracellular water to the ECF when cells are catabolized (5-25ml/100 Cal/day), and minus the quantity of water given as a vehicle for administering drugs. (17) In short, basal water requirements in the child with oligoanuric ARF range between 25 and 30ml/100Cal/day metabolized. In the absence of significant renal function, with no source of significant electrolyte loss, this fluid is given as "free water" (5-10% dextrose in water). Urinary electrolytes should be measured and urinary losses replaced with the appropriate solution to maintain electrolyte balance.

Unless nitrogen balance can be maintained (this usually requires hyperalimentation), a daily weight loss of 0.5-1.5% of lean body mass should be anticipated, and verified by monitoring the patient's weight once or twice daily. The failure to loose weight by a patient provided with minimal calories indicates an ongoing accumulation of extracellular fluid which, if progressive, can lead to hyponatremia, hypertension, and cardiovascular overload.

CARDIAC FAILURE AND PULMONARY EDEMA

Cardiac failure and pulmonary edema are usually due to volume overload in children with ARF, and often are complicated by hypertension or pneumonitis. Although children with these conditions require management in an intensive care unit, the degree to which invasive monitoring is indicated depends not only upon the magnitude of the problem but also upon the response of the patient to initial therapy.

Initial steps to treat acute volume overload include placing the child in a sitting position, using intravenous furosemide (2-4mg/kg), providing oxygen by mask, possibly rotating tourniquets, and performing phlebotomy, with or without replacement of red cells. If an immediate response is not observed, additional steps should include the use of low dose morphine (0.1 mg/kg, with a maximum dose of 5.0 mg), intubation with positive pressure ventilation if respiratory failure develops, and the insertion of catheters to monitor central venous, pulmonary wedge, and systemic arterial pressure.

Conventional x-ray films of the chest, combined with ultra-sonography, EKG and echocardiographic studies, obtained shortly after admission and at appropriate intervals thereafter will aid in defining the patient's initial cardiopulmonary status and in monitoring changes occurring over time. When cardiac or pulmonary function is reduced because of pericardial or pleural effusion(s), drainage should be considered. Unless intrinsic myocardial dysfunction is shown to be a major factor in a child's impaired cardiac status, digitalis should not be given to children with ARF, as this drug demonstrates altered pharmacokinetics in renal failure and is associated with an increased incidence of arrhythmias. Acute dialysis is often the treatment of choice, because the rapid fluid removal achieved usually will reverse cardiac failure or pulmonary edema.

HYPERTENSION

Mild to moderate hypertension as well as acute hypertensive emergencies frequently occur in children with acute renal failure. Severe hypertension occurs more commonly in children with renal failure due to glomerular lesions, and may contribute to the development of cardiac failure and pulmonary edema.

The hypertensive process is mediated by a combination of volume overload, abnormal renin release, and perhaps inhibition of vasodepressor substances. The specifics of treating acute hypertensive emergencies in children with renal disease (29) are detailed elsewhere in this volume.

CENTRAL NERVOUS SYSTEM INVOLVEMENT

Seizures and altered levels of consciousness may be manifestations of urémia per se, or of the hyponatremia, hypocalcemia or hypertension associated with acute renal failure. Symptomatic therapy is indicated to treat the seizures and prevent status epilepticus while attempting to identify etiologies for which specific therapies are available. There is no general agreement about which anticonvulsant to use first. Some prefer to use phenobarbital initially while others believe that diazepam is more effective.

Prompt control of seizures in children, especially those in status epilepticus, may be achieved through the use of intravenous diazepam which is given in a dose of 0.25 mg/kg IV at a rate not to exceed 1 mg/min. A second dose may be given 2-5 minutes later if the first is unsuccessful in achieving seizure control. Parenteral diazepam may transiently depress respirations, especially when given in addition to barbituates; therefore, facilities and equipment should be available for performing endotracheal intubation and mechanical ventilation. Suppression of all evidence of seizure activity is unnecessary, as this increases the risk of respiratory depression. Because its duration of action is only 10-20 minutes, diazepam, when used as the first drug for seizure control, should be followed by a longer acting anticonvulsant such as phenobarbital or phenytoin.

The initial dose of phenobarbital for seizure control is 10 mg/kg with a maximum dose of 200-300 mg given intramuscularly, or 5.0-7.5 mg/kg by slow IV injection. If seizures are not controlled, two additional doses of 2.5-3.0 mg/kg may be administered at 20 minute intervals. Peak blood levels occur more rapidly after intravenous (20 minutes) than intramuscular administration, but the intravenous route carries with it a greater risk of respiratory depression. The usual maintenance dose is 4-6 mg/kg/day, adjusted to keep the serum concentrations within a therapeutic range of 15-40 mcg/ml. Dose related toxicity includes sedation, nystagmus, and ataxia.

The loading dose of phenytoin is 10-15 mg/kg given intravenously, at a rate not to exceed 50 mg/min because of the potential induction of cardiac arrhythmias, leading to cardiovascular collapse. A rhythm strip should be checked prior to administration and along with BP, monitored during the infusion. The presence of a significant arrhythmia is a contraindication to the use of phenytoin. Other major side effects include central nervous system depression, and hypertension which may occur when the drug is infused too rapidly. The maintenance dose ranges from 3-8 mg/kg/day. Levels should be monitored after the initial loading dose (therapeutic range = 5-20 mcg/ml), and periodically thereafter; the best time to measure serum concentrations in a child receiving phenytoin twice daily is 8 hours after the last dose. (30) Children undergoing hemodialysis should have drug levels monitored pre and post dialysis. The percent plasma protein binding of phenytoin is reduced by up to 10-25% in patients with uremia. Thus the fraction of the total circulating drug concentration which is free and available for binding to cerebral tissue receptors is increased at any serum level. Moreover, serum phenytoin levels are reduced at any given dose of the drug in patients with chronic renal insufficiency, possibly due to an increased volume of distribution. (31, 32) The net effect of these two observations may be that therapeutic efficacy is achieved at lower total serum concentrations of phenytoin. (33) Therefore, in children with renal failure, drug levels should be monitored and maintained near the lower end of the therapeutic range (5-10 mcg/ml).

Both phenytoin and phenobarbital have been noted to cause transient elevations of hepatic transaminases, particularly GGTP. (34) These changes appear to be related to hepatocellular hypertrophy and are not a contraindication to continuation of drug therapy.

Should a combination of the above agents fail in treating status epilepticus, paraldehyde may be given rectally in a dose of 0.3 cc/kg. Equal volumes of paraldehyde and mineral oil should be used. Paraldehyde must be freely prepared as decomposition to acetaldehyde and then to acetic acid occurs on exposure to light and oxygen, and must be administered using glass syringes, as it forms toxic substances upon contact with plastic. Paraldehyde may also be given as a continuous intravenous infusion, in a dose of 0.15 cc/kg (maximum dose, 0.3 cc/kg/hr), following its dilution in dextrose water or saline, in a 1:10 ratio. Paraldehyde is excreted via the lungs, and is contraindicated in the presence of pulmonary disease. Overdosage may cause respiratory depression, hypotension, and metabolic acidosis.

If all of the above measures fail to control seizures, induction of general anesthesia may be necessary. This should only be performed following endotracheal intubation, and by an experienced anesthesiologist. The drug of choice is the ultra-short acting sedative-hypnotic, thiopental, which is administered by intravenous drip titration.

Once anticonvulsant therapy is started it has been our practice to continue therapy for 1 1/2 - 2 years, beyond the last seizure even when the seizures are thought to be "purely metabolic," and then to taper the dose gradually until a sub-therapeutic blood level is achieved at which time the drug is discontinued. An EEG should be obtained and repeated prior to discontinuing therapy.

ANEMIA

Anemia commonly develops in patients with ARF, with hemoglobin concentrations in the range of 7.0 - 9.5 gm/dl (35). Blood transfusions are required when ARF is associated with acute blood loss, when hemolysis occurs as in the hemolytic uremic syndrome, or when the patient has a pre-existing anemia. We give transfusions when symptoms of anemia develop or the hemoglobin falls to less than 6.0 gm/dl. Unless rapid blood loss has occurred, packed red cell transfusions are utilized. The number of grams of hemoglobin required may be calculated as follows: (17)

gm. Hgb required = (wt kg x 0.07) x (desired-observed Hgb in gm/liter)

The term 0.07 is equal to the percentage of body weight which is blood volume and the hemoglobin value is in gm per <u>liter</u> and not gm per dl as most laboratories report. The actual volume of blood required depends on the hemoglobin concentration of the blood product used; whole blood and packed cells contain 11-13 mg/dl and 20-25 gm/dl, respectively. A more useful formula to determine the volume in ml, of packed red cells is:

4 x wt kg x (desired - observed Hgb in gm/dl) (36). This formula assumes that the hematocrit of the packed cells is between 72 and 75%.

Patients with ARF may become acutely hypertensive from transfusions of even small volumes of blood. Blood should be given slowly, at a rate of 2 cc/kg per hour and blood pressure monitored at frequent intervals. Children undergoing dialysis should be transfused during dialysis while extracellular volume is simultaneously being removed. Occasionally, partial exchange transfusions are necessary to alleviate acute volume overload and simultaneously correct anemia.

CONTROL OF BIOCHEMICAL ABERRATIONS

Acidosis

The development of acidosis is common in ARF because the kidney can no longer excrete the 1-2 mEq/kg/day of hydrogen ion normally generated, and many of the disorders giving rise to ARF are associated with an increased rate of hydrogen ion production. While mild acidosis (CO_2 > 15 mM/L) does not generally require treatment, alkalinizing agents should be considered when the CO_2 is less than 14 mM/L. The formula used to determine the amount of alkali required to raise the serum bicarbonate over a 30-90 minute interval follows: (mEq HCO_3^- required = wt (kg) x 0.6 x (desired - observed serum HCO_3^- mM/L) (17). Doses based on this formula often will be insufficient in the presence of ongoing production of hydrogen ion and consumption of available bicarbonate. The ultimate quantity of bicarbonate used should be determined by repeated monitoring of serum levels and the monitoring of changes in ECF.

Supportive therapy to reduce hydrogen ion production includes protein restriction, provision of adequate non-protein calories, control of infection, and removal of devitalized tissue. (37) Dialysis, which can simultaneously correct acidosis and volume overload, needs to be considered when severe acidosis is present and additional sodium cannot be given because of volume overload.

Hyponatremia

The hyponatremia of ARF is usually due to a combination of hypotonic fluid intake during the time that the GFR is falling and extrarenal losses of solute, usually GI in nature, resulting in hyponatremic extracellular volume expansion. Hyponatremic extracellular volume depletion may occur if the child has been vomiting excessively. (38) Serum sodium concentrations above 125 mEq/L do not warrant therapy with iso or hypertonic saline; indeed in the absence of seizures hyponatremia with volume expansion is best treated by water restriction. In contrast, consideration should be given to acutely raising the serum sodium concentration even in the asymptomatic child when the serum sodium concentration is less than 120 mEq/L. Treatment is mandatory when seizures or other significant symptoms attributable to hyponatremia have developed. The quantity of sodium needed to raise the serum sodium concentration can be approximated by the following formula: number of mEq sodium required = (desired serum [Na+]) - observed serum [Na+] x body weight in kg x 0.6). Administration of 1.2 ml/kg of 3% NaCl (0.6 mEq/kg) will raise the serum sodium concentration by 1.0 mEq/L. A reasonable end point of such therapy is an increase in the serum sodium concentration to approximately 125 mEq/L over 60-180 minutes, depending upon the initial serum sodium concentration and the severity of symptoms. Gradual progressive increases in the serum sodium concentration are preferred over rapid "acute" elevations. In patients capable of responding to a diuretic, correction of hyponatremic hypervolemia may be achieved with diuretic-induced fluid loss and simultaneous replacement of sufficient quantities of solute to raise the serum sodium concentration to the desired level.

Raising the serum sodium concentration in any patient with ARF carries the potential risk of iatrogenic hypervolemia, acute hypertension, cardiac failure, or pulmonary edema. Any child with ARF who is treated with hypertonic saline needs frequent monitoring. If hypervolemia is present or develops, and diuretics are ineffective, dialysis is the preferred mode of therapy with which to reduce ECF volume and increase the serum sodium concentration.

Hyperkalemia

Hyperkalemia is the most feared electrolyte abnormality occurring in ARF. The acute loss of renal function in conjunction with infection, acidosis, malnutrition, hemolysis or a hypercatabolic state may result in a rapid, often unexpected, increase in extracellular potassium concentration. Coincident hypocalcemia or hyponatremia may exacerbate the effects of hyperkalemia. (39) Children with developing ARF should be monitored at frequent intervals by EKG as well as with repeated determinations of serum potassium concentrations until the patient has been stable for a period of time. EKG changes associated with increasing levels of serum potassium consist of peaked T waves, prolonged PR interval, widening of the QRS complex with disappearance of P waves, and finally nodal and ventricular arrhythmias.

The treatment of hyperkalemia in a child with ARF should proceed simultaneously along complementary paths: reduction of potassium input into the extracellular compartment and correction of elevated extracellular concentrations already present, and removal of potassium from the body. Steps to reduce the input of potassium should include the elimination of all external sources of potassium, (e.g., diet, potassium salts used in compounding drugs), treatment of infection, provision of calories, and removal of devitalized tissue including accumulated collections of blood.

Emergency maneuvers to mitigate the cardiac effect of hyperkalemia are indicated when the serum concentration of potassium exceeds 7.0 mEq/L. Myocardial excitability may be stabilized without lowering serum potassium by the intravenous infusion of 0.5 ml/kg of 10% calcium gluconate (40) or 0.25 ml/kg calcium gluceptate (1, 17, 41) over 2-4 minutes. Such infusions need to be monitored by EKG as the rapid infusion of calcium may cause bradycardia, ventricular fibrillation and cardiac arrest. If the pulse rate falls by more than 20 beats per minute the infusion should immediately be slowed or stopped. (42)

If the child can tolerate sodium, an intravenous infusion of 3.0 mEq/kg of sodium bicarbonate (3.3 ml/kg of 7.5% sodium bicarbonate) over a period of 5-10 minutes will shift potassium into cells by raising blood pH. This effect is only transient because as the bicarbonate is buffered, pH will again fall and potassium ions will move back into the ECF.

Glucose infusions accelerate glycogen synthesis and increase the intracellular uptake of potassium. Glucose infusions alone may elicit an appropriate insulin response and facilitate the transcellular transport of glucose and potassium. Insulin, if needed, may be added to the infusion or given separately. Recommended schemes include an intravenous infusion of glucose at 0.5 g/kg per hour for one to two hours with the addition of 1 unit of insulin per 5 gms of glucose, (40) or 1 ml/kg 50% glucose containing 1 unit of insulin per ml, (39) or an infusion of 14% glucose to which 0.5 units of insulin is added for each gram of glucose to be given. (17) Insulin can be added to the dialysate if peritoneal dialysis is being performed. Frequent monitoring of blood sugars both by Dextrostix(R) or Chemstrip(R) and by serum determination are needed to insure that hyperglycemia does not develop.

In order to facilitate potassium removal from the body Kayexalate(R), an ion exchange resin which exchanges sodium for potassium in a 1.5 to 1.0 ratio (18, 43) may be given rectally or orally. The rectal route should be used when the serum potassium needs to be lowered acutely, for the colon is the site in which the highest rate of potassium sodium exchange occurs within the gastrointestinal tract. (44) Although the retention of a Kayexalate(R) enema for 30 minutes allows for a reasonable exchange of potassium for sodium, retention of the enema for several hours (44) is required for maximal exchange. Most children do not retain enemas for such long periods of time, thereby limiting the effectiveness of rectal Kayexalate(R) in the treatment of hyperkalemia. The rectal dose of Kayexalate(R) is 1.0 gm/kg dissolved as 1 gm per 4 ml of 10% dextrose in water or 10% sorbitol. A similar dose may be given orally. When Kayexalate(R) is given orally the addition of 0.2 ml/kg of 70% sorbitol will enhance its transit time throughout the bowel, increase exchange efficiency, and reduce the development of constipation. (17) Oral resin therapy works slowly and may need to be given every 4-6 hours.

Potassium free dialysis is indicated when the above maneuvers are ineffective in lowering serum potassium and maintaining acceptable levels;when peritoneal dialysis is used, hypertonic dialysate exchanges will enhance potassium removal. (45)

Hyperuricemia

Hyperuricemia may result in renal and interstitial deposition of uric acid, and may increase renal vascular resistance. Low intratubular pH and low urine flow rate predispose to urinary precipitation of uric acid. Hyperuricemia may occur in association with non renal disorders and cause ARF, or may develop as a consequence of intrinsic ARF.

The best therapy is preventative and depends upon recognizing diseases such as leukemia or large tumor masses which, because of rapid cell turnover rates or the use of chemotherapy, give rise to hyperuricemia. Uric acid nephropathy may be anticipated in patients who have a urinary uric acid to creatinine ratio greater than 1.0. (46) ARF can often be prevented in such patients by treating them with allopurinol in a dose of 10-20 mg/kg/day (maximum of 300 mg), especially prior to the initiation of chemotherapy. (47,48) In patients in whom pretreatment with allopurinol is not possible and renal insufficiency is anticipated, volume expansion with a solution containing sodium bicarbonate to induce an alkaline diuresis may prevent uric acid deposition. Sodium bicarbonate, not sodium lactate, should be used because lactate inhibits uric acid secretion by renal tubular cells. Uric acid has a pK of 5.1;hence, if the urine pH can be kept above 7.0 (preferably above 7.5), most of the urate will remain in solution. The urine pH should be monitored frequently and kept above 7.0. If necessary, a single dose of acetazolamide may be given to alkalinize the urine acutely. The rate of infusion of intravenous fluids should be adjusted so that a urine flow rate of 2-3 times the maintenance urine output is obtained.

Patients with developing uric acid nephropathy should have their GFR monitored two to three times a day when a forced alkaline diuresis is undertaken, to help prevent iatrogenic volume overload. Measured ongoing urinary water losses should be replaced every 1 to 2 hours to perpetuate diuresis. In patients with already established mild to moderate renal failure, an attempt to induce such a diuresis may succeed but careful monitoring is critical. Some patients may be slow to respond to attempts to induce a diuresis because they are already volume depleted. Replacement of any volume deficits is required before a significant increase in urine flow can occur. Finally, when the load of uric acid exceeds the ability of an adequately functioning kidney to excrete it, or when renal insufficiency is severe, dialysis is indicated for its capacity to remove large quantities of uric acid. (49)

DIVALENT ION ABNORMALITIES

Hyperphosphatemia and hypocalcemia are the two major divalent ion abnormalities in children with ARF; occasionally, abnormalities occur in magnesium metabolism as well. Hyperphosphatemia generally develops to a greater extent than does hypocalcemia, resulting in an abnormally high calcium-phosphorous product. At a calcium-phosphorous product levels above 70 there is an increased danger of calcium precipitation in blood vessels, lung, and brain. In order to minimize the risk of metastatic calcification, hyperphosphatemia should be reduced prior to administering agents which might increase serum calcium.

Serum phosphate levels may be lowered by reducing both dietary intake and endogenous production of phosphate. (i.e., by controlling infection, hemolysis, etc.). Oral phosphate binding gels are helpful in reducing serum phosphate concentrations even when patients are not eating. Aluminum gels are the agents usually recommended for control of serum phosphate levels; the recommended dose of aluminum hydroxide is 60-150 mg/kg/day (17,40,41). The use of such agents in high doses over prolonged periods of time may be associated with the development of aluminum toxicity - encephalopathy or bone disease. (50) The use of magnesium containing antacids may increase serum and CSF levels of magnesium resulting in central nervous system depression.

After lowering serum phosphate levels, if the serum calcium level has not already spontaneously risen, calcium therapy may be started. In the absence of tetany or seizures, hypocalcemia can be corrected with oral calcium supplements starting at a dose of 50 mg/kg/day (51) given as calcium gluconate, calcium lactate, or calcium carbonate. These drugs have the advantage of also supplying extra base. Vitamin D therapy, as Dihydrotachysterol (DHT)(R) 0.125 - 0.5ug/day, 1-25 dihydroxy cholecalciferol (Rocaltrol[R]) 10-30 ng/kg, or 25 hydroxyvitamin D_3 (Calderol[R]) 1-2 ug/kg/day may be required to raise serum calcium levels even when oral calcium is provided. Serum calcium and phosphate levels should be monitored frequently until divalent ion metabolism stabilizes.

Patients with tetany or seizures should be treated with intravenous calcium salts, either gluconate or gluceptate, at doses similar to those discussed in the section on hyperkalemia. An intravenous infusion which provides elemental calcium at a rate of 4 mg/kg per hour will generally raise serum calcium levels by about 1 mg/dl per hour. Unremitting hyperphosphatemia or the inability to return the calcium phosphorous product towards normal are indications for initiating dialysis.

INFECTION

Infection may occur in three clinical settings in children with ARF: 1) infection may be a cause of ARF (sepsis); 2) infection may be a consequence of the primary cause of ARF (obstructive uropathy, devitalized tissue); or 3) infection may be a complication of the therapy for ARF (bladder catheterizations, indwelling lines, effusions or ascitis, and malnutrition). Infection leads to an increase in catabolism and thereby affects potassium, phosphate, and acid base balance, azotemia, and nutrition. These abnormalities retard wound healing and, perhaps, recovery of renal function. (52) The most common site of infection during the course of ARF is catheter-related urinary tract infection, (53, 54) and progression to pyelonephritis may further compromise GFR. (53) Sepsis, pulmonary, and wound infections also occur commonly in the child with ARF.

Infection remains a major cause of morbidity and mortality in children with ARF, and control of infection in these patients should include preventative (Table IV) and therapeutic measures. Specific antibiotic therapy should be based on the results of cultures taken to identify specific organisms. Decisions made prior to receiving culture reports are based on an appreciation of the usual organisms associated with the conditions leading to ARF or associated with its therapy. The organisms most commonly isolated from septic children are Staph aureus, and E Coli. We usually treat with Nafcillin, Gentamicin and possibly Ampicillin while awaiting the initial culture results. Dosages and/or intervals for administering antibiotics should be adjusted according to the level of renal function. (55)

Table IV: GENERAL PRINCIPLES OF INFECTION CONTROL IN THE CHILD WITH ARF

Ambulation
Avoidance of prophylactic antibiotics
Avoidance of bladder catheters
Early dialysis
Frequent replacement of indwelling lines
Provision of adequate nutrients
Pulmonary physiotherapy
Removal of devitalized tissue
Systematic cultures of urine, peritoneal fluid, etc.
Use of aseptic techniques
Use of closed system urinary drainage bags

NUTRITION

Successful provision of required nutrients may reduce catabolism and retard the development of the biochemical aberrations, malnutrition, and alterations in immunologic processes associated with ARF, thus improving overall healing and perhaps even increasing the rate of repair of renal tissue. Providing adequate nutrition for a child with ARF is difficult to achieve in most cases. Some of the many approaches to the nutritional management of these patients include: conservative dietary management alone; a combination of a liberalized diet plus dialysis; central parenteral alimentation;

peripheral alimentation alone or with oral intake, and dialysis with central or peripheral parenteral alimentation.

Unless dialysis is to be performed, in which case the volume of the child's diet can be liberalized and adjusted according to the volume ultrafiltrated, the fluid content of the diet should not exceed insensible (approximately 30 ml/100 cal metabolized/day or 400-500 ml/m^2) plus measured urinary losses. The provision of at least 30 Kcal/100 Kcal metabolized/day (400 Kcal/m^2/day) will minimize protein catabolism. A variety of diets that provide adequate calories with limited amounts of high biologic value protein have been designed for infants, children, and adults for conservative management of renal failure. (4, 42, 56) These diets are best prepared and administered with the help of a skilled pediatric nutritionist.

The use of essential amino acids provides alpha amino nitrogen for the biosynthesis of non essential amino acids. A high-calorie, reduced protein intake containing small amounts of essential amino acids, 1 - 1.5 gm of nitrogen and 2000 - 3000 Kcal in the adult (the Giovanetti diet), (57) decreases urea production, reduces the incidence of uremic symptoms and results in positive nitrogen balance. (58) Indeed the appropriate management of protein intake can reduce the need for dialysis (59).

The wide availability of peritoneal dialysis and hemodialysis has modified the approach to the dietary management of ARF. The issue now is to what degree unpalatable diets should be forced upon anxious, frightened children prior to starting dialysis. It is our belief that dialysis (which would allow a more liberal intake of nutrients and fluids) should be employed with the aim of maximizing nutrition when unpalatable diets will be needed for more than a few days. Our experience has been that when a liberalized diet is combined with dialysis, the nutritional management of ARF is more successful because it is more acceptable to the child, the family and the nursing staff. Once dialysis is begun, the dialytic losses of amino acids and protein (60,61) need to be considered in the child's nutritional prescription.

In the past few years dietary management of acute renal failure has been expanded to include parenteral nutrition, both peripheral and central. Peripheral hyperalimentation using various combinations and concentrations of glucose, lipids and amino acids has been used successfully to replace or to supplement oral intake although the use of peripheral hyperalimentation always requires adjunctive dialysis because of the large volumes involved. If full nutrition can be provided peripherally this regimen may obviate the need for central lines with their attendant complications.

Central alimentation, using volumes tolerable to an anuric patient, has been studied extensively in adults with ARF. In uncontrolled studies it has been shown that post-operative acute renal failure could be improved with central hyperalimentation using an intravenous infusion containing 8 essential amino acids and 50-70% glucose. (62) Subsequently, a prospective controlled clinical trial in adults comparing the advantages of a centrally infused solution containing hypertonic glucose with vitamins and amino acids to those of an isocaloric, isovolemic solution containing only glucose was reported. Although the ultimate survival rates were not different in the two groups of patients, a clear benefit from amino acid treatment, was evident by enhanced recovery from acute renal failure. (63) In another study, patient survival was improved in those 129 adults with post-operative ARF who received an infusion of hypertonic glucose with a fibrin hydrolysate. (64) Improved survival was noted in this study even in high-risk patients, with sepsis and hypertension. Other studies have shown that amino acid infusions in the experimental animal with acute renal failure may hasten the repair of the renal lesion itself. (65, 66)

Few data are available on the role of parenteral nutrition in acute renal failure in children. In one study in which it was used to provide nitrogen and to increase the caloric intake from 20 to 70 Kcal/kg/day, positive nitrogen balance was achieved in malnourished anuric children. (67, 68) We have used both peripheral and central nutrition successfully to retard the development of malnutrition as well as to reverse severe malnutrition in a limited number of children. We treated one six month old infant with combined central hyperalimentation and peritoneal dialysis, and achieved an increase in body mass of 35-40% over a period of 4 1/2 months. The benefits and risks (Table V) of hyperalimentation in ARF have recently been reviewed in depth by Toback. (68)

Table V: PARENTERAL NUTRITION IN ACUTE RENAL FAILURE

BENEFITS	COMPLICATIONS
Biochemical	Biochemical
Less Hyperkalemia	Hyperglycemia
Less Acidosis	Hypokalemia
Less Hyperphosphatemia	Hypophosphatemia
	Hypermagnesemia
Nutritional	
Positive Nitrogen Balance - Protein Sparing	
Nitrogen Balance - Protein Sparing	Surgical
Positive Caloric Balance	Anesthetic problems
Slows Catabolism	Placement injuries
Statistics	Catheter-Related
Improved Rate of Recovery of Renal Function	Thrombosis
Improved Patient Survival	
Reduced Requirements for Dialysis	

DIALYSIS THERAPY

There are no data on the frequency with which dialysis is indicated in children with various forms of ARF. In adult populations, 34% of patients with non-oliguric and 84% with oliguric ARF required dialysis, with mortality rates of 20% and 50% respectively. (69) Either peritoneal or hemodialysis can be used to treat ARF. The decision to begin dialysis should be based on a number of factors including volume status, biochemical derangements, cardiac impairment, and uremic symptomatology (Table VI).We often initiate dialysis for progressive azotemia in an oligo-anuric child, even in the absence of uremia or severe biochemical derangements. Early dialysis may allow for enhanced revovery by preventing severe uremic symptomatology, protecting against life threatening electrolyte disturbances, and allowing better nutritional support.

Table VI: INDICATIONS FOR CONSIDERING DIALYSIS THERAPY IN ACUTE RENAL FAILURE

Biochemical	Expansion of Extracellular volume
Acidosis (CO_2 <11 mM/L)	Hypertension (severe)
Hyperkalemia (persistently >7.0mEq/L, or ECG changes)	Pulmonary Edema
Hyperuricemia	Peripheral Edema (marked)
Hyponatremia (<125 mEq/L)	**Central Nervous System**
Hyperphosphatemia	Encephalopathy
	Impaired cognition
Cardiac	Behavioral disturbances
Arrhythmias	Decreased consciousness (lethargy, stupor, coma)
Pericarditis	Asterixis, myoclonus
Gastrointestinal	Seizures
Nausea	
Hemorrhage	
Vomiting	

Unless a child is very hypercatabolic ie., BUN increasing at a rate greater than 60-70 mg/dl/day (as may occur in patients with sepsis, often surgery, or with extensive tissue breakdown from burns, rhabdomyolysis, or trauma), we prefer to treat ARF with peritoneal dialysis. Peritoneal dialysis offers a safer and smoother approach to controlling uremia. Peritoneal dialysis can be instituted within 30-60 minutes of making the decision to dialyze, unless a more permanent type of peritoneal catheter is desired.

We have used several forms of peritoneal dialysis, to treat different phases of ARF; these include manual, automated cycler, and CAPD. We prefer to start with manual peritoneal dialysis because ultrafiltration can be measured after individual exchanges, and the dextrose or electrolyte composition quickly changed. Once the uremic process has been stabilized,an alternative, more chronic form of peritoneal dialysis may be started.

Hemodialysis with its rapid clearances may be the preferred method of treating ARF due to the toxic ingestion of agents such as ethylene glycol or methanol, and of treating children with severe abdominal trauma. The recent development of subclavian catheters has made it technically easier to perform acute hemodialysis. However, because relatively few children develop ARF, most pediatric services and hemodialysis units are not accustomed to the mechanics of initiating an acute hemodialysis. Our experience has been that children and families are terrified of the initial hemodialysis treatments and are often very difficult to manage.

The frequency of any form of dialysis should be set at a rate which permits satisfactory control of uremia, blood pressure, cardiorespiratory status and biochemical abnormalities. The more hypercatabolic the patient, the more frequently dialysis is needed. In some patients daily hemodialysis or continuous peritoneal dialysis may be required.

PROGNOSIS

The prognosis for children with ARF depends upon underlying illness or cause. Children whose ARF is due to acute dehydration or post infectious nephritis have a good to excellent prognosis. Children with HUS, RPGN, and a few with post infectious nephritis may be left with residual renal impairment. Their ultimate prognosis depends upon the level of GFR reached during recovery. Should maximal compensatory hypertrophy occur in infants during the period of recovery from ARF and the absolute GFR remain low, further "normal growth" may be associated with the ultimate development of chronic renal insufficiency leading to the need for dialysis and transplantation. Mortality is higher in patients when renal failure is related to surgery. (70) The overall recovery rate for children with ARF is approximately 75-80%. (40, 71)

REFERENCES

1. Chan, J.C.: Acute renal failure in children: principles of management. Clin Pediat. 13: 686, 1974.

2. Kaplan, B.S., and Drummond, K.H.: Acute Renal Failure. In: Rubin, M.I. and Barratt, T.M., eds. Pediatric Nephrology. Baltimore: Williams and Wilkins Co., 1975, p. 374.

3. Gordillo-Paniagua, G. and Velasquez-Jones, L.: Acute renal failure. Ped. Clin. N. Amer. 23: 8107, 1976.

4. Royer, P., Habib, R., Mathieu, H., Broyer, M., Walsh, A.: Acute Renal Failure.In: Pediatric Nephrology; Vol II, Major Problems in Clinical Pediatrics, 1974. W.B. Saunders Co., p 343.

5. James, J.A.: Acute Renal Failure.In: James, J.A., ed. Renal Disease in Childhood, 3rd edition. C.V. Mosby Co., 1976, p. 259.

6. Anand, S.K.: Acute Renal Failure in the Newborn. Ped. Clin. N. Amer. 79:791, 1982.

7. Norman, M.E., and Asadi, F.K.: A prospective study of acute renal failure in the newborn infant. Pediatrics, 63: 475, 1979.

8. Rahman, H., Boineau, F.G., and Lewy, J.E.: Renal failure in the perinatal period. Clin. Perinatol., 8: 241, 1981.

9. Cronin, R.E.: The patient with acute azotemia. In: Schrier R.W., ed.Manua of Nephrology, Diagnosis & Therapy., Boston: Little Brown, 1981, pp.135-150.

10. Bolton, W.K., and Couser, W.G.: Intravenous pulse methylprednisolone therapy of acute crescentic rapidly progressive glomerulonephritis. Am. J. Med. 6: 495, 1979.

11. Fauci, A.S., Katz, P., Haynes, B.F., and Wolff, S.M.: Cyclophosphamide therapy of severe systemic necrotizing vasculitis. N. Eng. J. Med. 301: 235, 1979.

12. Lockwood, C.M., Rees, A.J., Pinching, A.J., et al: Plasma-exchange and immunosuppression in the treatment of fulminating immune complex crescentic nephritis. Lancet. 1: 63, 1977.

13. Madias, N.E., Kwon, O.J., Millan, V.G.: Percutaneous Transluminal Renal Angioplasty: A potentially effective treatment for preservation of Renal Failure. Arch. Intern. Med. 142: 693, 1982.

14. Schrier, R.W.: Acute renal failure: Pathogenesis, diagnosis, and management, Hosp. Practice. 16: 93, 1981.

15. Schrier, R.W., Conger, J.D.: Acute renal failure: Pathogenesis, diagnosis, and management. In: Schrier R.W., ed. Renal and Electrolyte Disorders, 2nd ed, Little Brown, and Co., 1980: pp. 375-408.

16. Miller, T.R., Anderson, R.J., Linas, S.L., et al.: Urinary diagnostic indices in acute renal failure. A prospective study. Ann. Intern. Med. 89: 47, 1978.

17. Gruskin, A.: Parenteral Fluid Therapy and Treatment for Electrolyte Disorders in Children with Genitourinary Disorders. In: Kendall, A.R. and Karafin, L., eds. Practice of Surgery: Urology., Harper & Rowe, Chapt. 23B, 1981.

18. Grossman, R.A.: Oliguria and Acute Renal Failure. Med. Clin. North Am. 65 (2): 413-427, 1981.

19. Burke, T.J., et al: Ischemia and tubule obstruction during acute renal failure in dogs: Mannitol in protection. Am. J. Physiol. 238, 305, 1980.

20. Blantz, R.C.: Effect of mannitol on glomerular ultrafiltration in the hydropenic rat. J. Clin. Invest. 54: 1135, 1968.

21. Peters, G., and Brunner, H.: Mannitol diuresis in hemorrhagic hypotension. Am. J. Physiol. 204: 555, 1963.

22. Flores, J., DiBona, D.R., Beck, C.H., and Leaf, A.: The role of cell swelling in ischemic renal damage and the protective effect of hypertonic solute. J. Clin. Invest. 51: 118, 1972.

23. Mannitol and renal function. Lancet 1: 1183, 1968.

24. Bailey, R.R., Natale, R., Turnbull, D.I., and Linton, A.L.: Protective effect of furosemide in acute tubular necrosis and acute renal failure. Clin. Sci. Mol. Med. 43: 1, 1973.

25. Montoreano, R., Mouzet, M.T., Cunarro, J., and Ruiz-Guinazu, A.: Prevention of the initial oliguria of acute renal failure by the administration of furosemide. Postgrad. Med. J. [Suppl.] 47: 7, 1971.

26. Ludens, J.H., Hook, J.B., Brody, M.J., and Williamson, H.E.: Enhancement of renal blood flow by furosemide. J. Pharmacol. Exp. Ther. 163: 456, 1968.

27. Ng., R.C.K. and Suki, W.D. Treatment of acute renal failure. In: Brenner, B.M., and Stein, J.H., eds. Comtemporary Issues in Nephrology: Acute Renal Failure. Churchill, Livingstone, 1980: p. 229.

28. Anderson, R.J., Linas, S.L., Berns, A.S., et al: Nonoliguric Acute Renal Failure. N. Engl. J. Med. 296: 1134, 1977.

29. Gruskin, A.B., Baluarte, H.J., Polinsky, M.S., et al: Treatment of severe hypertension in children with renal diseases. In: Strauss J., ed. Acute Renal Disorders and Renal Emergencies. Boston: Martinus Nijhoff, 1984, p. 143.

30. Dodson, W.E.: Phenytoin kinetics in children. Clin. Pharmacol Ther. 27: 704, 1980.

31. Letteri, J. M., Mellk, H., Louis, S., et al: Diphenylhydantoin Metabolism in Uremia. N. Engl. J. Med. 285: 648, 1971.

32. Borga, O., Hoppel, C., Odar-Cederlof, I., et al: Plasma levels and renal excretion of phenytoin and its metabolites in patients with renal failure. Clin. Pharmacol. Ther. 26: 306, 1979.

33. Burgess, E.D., Friel, P. N., Blair, A.D., Jr., et al: Serum Phenytoin Concentrations in Uremia. Ann. Intern. Med. 94: 59, 1981.

34. Aiges, H.W., Daum, F., Olson, M., et al: The effects of phenobarbital and diphenylhydantoin on liver function and morphology. J. Pediatr. 97: 22, 1980.

35. Bozzini, C.E., Devoto, F.C.H., and Tomio, J.M.: Decreased responsiveness of hematopoietic tissue to erythropoietin in acutely uremic rats. J. Lab. Clin. Med. 68: 411, 1966.

36. Naiman, J.L.: Personal communicative

37. Lordon, R.E., and Burton, J.R.: Post-traumatic failure in military personnel in Southeast Asia. Experience at Clark USAF Hospital, Republic of the Philippines. Am. J. Med. 53: 137, 1972.

38. Gruskin, A.B., Baluarte, H.J., Prebis, J.W., et al: Serum sodium abnormalities. An overview. Ped. Clin. N.Amer. 29: 907, 1982.

39. Trainin, E.B. and Spitzer, A.: Treatment of Acute Renal Failure. In: Edelman, C.M.,Jr., Pediatric Kidney Disorders, Vol. 1, Little Brown, 1978: 466.

40. Hollerman, C.E.: Acute renal failure, Ped. Nephr. Med. Exam. Publ. Co., Inc., Garden City, NY , 1979, pp. 409-425.

41. Boichis, H., and Winterborn, M.H.: Acute renal failure in childhood. Pediatr. Ann. 3: 58, 1974.

42. Lieberman, E.: Management of Acute Renal Failure in Infants and Children. Nephron, 11: 193-208, 1973.

43. Berlyne, G.M., Janabi, K., Shaw, A.B.: Dangers of resonium A in the treatment of hyperkalemia in renal failure. Lancet 1:167,1966.

44. Fleisher, D.S.: Cation exchange resin therapy for hyperkalemia in infants and children. J. Pediatr. 58: 486, 1961.

45. Gruskin, A.B., Morgenstern, B.Z. and Perlman, S.A.: Kinetics of Peritoneal Dialysis in Children. In: Fine, R.N., & Gruskin, A.B., (eds.) End Stage Renal Disease in Children; W.B. Saunders. In Press.

46. Dobrin, R.S., et al.: Acute Renal Failure. In: Smith, C.A., ed.: The Critically Ill Child: Diagnosis and Management. Philadelphia: W.B. Saunders Co., 1972, p. 113.

47. Baehner, R.L.: Hematologic malignancies: leukemia and lymphoma. In: Miller, D.R., and Pearson, H.A., eds. Smith's Blood Diseases of Infancy and childhood. C.V. Mosby, 1978: p. 603.

48. Kelton, J., Kelley, W.N. and Holmes, E.W.: A rapid method for the diagnosis of acute uric acid nephropathy. Arch. Intern. Med. 138: 612, 1978.

49. Kjellstrand, C.M., Campbell, D.C., von Hartizsch, B., et al.: Hyperuricemic acute renal failure. Arch. Intern. Med. 133: 349, 1074.

50. Polinsky, M.S., Gruskin, A.B., Baluarte, H.J., et al: Aluminum in Chronic Renal Disease. In: Strauss, J., ed. Ped. Neph. Vol. VI., Plenum Press, 1981: p 315.

51. Dobrin, R.S., Larsen, C.D., and Holliday, M.A.: The critically ill child: acute renal failure. Pediatrics. 48: 286, 1971.

52. Elliot, W., Hill, M., Ken, D.N.S., et al: The management of acute renal failure. Postgrad. Med. J. 36: 230, 1960.

53. Zech, P., Bouletreau, R., and Moskovtchenko, J.F.: Infection in acute renal failure. Adv. Nephrol. 1: 231, 1971.

54. Cameron, J.S.: The management of acute and chronic renal failure in children. Turk. J. Pediatr. 15: 14, 1973.

55. Gruskin, A.B., Baluarte, H.J., Polinsky, M.S., et al: Usage of antibiotics in children with renal insufficiency: In: Strauss, J.,ed. Ped. Neph. Vol. VI. Plenum Press, 1981: p 391.

56. Chan, J.C.M.: Dietary management of renal failure in infants and children. Clin. Pediatr. 12: 707, 1973.

57. Giovannetti, S. and Maggiore, Q.: A low-nitrogen diet with proteins of high biological value for severe chronic uraemia. Lancet. 1: 1000, 1964.

58. Berlyne, G.M., Bazzard, F.J., Booth, E.M., Janabi, K. and Shaw, A.B.: The dietary treatment of acute renal failure. Q.J. Med. 36: 59, 1967.

59. Levin, S., and Winkelstein, J.A.: Diet and infrequent dialysis in chronic anuric uremia. N. Engl. J. Med. 277: 619, 1967.

60. Rubini, M.E., and Gordon, S.: Individual plasmafree amino acids in uremia: Effect of hemodialysis. Nephron 5: 339, 1968.

61. Blumenkrantz, M.J., Ghal, G.M., Kepple, J.D., et al: Protein losses during peritoneal dialysis. Kidney Int. 19: 593, 1980.

62. Dudrick, S.J., Steiger, E. and Long, J.M.: Renal failure in surgical patients. Treatment with intravenous essential amino acids and hypertonic glucose. Surg. 68: 180, 1970.

63. Abel, R.M., et al.: Improved survival from acute renal failure after treatment with essential L-amino acids and glucose. N. Engl. J. Med. 288: 695, 1973.

64. Baek, S.M., Makabali, G.G., Bryan-Brown, C.W., et al: The influence of parenteral nutrition on the course of acute renal failure. Surgery, Gynecology and Obstetrics. 141: 405, 1975.

65. Toback, F.G.: Amino Acid enhancement of regeneration after acute tubular necrosis. Kidney Int. 12: 193, 1977.

66. Toback, F.G., Teegarden, D.E. and Havener, L.J.: Amino acid-mediated stimulation of renal phospholipid biosynthesis after acute tubular necrosi Kidney Int. 15: 542, 1979.

67. Abitbol, C.L. and Holliday, M.A.: Total parenteral nutrition in anuric children. Clin. Neph. 5: 153, 1976.

68. Toback, F.G.: Amino Acid Treatment of Acute Renal Failure. In: Brenner, B.M., and Stein, J.H. eds. Acute Renal Failure. Churchill Livingstone, 1980: p. 202.

69. Schrier, R.W.: Acute renal failure. JAMA, 247: 18, 1982.

70. Chesney R.W., Kaplan, B.S., Freedom, R.M., et al: Acute renal failure. An important complication of cardiac surgery in infants. J. Pediatr. 87: 381, 1975.

71. Stott, R.B., Ogg, C.S., Cameron, J.S., and Bewick, M.: Why the persistently high mortality in acute renal failure? Lancet 2: 75, 1972.

Mailing Address: Section of Pediatric Nephrology, St. Christopher's Hospital for Children, Department of Pediatrics, Temple University School of Medicine, 5th & Lehigh Avenue, Philadelphia, PA. 19133.

Supported in part by Clinical Center Research Grant RR75 and NIH grants, HL 23511, HL 19869 and the Hoechst-Roussel Corporation.

SOME ASPECTS OF TREATMENT OF SEPTIC SHOCK

Heinz F. Eichenwald, M.D.

The word "shock" describes a complex pathophysiologic state of circulatory impairment sufficiently severe to affect delivery of oxygen and essential nutrients to tissues which, in turn, produces alterations in cellular metabolism. When the condition is associated with infection, the situation is further complicated by the various effects of endotoxin and/or other bacterial products; septic shock is caused not only by endotoxin-producing bacteria but also by other organisms such as staphylococci, streptococci and pneumococci. Furthermore endotoxin can be demonstrated in the blood stream of most patients with severe shock, no matter what its cause. Presumably this is the result of anoxic damage to the mucosa of the colon which allows bacterial products in the lumen to diffuse into the circulation. A self-sustaining process may then develop, with increasing severity of shock leading to further absorption of endotoxin which, in turn, accelerates the severity of the process.

It is common practice to divide the various shock syndromes into three types: a) hypovolemic, b) cardiogenic and c) distributive shock. This classification, while useful for purposes of discussion, is somewhat simplistic because elements of two or even all three types may coexist in a patient.

Hypovolemic shock results from a significant reduction in circulatory blood volume. Such a loss requires the body to make a number of homeostatic adjustments in order to maintain arterial and perfusion pressures in critical organs such as the brain and the heart. These adjustments may indeed restore cardiac output and systemic arterial pressure but this is often accomplished at the expense of the blood flow in various regional circulations.

Cardiogenic shock occurs when cardiac function is depressed to the point that the circulation can no longer meet the metabolic needs of tissues. This, almost by definition, means diminished cardiac output (Fig. 1).

Distributive shock is the result of faulty distribution of blood flow, produced by vasomotor paralysis or physiologic arterial-venous shunting past capillary beds. Among its causes are sepsis, anaphylaxis, central nervous system injury and drug intoxication.

Many of the thoughts in this paper are based on material prepared by Dr. Daniel Levin to whom I am also indebted for the figures and tables.

Figure 1. Self-perpetuating pathways in cardiogenic shock

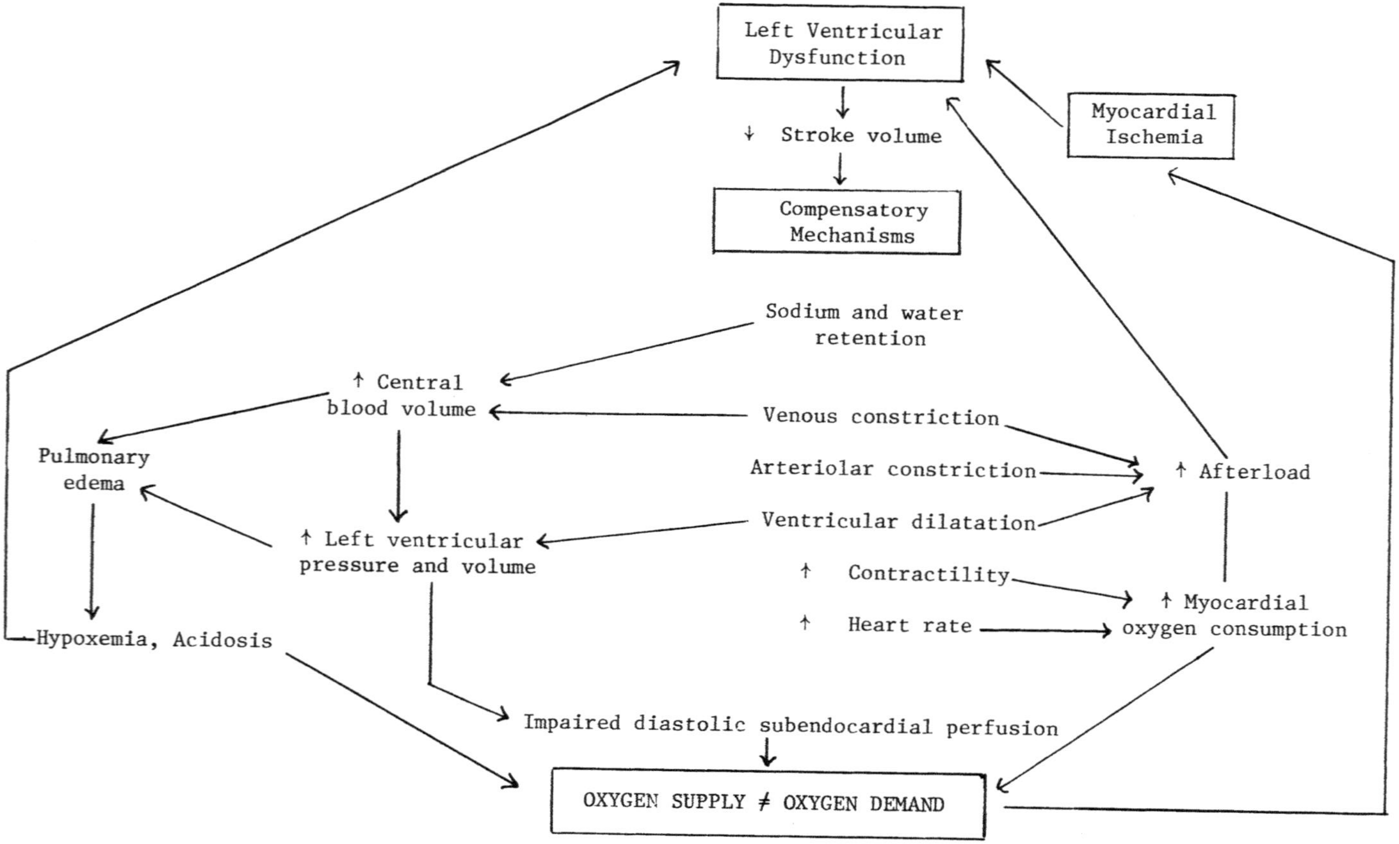

At present, the aspect of shock that can be treated most successfully is circulatory failure; it is often possible to support the circulation for long periods of time only to have the patient die of multiple organ failures such as "shock lung", gastrointestinal bleeding, acute renal failure or central nervous system damage so severe as to make meaningful life impossible.

THERAPY

Because of the complexity of the problem, only certain aspects of treatment will be discussed. Thus, no mention will be made of non-controversial therapeutic approaches, such as the administration of oxygen, or of specialized problems, such as burns, which require a somewhat different plan of action.

Successful treatment of even moderate degrees of shock requires the use of sophisticated monitoring equipment; the days are long gone when a patient's condition was judged on the basis of blood pressure and pulse rate. Because of the fact that individual children respond differently to shock as well as to various methods of therapy, and because treatment may involve the use of powerful pharmacologic medications, sophisticated measuring tools are absolutely essential to monitor the parameters listed in Table 1.

The most immediate goal of therapy is the maintenance or restoration of circulation. This is best accomplished by dealing with various aspects of ventricular performance.

Heart rate and rhythm are generally not treated directly since they respond to appropriate therapy of other determinants of ventricular performance. The preload to the ventricle can be returned to normal by the administration of various types of fluid to correct hypovolemia. If the patient has lost significant amounts of blood, normal red cell mass must be re-established with blood transfusions.

Solutions of crystalloids are often used to correct hypovolemia but there is little agreement about the ingredients these should contain or their relative concentration. Isotonic solutions such as lactated Ringers remain within the extracellular space, hypotonic solutions become more uniformly distributed throughout the body water and hypertonic fluids cause a shift of intracellular water into the extracellular space. In general, hypotonic solutions are never used in the immediate resuscitation of shock patients.

Colloid solutions, especially iso-oncotic ones such as 5% albumin in 0.9% sodium chloride, fresh frozen plasma, or plasma protein fractions produce consistently greater and more prolonged volume expansion than do similar amounts of isotonic crystalloid solutions.

Table 1. Common causes of hypovolemia in children

Whole Blood Loss

Hemorrhage
- External
- Internal - gastrointestinal bleeding, hepatic or splenic rupture, fractures, major vessel injury, intracranial bleeding, surgical complications.

Relative Loss
- Anesthetic agents (vasodilatation)
- Vasodilating drugs (e.g., phentolamine)
- Positive pressure ventilation
- Sepsis

Plasma Loss

Burns
Inflammation/sepsis (capillary leak syndrome)
Nephrotic syndrome
Intestinal obstruction
Hypoproteinemic syndromes

Fluid and Electrolyte Loss

Vomiting and diarrhea
Excessive sweating
Pathologic renal loss
- Altered intrinsic renal function
- Endocrine causes such as adrenal insufficiency, diabetes insipidus, diabetes mellitus

Synthetic plasma expanders have been widely used in developing countries as well as in Europe and include a number of different materials such as dextrans, starches, and gelatin but our own experience with these substances is limited. Aside from ready availability, they appear to possess no advantage over plasma or plasma-derived materials.

The treatment of hypovolemic shock thus includes the administration of isotonic crystalloid solutions, initially administered in amounts not exceeding 20 ml/kg (Fig. 2). If two such infusions fail to increase pulse pressure, correct metabolic acidosis or allow adequate urine output, further measures must be undertaken but require that central venous pressure be measured because otherwise cardiac failure from excessive fluid administration may occur. If central venous pressure is found to be low, a third fluid challenge may be attempted but should this also fail to produce improvement, the next step consists of pharmacologic therapy which has as its goal the improvement of cardiac function and vascular tone. This involves the use of inotropic and vasoactive drugs, such as the

FIGURE 2. Approach to fluid management in a child with hypovolemic shock

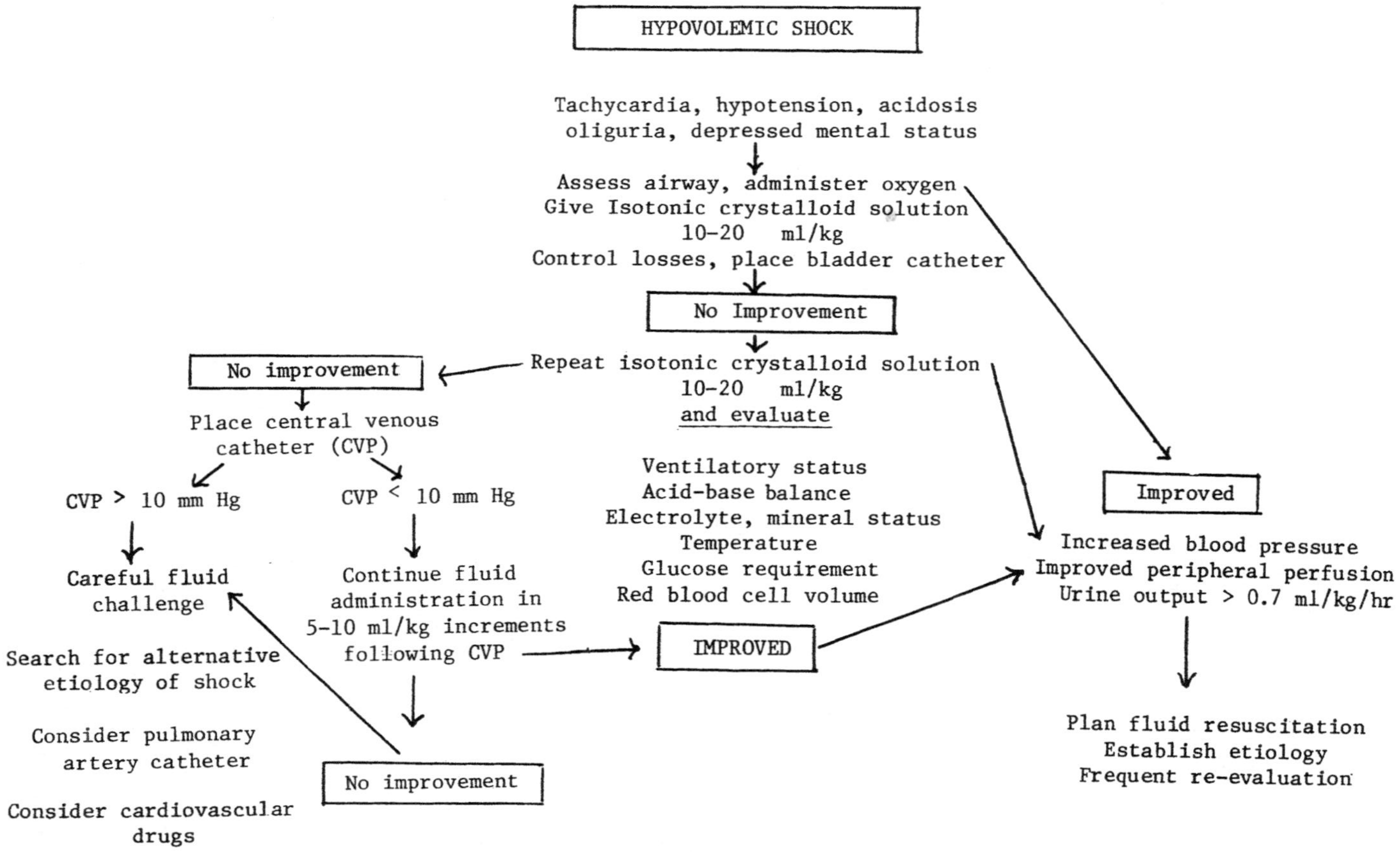

sympathomimetic amines norepinephrine, epinephrine, isoproterenol, dopamine and dobutamine. These drugs affect not only heart rate, but also produce a number of complex changes in the vascular bed of various organs which under certain circumstances, may further complicate the patient's course and thereby have a deleterious effect on his shock state (Table 2).

The sympathomimetic amines are administered continuously through a central catheter. There is no usual drug or usual dosage; the rate of administration is based on the patient's response. Because of their great potency and narrow margin of safety, these drugs must never be used without ongoing supervision by a physician familiar with their actions.

Survival in septic shock seems to depend greatly on the ability to maintain a hyperdynamic state. Nevertheless, mortality rates continue high in septic patients requiring pharmacologic intervention, perhaps due to the fact that such treatment improves the functioning of some organs at the expense of others.

Digitalis was once widely used to aid a failing heart by improving its muscular function. Most authorities now agree that this drug has no place in the early stages of management of shock.

Somewhat paradoxically, vasodilators are also useful when the contractile state of the ventricles is depressed. Various homeostatic changes in response to shock produce increased systemic vascular resistance, resulting in increased afterload along with ventricular dysfunction. Under such circumstances, a reduction in the afterload may result in improved cardiac output. The use of vasodilators in shock, therefore, is generally limited to those situations where cardiac dysfunctions exist, associated with elevated ventricular filling pressures, increased systemic vascular resistance, and normal or near normal systemic arterial blood pressure. The effects that vasodilators produce on the heart depend on their action on the arterial and venous systems. Those agents which dilate the arteriolar vessels will decrease arterial resistance with a resulting increase in ventricular stroke volume. Drugs which predominantly cause dilation of the venous sytem increase venous capacitance and thereby lower the filling pressures of both ventricles. The production of severe hypotension is the major risk of vasodilator therapy, but this danger can be reduced by careful hemodynamic monitoring and proper fluid therapy. The vasodilator drugs most frequently used include phentolamine, hydralazine, nitroprusside and nitroglycerin (Table 2).

Metabolic acidosis occurs commonly in shock and is especially severe in septic infants where, on occasion, it may prove impossible to restore a normal blood pH. In general, correction of inadequate tissue perfusion will result in relief of acidosis. Should the degree of acidosis be such that it affects ventricular response by depressing the myocardium, measures should be taken to correct the arterial blood pH to 7.25 or above.

To achieve this, sodium bicarbonate is usually employed. Before the exact base deficit is known, 1-2 mEq/kg may be administered but further dosage is calculated on the basis of measured base deficit. No attempt should be made to fully correct arterial pH levels because

Table 2. Stages of septic shock

Early: Hyperdynamic	Late: Cardiogenic
Bedside Observations	
Tachycardia	Tachycardia
Tachypnea	Respiratory depression
Febrile	Hypothermia
Warm extremities	Cool, pale extremities
Bounding pulses	Decreased pulses
Normal capillary refill	Prolonged capillary refill
Normal or elevated systemic systolic blood pressure	Hypotension
Wide pulse pressure	Narrow pulse pressure
Elevated cardiac index	Depressed cardiac index
Decreased systemic vascular resistance	Increased systemic vascular resistance
Adequate urine output or polyuria	Oliguria
Mild mental confusion, occasional hallucinations	Lethargy or coma
Laboratory Measurements	
Hypoxemia	Hypoxemia
Respiratory alkalosis	Respiratory acidosis
± Metabolic acidosis	Metabolic acidosis
Marked pulmonary shunt	Minimal pulmonary shunt
Narrow arterio-venous oxygen saturation difference	Wide arterio-venous O_2 saturation difference
Hyperglycemia	Hypoglycemia
Mild coagulation abnormalities	Marked coagulopathy
Normal or mild elevation of blood lactate	Markedly elevated blood lactate

too rapid administration of bicarbonate may cause paradoxical intracellular acidosis with extracellular alkalosis which impairs the delivery of oxygen and favors the development of hypokalemia or hypocalcemia. Larger doses may also result in hypernatremia with hypertonicity. If the patient has respiratory acidosis, any administered bicarbonate may increase the degree of acidosis because this ion is metabolized to carbon dioxide and water, producing further elevation of $PaCO_2$. When respiratory acidosis occurs in shock, it is usually related to such events as muscle fatigue, pneumonia, pulmonary edema, pneumothorax or incorrect mechanical ventilation. Under these circumstances, adequate ventilation must be established.

One of the organs most profoundly affected by shock is the kidney. In general, adequate restoration of plasma volume and improvement in left ventricular dysfunction will prevent acute renal failure. In patients whose fluid replacement appears adequate but who continue to have poor urine output, an injection of mannitol and/or furosemide may convert oliguric renal failure to high output renal failure. Should these measures not induce a diuresis, it is likely that the child has acute renal failure, which must be treated by careful fluid, electrolyte and acid-base control. Should hyperkalemia, acidosis, etc. follow, dialysis may be required.

The liver is also affected by shock but the degree of dysfunction is determined to a considerable extent by the nutritional support that the patient receives. Short periods of starvation are tolerated reasonably well by adequately nourished older children but younger ones are more profoundly affected by the massive catabolism of shock. Poorly or malnourished youngsters require almost immediate nutritional support to protect the liver.

The gastrointestinal tract also becomes involved but while stress ulceration occurs commonly, the frequency of bleeding or perforation is low. These complications can be prevented by continuously neutralizing gastric acidity to levels of pH of 4 or higher.

One obvious aspect of therapy in septic shock is the control of the infection. This represents a chapter all of its own and requires expert management by an individual schooled in the use of antimicrobial agents. Because of the circulatory disturbances and organ damage associated with shock, the excretion, metabolism and toxicity of most antimicrobial agents are profoundly altered. Adequate management of the patient's infection require frequent monitoring of serum and/or urine levels of antibiotic.

Recently the use of an anti-endotoxin antiserum was shown to alter favorably the outcome of septic shock in adults; it seems likely that in the future such material may become part of standard therapy but at this point in time, its use must be considered experimental.

The routine use of heparin and of corticosteroids, has been advocated by some investigators but is decried by others. Evidence exists that large, so called "pharmacologic doses" of corticosteroids have some beneficial effects on the clinical course of adults with shock. In children, no similar studies have been performed, so this form of therapy remains controversial. The usual reason that corticosteroids are administered is based on the physician's belief that severe infections produce a hypoadrenal state. This rarely occurs; cortisol levels are usually increased, even in children with meningococcal sepsis.

The use of heparin also had its supporters because it was believed that this drug would prevent disseminated intravascular coagulation (DIC) which occurs to some degree in all shock patients. It is now known that heparin is usually ineffective and that DIC can be managed and prevented more successfully by controlling the infection, and by improving the circulation, hypoxia, and acidosis.

In summary then, successful therapy of septic shock consists of an individualized approach to each patient, the management of the pathophysiologic states as they occur, and the availability of those resources required to monitor the contantly changing clinical parameters of the patient (Figures 3,4 and Tables 3-5).

Table 3. Monitoring Aids for Shock

Bedside

- Electrocardiographic display of heart rate and rhythm
- Skin and/or core temperature
- Intra-arterial systemic blood pressure and pulse wave
- Central venous blood pressure
- Pulmonary arterial and wedge pressure
- Thermodilution cardiac output
- Fluid intake and output

Laboratory

<u>Hematologic</u>:	hemoglobin, hematocrit, white blood cell count, platelet count, coagulation studies
<u>Metabolic</u>:	sodium, potassium, chloride, calcium, phosphorus, osmolality (serum and urine), blood lactate, arterial and mixed venous pH, pCO_2, PO_2 and O_2 saturation, colloid oncotic pressure or total serum protein
<u>Bacteriologic</u>:	appropriate cultures and gram stains

Complementary measurements

- Chest roentgenogram
- Echocardiogram
- Electroencephalogram
- Ultrasonogram
- Computerized tomographic scan
- Intracerebral pressures and blood flows
- Respiratory measurements

Derived data

Cardiac index (CI)

$CI = CO/BSA$

Normal values = 2.8 - 3.5 $l/min/m^2$

Stroke index (SI)

$SI = CI/HR$

Normal values = 35-40 ml/m^2

Systemic vascular resistance index (SVRI)

$$\frac{(MAP - CVP)\ 80}{CI}$$

Normal values = 1700 - 2200 $\frac{\text{dyne sec}}{\text{cm}^5\ \text{M}^2}$

Derived data (Cont.)

Pulmonary vascular resistance index (PVRI)

$$\frac{(MPAP - PCP)\ 80}{CI}$$

Normal values = 100 - 200 $\frac{\text{dyne sec}}{\text{cm}^5\ \text{M}^2}$

Where BSA - body surface area (M^2)
CO - cardiac output (L/min)
HR - heart rate (beat/min)
MAP - mean systemic arterial blood pressure (mm Hg)
MPAP - mean pulmonary arterial blood pressure (mm Hg)
CVP - central venous blood pressure (mm Hg)
PCP - pulmonary capillary pressure (mm Hg)

Figure 3. Fluid challenge for patients in shock

Observe CVP or PWP for 5 - 10 minutes

If CVP	or PWP	Then give following fluid
< 6 mm Hg	< 8 mm Hg	10 ml/kg or 200 ml over 10 min
< 10 mm Hg	< 12 mm Hg	5 ml/kg or 100 ml over 10 min
≥ 10 mm Hg	≥ 12 mm Hg	3 ml/kg or 50 ml over 10 min

Observe CVP or PWP for 10 minutes after challenge

If the CVP returns to within 2 mm Hg or the PWP returns to within 3 mm Hg of preinfusion value then the fluid challenge is resumed. In each instance the pressure value immediately preceeding the fluid challenge serves as the reference measurement. Fluid is administered until either the hemodynamic signs of shock are corrected or the CVP persistently exceeds 2 mm Hg or the PWP persistently exceeds 3 mm Hg of the starting values.

Figure 4. Pharmacologic measures to improve cardiac function in patients with shock syndrome.

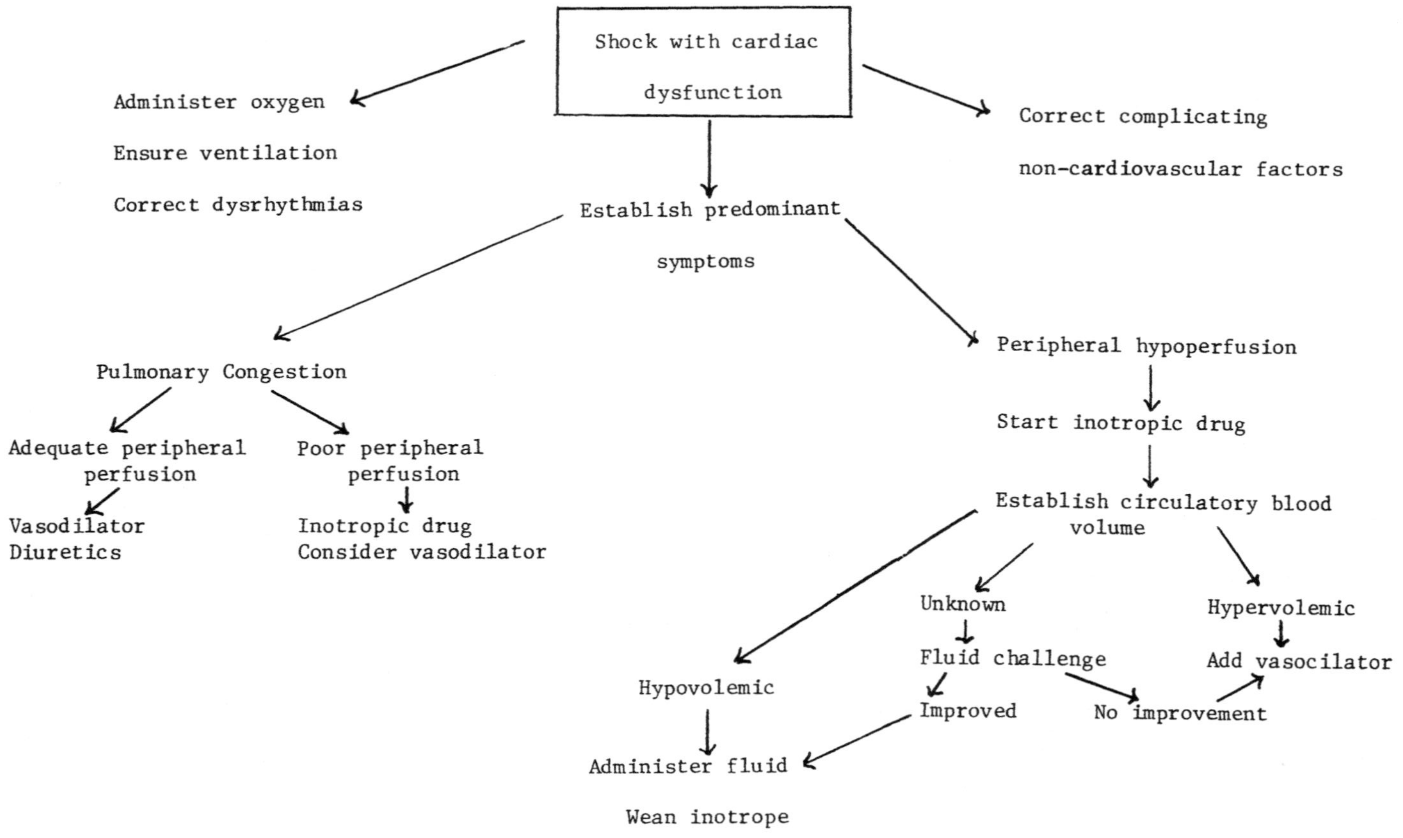

Table 4. Common cardiovascular drugs used in shock

DRUGS	MECHANISM	USUAL DOSE	COMMENT
Norepinephrine	α and β agonist	0.05-1.0 mcg/kg/min	Intense α vasoconstriction may mask the myocardial stimulating effect. May dramatically compromise peripheral tissue and organ perfusion. With systolic arterial blood pressure above 90 mm Hg is usually not indicated.
Epinephrine	α and β agonist	0.05-1.0 mcg/kg/min	Positive inotropic and chronotropic effects. Intensity of stimulation increases with increasing dose. May lead to renal and mesenteric ischemia. Causes tachydysrhythmias and increases myocardial oxygen consumption. Has potent metabolic effects (↑FFA, ↑glucose).
Isoproterenol	β agonist	0.05-0.5 mcg/kg/min	Positive inotropic and chronotropic effects. Peripheral vasodilator which diverts cardiac output to noncritical tissue (skeletal muscle). Dysrhythmogenic.
Dopamine	α and β agonist dopaminergic receptor agonist	1-20 mcg/kg/min	Stimulates cardiac beta receptors by direct and indirect mechanisms. At low doses (< 10 mcg/kg/min) a selective dilation of renal and mesenteric beds occurs. Alpha adrenergic effects predominant at higher doses. May increase pulmonary vascular resistance. Value in newborns and infants is debatable. Dysrhythmogenic.
Dobutamine	Selective β_1	1-10 mcg/kg/min	Positive inotropic effect with minimal chronotropic effect. Mild β_2 activity. Benefit in children is under investigation.

DRUGS	MECHANISM	USUAL DOSE	COMMENT
Sodium Nitroprusside	Smooth muscle relaxation	0.5-8.0 mcg/kg/min	Balanced arterial and venous dilator. Rapid onset, short duration (2-4 sec). May increase pulmonary ventilation / perfusion mismatch. Thiocyanate toxicity. Methhemoglobinemia.
Phentolamine	α antagonist	1-20 mcg/kg/min	Dilation of arterial and venous beds. Indirect inotropic effect. Duration of action 20-40 minutes. May cause tachycardia. Expensive.
Hydralazine	Smooth muscle relaxation	0.1-0.5 mg/kg IV q 3-6 hrs	Duration of action 2-6 hours. Pure arterial dilator. May produce tachycardia. Not for continuous infusion.
Nitroglycerin	Smooth muscle relaxation	N/A	Venodilator. Uncommonly used in children. Exact dosage requirements unknown.

Table 5. Suggested mechanisms or corticosteroid protection in shock*

Circulatory
- Positive inotropic effect
- Vasodilation and improvement in regional blood flows
- Decreased production of vasoactive hormones

Metabolic
- Improved gluconeogenesis
- Antagonism of proteases

Cellular
- Increased neutrophil count
- Stabilization of cellular and intracellular membranes
- Promotion of type II pneumocyte proliferation
- Inhibition of granulocyte and platelet aggregation
- Protection against mast cell disruption
- Preservation of capillary endothelium
- Prevention of formation of toxic factors

*Modified from Lefer AM, Spath JA: Pharmacologic basis of the treatment of circulatory shock, in Cardiovascular Pharmacology, edited by Antonaccio M. Raven Press, New York, 1977.

BIBLIOGRAPHY

1. Bachbinder, N. and Ganz, W.: Hemodynamic monitoring: invasive techniques. Anesthesiology 45:146, 1976.
2. Benotti, P. and Blackburn, G.: Protein and caloric or micronutrient metabolic management of the critically ill patient. Crit. Care Med.7:520, 1979.
3. Cohn, J.N. and Franciosa, J.A.: Selection of vasodilator, inotropic or combined therapy for the management of heart failure. Am. J. Med. 65:181, 1978.
4. Mammond, G.L.: Acute respiratory failure. Surg. Clin. North Am. 60:1133, 1980.
5. Hazard, P.B. and Griffin, J.P.: Sodium bicarbonate in the management of systemic acidosis. Southern Med. J. 73:1339, 1980.
6. John, E.G., et al.: Management of acute renal failure complicating cardiac surgery in infants and children. Crit. Care Med. 8:562, 1980.
7. Lappas, D.G., et al.: Cardiac dysfunction in the perioperative period: pathophysiology, diagnosis, and treatment. Anesthesiology 47:117, 1977.
8. Lucas, C.E.: Resuscitation of the injured patient: The three phases of treatment. Surg. Clin. North Am. 57:3, 1977.
9. Perkiñ, P.M., and Levin, D.L.: Common fluid and electrolyte problems in the pediatric intensive care unit. Pediatr. Clin. North Am. 27:567, 1980.
10. Shoemaker, W.C., and Hauser, C.J.: Critique of crystalloid versus colloid therapy in shock and shock lung. Crit. Care Med. 7:117, 1979.

11. Siegel, J.H., et al: Ventilation: perfusion maldistribution secondary to the hyperdynamic cardiovascular state as the major cause of increased pulmonary shunting in human sepsis, J. Trauma 19:432, 1979.
12. Siegel, H.H., et al: Physiological and metabolic correlations in human sepsis. Surgery 86:163, 1979.
13. Tarazi, R.C.: Sympathomimetic agents in the treatment of shock. Ann. Intern. Med. 81: 364, 1974.
14. Zweifach, B.W., and Fronek, A.: The interplay of central and peripheral factors in irreversible hemorrhagic shock. Prog. Cardiovasc. Dis. 18:147, 1975.

PANEL DISCUSSION: ACUTE RENAL FAILURE

MODERATOR: José Strauss, M.D.

QUESTION: I want to present very briefly the history of a child with minimal lesion nephrotic syndrome whom I took care of recently. A year ago she presented with minimal lesion nephrotic syndrome, did not respond to prednisone, and therefore was given a course of chlorambucil. Eventually, she responded and eventually she was taken off prednisone. About a year after her initial presentation, she had a relapse and we elected to watch her a few days before starting therapy again whereupon she began to feel slightly ill in the afternoon, and by the evening was admitted to our intensive care unit in a state of shock. A diagnosis of peritonitis was made and subsequently streptococcus pneumoniae was cultured from the blood. Her shock was treated with administration of normal saline, Ringer's lactate, and antibiotics were given; methylprednisolone in large doses was administered. She appeared to be responding but not all that well. So, I began to give her albumin. After a few hours her blood pressure normalized; her sensorium was normal; her urine output was normal; she was eating well. We were planning to send her down to the ward. Eight hours after she had begun to feel well, she very suddenly collapsed, had massive pulmonary edema, and was put on a respirator; resuscitation was attempted but she died. At post-mortem she had massive pulmonary edema and minimal, hardly significant, peritonitis. Now, her serum albumin at the time of admission was around 1.5 g/dl and at the time of death was 2.6 g/dl. Listening to you, I began to remember that perhaps she had received chloramphenicol: that two-gun salute to an unknown organism or an organism of unknown sensitivity. She probably got chloramphenicol and ampicillin. I'm going to check that when I go back. It is interesting that her sudden death occurred about an hour after she was given her second dose of antibiotics. But, a great deal of anxiety was provoked in myself by accusations by many people that I had contributed toward the death of this child by the administration of albumin. Papers were found in the surgical literature, quite a few, pointing to the development of shock lung consequent to the administration of albumin. I really would like to hear your views on this subject. Secondly, I would like to know how you feel about putting a patient on a respirator when he comes in with quite severe lung disease but doesn't appear to have a good indication for respirator support at the time.

RESPONSE: This is the sort of unfortunate patient that happens to all of us and I don't think you did anything wrong. Obviously, no matter what you do, there are going to be some bystanders who are going to say you did the wrong thing. They probably would say that even if the patient had done extremely well. This is the nature of things. I think it is possible that chloramphenicol was related to the problem. I am very concerned about the use of chloramphenicol and there is no longer any reason to use it except out of habit which is what's going on now. Secondly, albumin, interestingly enough, is associated more commonly with shock lung than plasma or fresh frozen plasma. The reason for that may be related to the fact that albumin is a fraction product. It has been subjected to cold ethanol precipitation and you can show that there are particles in it which block particular endothelial cells and pulmonary macrophages. What sort of situation leads to the development of pulmonary edema, I do not know. I probably would have given the child albumin also, and in fact I have treated patients somewhat similarly, perhaps like this, without having the severe pulmonary edema and shock lung develop. It's hard to say, I don't really know. I think you did what needed to be done. I would probably not have used the steroids because you then have at least two possible provoking factors of shock, the steroids which might produce a Schwartzman-like phenomenon, and chloramphenicol (in itself pharmacologically active). But otherwise, I'm sure that all of you have treated very similar patients with great success.

COMMENT: We are in a double bind with respect to steroids in a patient who has been on long-term steroid therapy, but I take your point.

COMMENT: I would use only physiological doses.

RESPONSE: Yes, of course, physiological doses. In reviewing this unfortunate patient, I noticed that in the series of nephrotics in the International Study of Kidney Disease in Children, there was at least one other similar case.

COMMENT: I really don't know why the patient died. I don't know whether there was anything you did that was responsible. I doubt it. But the same patient at some other time under the same circumstances might have done very well.

MODERATOR: I wonder whether this is the time to bring back the subject of crystalloid versus colloid. At various times the subject did come up during the Seminar. The point that was made I think is very important. It was said that going from one to the other does not make as much sense as introducing a pharmacologic agent. Can we agree on a general approach as to why albumin versus sodium lactate, sodium chloride, or other solutions? Does it actually make any difference? What are the specific situations, other than hemorrhagic shock, when you would give blood? Are there any comments or thoughts that the panelists would like to express in this regard?

RESPONSE: The particular recommendation I make is that you could use three fluid challenges, the last one only if you can measure central venous pressure. Then, you go to pharmacologic therapy simply based on experience - experience of quite a few intensivists who have found that after the three fluid challenges if you then go on to a colloid, you will overload the child and you will get into problems. If you use the colloids earlier, you also produce some problems. Now, I used to be a very big colloid man. I initially felt that you started with plasma right away but the various physiologic measurements that we can now do in the intact patient indicate that that is not the way to go -- that the initial correction of whatever this complex of physiologic parameters that shock is, is best achieved with the electrolyte solutions. But, I don't know which electrolyte solution is best. That evidence, no one has. No one has done "controlled studies" of one electrolyte solution versus another. To go from colloids to pharmacologic therapy, particularly in septic shock where you have to produce a hypermetabolic state in order to get survival, is the most logical way. It may not be the best way but it's the best we can do at this time.

COMMENT: I have personally never been too enamored with the use of colloid. In my own simplistic way of thinking about it, the body is a box of a number of compartments. And whether or not one is shocky, the reflection of that is the intravascular volume. How is that held in place by the interstitial volume? What happens when the intravascular volume is acutely changed by Central Nervous System activity, circulating catecholamines, etc.? One of the things at least I've thought about is, if you put colloid into the intravascular compartment, and for the sake of argument say it can't move out very well, when the vascular tone starts changing, the fluid overloads the circulation, and the patient runs into problems whereas if you use pure crystalloid you are much more able to adapt to those rapid changes. My own personal approach has been pretty much to use crystalloid. I think one of the best examples of the use of crystalloid alone has to do with the massive amounts used to treat burn shock where, without much colloid, one can do very well. So, I think it's a matter of getting back to first order principles. With the newborn and the prematures, people giving colloid have found that they are overloading and getting intravascular hemorrhage. The other problem is, if you give it, you can't get it out. It's a problem. And crystalloid is easier to deal with; so, perhaps it is more practical.

MODERATOR: This has application to other areas. I remember in Latin America being asked very often the question, what type of fluid do you give to a patient that has diarrhea? And everybody has a fancy formula. So, it has application to a number of areas, not only shock or acute renal failure.

COMMENT: The other point just worth mentioning because we were going to do an albumin-peritoneal dialysis last week, is that the albumin is extraordinarily expensive. I'm sure one can use it, but again the question is, does it really work or where does it really work?

COMMENT: It looks and feels and acts like fish glue which tends to make me shy away from it. It is not pure albumin. We talk about it as one thing, but it has changed. And, if you radio-label it, you can see that it is selectively picked up by the endothelial system as a foreign substance. The cold ethanol precipitation used in its production physically changes the initial protein molecule which makes much of it; then it is considered by the body to be a foreign substance and it is picked up. I don't think blockage of a particular endothelial system is a good thing in a patient who is in shock.

COMMENT-QUESTION: The other question just worth asking in passing is: what is the osmolality of the solution? As everyone knows, one often uses 5% dextrose and half-normal saline to initially rehydrate children with gastroenteritis. Yet, when you run that down a little bit (and indeed 10% dextrose alone has been used to treat shock, although I would not personally use it), you are providing a hyper-osmolar solution into the intravascular compartment. Or if you are giving normal saline or Ringer's lactate, at least it is iso-osmotic but when you put in, at least transiently, something that is hyperosmotic, you get fluid movement from intra- to extra-cellular compartments. Again, this may impact upon the rapidity with which you reverse a shock-like state. On the other hand, one always has to keep in mind, when you subsequently change the composition of the solution, if you put in something that is less hyperosmotic than what you have been infusing, the fluid will, by definition, move in the other direction and if you don't provide enough osmols you can run into fluid shifts and hypovolemic problems once again.

COMMENT: Pertaining to the case just presented, I wanted to introduce another question, and that is, maybe some patients with nephrotic syndrome are different birds and we are seeing more and more patients with full blown nephrotic syndrome, hypoalbuminemic, who we presume are hypovolemic; we give them albumin and they do not have an appropriate diuretic response. Recent data from adult populations suggest that our whole concept of the pathophysiology of nephrotic syndrome probably cannot be applied to all the patients. There are some patients who, despite being hypoalbuminemic, have hypervolemia, and suppression of renin-aldosterone. This is completely contrary to the orthodox concept. And we wonder if other things might not have played a role in the generation of pulmonary edema in that particular patient; it may be similar to the capillary permeability in nephrotics.

RESPONSE: I think the point is well taken in the child who comes off the street with nephrotic syndrome. However, if the patient comes in with very low blood pressure and poor peripheral perfusion, and metabolic acidosis, I think it would be not unreasonable to assume that the patient is hypovolemic and has poor distribution of whatever circulating volume he has. I think that is a different circumstance. And there is the danger in those patients of acute tubular necrosis developing. Acute tubular necrosis in adults certainly can be irreversible. So, one is caught between the devil and a hard place when one is dealing with a nephrotic who is in shock.

COMMENT: I agree entirely. But I think that even if he is hypovolemic and in shock this does not negate the possibility that there is also increased capillary permeability. So, obviously, both things can coincide.

QUESTION: I wonder how could you be sure that this pulmonary symptom did not belong to extensive hemorrhagic pneumonia in a septic nephrotic with a bacteremia and streptococcal pneumonia? I wonder because we see that in our place and it is not easy any time to distinguish between infectious problems.

RESPONSE: Again, the point is well taken. There weren't extensive areas of hemorrhage on post-mortem examination. There was massive pulmonary edema. The time sequence was what bothered me so much- that the patient was theoretically getting better and certainly had been given appropriate antibiotic therapy, and then ZAP! So, what I have agonized about is, what was the ZAP? I think if the child were on chloramphenicol - I have to check on that - that might have been it. One has to look for another factor. But the adult respiratory distress syndrome with shock lung, can occur several hours later when the patient is in fact doing well. It's not clear to me why that occurs. Maybe it is because there is damage to the lung early on but the results of it are only seen later. It puzzles me, this adult shock lung syndrome.

COMMENT: I did refer to this peripherally in one of my comments when I was talking a while ago. We do see patients in whom we are able to correct the cardiovascular problems completely - at least as far as we can measure-but who still die of shock lung. As you say, this happens later. Why this develops, I don't know. The reason I made the statement is that we are so capable of dealing with cardiovascular problems that they die of other causes at the present time.

QUESTION: You mentioned in terms of your priorities, rehydrating the patient first, and then giving antibiotics. I was wondering if you could be a bit more specific in terms of time. Are you talking about waiting an hour, two hours, 30 minutes before giving antibiotics? The other half of the question would be, in a patient presumed to be septic, would you alter your first dose of antibiotics, give a bit less?

RESPONSE: To answer the second question first, no, I would not alter the dose because I wouldn't know what to alter it to. You could say, well I ought to use less, maybe, but I don't know how much less one would use. To answer the first part of the question, I think that is an individual decision made for an individual patient. I would like to see the patient reasonably "stabilized" before I start antimicrobial therapy. Patients don't die that quickly from infection. The reason they die from infection, generally,is because they go into shock, because they become hypoxic or whatever. We are controlling that part of the illness at that point, and some of the patients whom we can take care of relatively rapidly - the meningococcemia is a good example - can start on antimicrobial therapy within a half-hour to an hour after management has been begun. On the other hand, a patient with Rocky Mountain Spotted Fever in shock probably should not be treated, mostly because of the two drugs that are involved (either tetracycline or chloramphenicol),until his shock state has been well controlled and then you can start worrying about the rickettsia. This is heresy. I realize that. And it is very difficult to prove that what I am saying is correct but we do have these human models, meningococcemia, plague, pseudomonas,bacteremias and septicemias, and so forth. There is no reason why these general things which can be observed over and over again clinically should not be generally true. Certainly, our mortality rate of patients who come to us with severe infections is at least as low as anybody else's. While we do things this way, our mortality rates certainly are not increased and, in fact, have diminished in recent years probably primarily because of our greater ability to deal with the physiologic parameters rather than because of any sudden improvement in antimicrobial therapy.

QUESTION: I wanted to ask you, if you would, to amplify a little bit or perhaps to evaluate for us through the perspective of your experience, this paper which you alluded to in the New England Journal where a J strain of E. Coli was used to produce antibody to endotoxin and where the results in that article look so startlingly good. I felt as though if I were faced with a patient with endotoxic shock, the first thing I would want to do is send somebody to make a call to San Diego where they had this available and get it as quickly as I could. Can you put that in a little bit of perspective for us. How valuable do you think this is going to be in the future?

RESPONSE: I think it's going to be a supplementary thing. I don't think it's going to produce a profound change in our management of these patients. Interestingly enough, there has been an experimental method which goes about it in the diametrically opposite manner. We have used it under very careful circumstances and that polymyxin B, which as I indicated is a useless antibiotic, has the interesting property of binding endotoxin. The bound polymyxin B-endotoxin, at least in animal models, is less toxic than either polymyxin B or endotoxin on its own. So, in some profoundly endotoxemic children, we have used this approach. It is hard to control, of course. It's the impression that it probably does do some good. I believe that the anti-endotoxin anti-serum will be very much in that category. It may make the difference in some patients between death and survival, which is the way I would interpret the data that they showed. But it will not have a profound effect in children, I believe, to reduce the mortality from endotoxemia, and it will not negate all the other things that we should be doing. What I am afraid of, and this almost invariably happens when a new material appears on the market, is that people will get it and then step back and wait to see if a patient isn't going to get miraculously well. That's not the way to go at it.

COMMENT: Of course, giving something like an antibody to endotoxin does not mitigate against giving good supportive care which has to be the mainstay of therapy. But the mortalities, as I remember, in that multicenter study were 70% for the control group which did not receive that antibody and 50% for those that did. That's quite a significant difference it seems, if they were truly comparable. It appears that they were.

COMMENT: I should have said something which I omitted to say. Adults have much more trouble with endotoxin, older adults - of which there were a lots in this study - than do children. In fact, until about ten years ago there was a huge argument among the endotoxologists as to whether indeed endotoxemia was of any profound clinical significance in children. In animal models one can show that the young of a species may be considerably more or considerably less susceptible to endotoxin effects than a mature member of that species. You can change that around depending upon which animal species you use. There are, of course, only indirect data that would bear on this problem in humans. If you have a child with endotoxemia and in shock, our present cure rates are so high - completely different. We don't lose 70% of the children. We lose maybe 10% if that. So, that's the introduction of another method. It's probably going to have some effect but it won't be as great as it is in these adults, mostly old people.

MODERATOR: Before we leave that subject, somebody wants to ask you to tell us what is your experience with exchange transfusion in septic shock with and without DIC.

RESPONSE: Septic shock is like so many other things. Exchange transfusions have been used for an awful lot of things. Whenever people talk about a toxin, exchange transfusion seems to make sense. It might even be better if we had some human "sani-flush" to rinse the patient out for whatever ails him. The problem with endotoxin is that it binds to tissue immediately. It's a very acid material. To me it doesn't make any logical sense to use exchange transfusions under those circumstances and it introduces another whole set of problems. The child who is in shock does not need another set of problems, which I think exchange transfusion does introduce. It's the same business as with the Reye Syndrome. After the initial enthusiasm, it became evident that this approach was really not life-saving as had been proposed. I personally don't use it. I'm not impressed by the data which people have presented to show that it does lower mortality rates. I don't think it does. I don't think anyone has proven that it does. I simply have never used it and I would not use it until such a time as there is a good study which proves that it is of benefit. I would venture to predict that it is going to be of benefit in some small, definable subgroup of children rather than in the general sense - all children with septic shock. Incidently, we do not exchange infants either for that reason although this has been widely advocated by others. They are reporting mortality rates of 25% or so with group B or E. Coli septicemias. Ours are much lower than that without an exchange.

COMMENT: We don't quite have a "sani-flush" system but we have a sanitized system called dialysis that's been used for virtually everything under the sun and hasn't turned out to be too useful for much of anything else other than controlling uremic symptomatology. But the other point I would make for those who wander in and out of intensive care units, as soon as you add a new therapy, dialysis, exchange transfusion, etc., etc., etc., what people forget to do while they are trying to get all these things going, is to monitor the basic support systems of the patient, and the patients invariably have more trouble, the more modalities one adds. Unless one can clearly show a therapeutic benefit ratio for some of these things, one ought to be very skeptical about using them.

COMMENT: You just stated beautifully what I have tried to say in a much less succinct manner. He is perfectly right.

MODERATOR: I agree. I think it is our resposibility truly to be more selective so that we don't provide our dialysis services indiscriminately. We have grown in that respect and should feel quite within our rights in having a medical as well as a technical opinion.

COMMENT: We forget that as nephrologists, we have the right to dialyze or not to dialyze. You run into this all the time with the surgeons who say I won't operate because of such and such. People who do all these techniques have the right to say they won't do them. More importantly, you have the moral obligation to be sure that what you are doing is going to offer some benefit.

MODERATOR: In addition, I think that as we have evolved in our Division, the Dialysis Unit nurses have played a more important role and what I require now is that the nurses understand and accept why we are doing the procedure. If there are any questions,we get together and kick it around and sometimes don't do it. As a matter of fact, the reason all the nurses, or most of them are here now is because we were discussing yesterday the lack of need for a so-called "emergency procedure" that had to be done today because somebody else made that decision. We are taking a more responsible approach and challenging some of the demands.

COMMENT: As I get older,I get more and mor away from what is one of the problems of American medicine which is that it is an activist medicine. We feel we must do something. As I get older, I get more passive, contemplative. In my "middle age" I am more of a contemplative physician than activist. This is based on the fact that many things that were said to really do beautifully, within a few years were shown to be of no value or of negative value. So, like most of you, I'm sure, I've become increasingly skeptical of some of the easy solutions to difficult problems.

MODERATOR: The work of one of my heroes, Bill Silverman, one of the greats of Babies Hospital, is taken as the model for many study designs. He has a very keen mind and lived through hyperoxygenation in Neonatology and helped in calling attention to its dangers. He used to say, "DON'T do something!" He wanted people to do what they could document as being useful.

QUESTION: In the lists of acute renal failure, pyelonephritis was included. In adult nephrology I can't ever recall seeing it, and some of my mentors have said they have never seen it. Is there something unique about pediatrics or does this also not occur? Obstruction with papillary necrosis and acute renal failure with infections are one thing, but just pure pyelonephritis, say without sepsis? I'd like some comments on that.

RESPONSE: Yes, I would agree that so-called fulminant pyelonephritis in the absence of papillary necrosis is not responsible for acute renal failure. But you will find it traditionally listed in many references. I think that it is a lack of understanding of what is going on in patients who appear to have pyelonephritis. I think most of them are in septic shock, particularly in the perinatal period. The newborn infant who is septic may have renal involvement and may, at one time, have been thought to have fulminant pyelonephritis. But, actually, the acute renal failure is more likely to have a vasomotor type of pathogenesis, secondary to sepsis.

MODERATOR: I just finished looking at the literature for a chapter we are writing about the Intensive Care Unit situation, particularly for the neonate, and I quoted Gustavo Gordillo's experience. I think he has the largest series of Acute Renal Failure in infants. Do you think that those patients that he reported as having acute renal failure secondary to pyelonephritis did not truly have acute renal failure?

RESPONSE: I have trouble in the absence of a papillary necrosis kind of situation, ascribing an acute renal failure simply to a pyelonephritis, however fulminant it might be. I don't have any proof for it, and I know it is in all the references and texts. There are lots of times we'd like to say I don't believe something, but first I've got to prove it before I break with tradition.

MODERATOR: Since the subject has been brought back to acute renal failure, in that review I zeroed in on another review that to me was rather confusing, and I got a little bit (but I hope not excessively) nasty in my comments. The review I was covering stated that acute renal failure could be pre-renal, renal, or post-renal. If you take pre-renal problems and you have severe dehydration with decreased circulating volume and you have a kidney that is not producing a lot of urine, that is not "functioning", is that dysfunction? Is that failure, or is it, in fact, appropriate function, appropriate response to the body needs? Can we put them together and say all three are acute renal failure when in fact we may have a functioning kidney in the pre- and the post-, but a truly dysfunctioning kidney in the real acute renal failure. That review article in one of the distinguished journals failed to separate those three components. In my comments I disagreed with that approach. What is the reaction from the group? Can we agree on the concepts?

COMMENT: You perhaps are talking about definitions. People use the phrase "pre-renal azotemia" to signify an increase in BUN, often without a demonstrable change in GFR. On the other hand, we have seen a few children with gastroenteritis who have had BUN's in the 60, 80, 100's and serum creatinines that were 5 or 6, not below 2, as is usually bantered around. Yet, with hydration, in 48 hours their creatinine is down to 1 mg. Now, is that true pre-renal renal failure? I think it's a matter of semantics. Now certainly if you get enough volume depletion, pre-renal volume depletion will lead to intrinsic renal failure. Where does the line get crossed, I don't know. I don't worry about it.

MODERATOR: Is it renal dysfunction, renal failure as such? A failure of the kidney to perform the function that the body needs? Renal function, the way I define it, is the performance of a certain role that would lead towards health.

RESPONSE: Obviously, it is doing its job properly physiologically.

COMMENT: I think it is more than semantics because I think that the way we use language indicates the way our minds are processing thoughts. And I have considered pre-renal azotemia to be a much more accurate designation. If there is a patient with gastroenteritis whose creatinine is 5 and who returns to normal within 24 hours with fluid replacement, obviously that patient didn't have acute tubular necrosis, and unless you can show that the urinary indices indicated that the patient had acute tubular necrosis, then I don't think that patient was in renal failure. What we are dealing with is pre-renal success. I think one has to keep saying to residents: "a child with decreased urine output is not in renal failure until you have shown that the patient is in renal failure." I would go further than you have gone. I would say that the inclusion of posterior urethral valves and other forms of obstructive uropathy under the designation of acute renal failure is not really correct either because those patients have chronic renal failure. I think that what we need to say is that in any child who presents with acute or chronic renal failure, one should rule out an obstructive uropathy right at the beginning in order not to be caught. But to say that an obstructive uropathy is the cause of renal failure in children, I think is taking it a little bit too far.

QUESTION: Would you argue that a persisting obstructive uropathy is not going to lead, in time, to renal failure?

RESPONSE: The definition of acute renal failure is an abrupt cessation or reduction of renal function. Most cases of PUV tend to occur in utero. So, when the patient presents, he has already had several months of obstructive uropathy; the same is true for most of the other causes that I can think of in children. I think the point is, one has to rule out the PUV in a child who presents with what looks like acute renal failure.

COMMENT: Yes, the point is well taken. I think you are right about the concepts reflecting the way we think. Traditionally, this has been the way we organize our thoughts about the problem of acute renal failure. It has its faults. Most systems do tend to have overlaping and problems with them and you are bringing them up.

MODERATOR: In a way it reminds me of the problem which at times we used to face when I was playing with the earlobe oximeter - the PO_2 electrode that we designed in the 60's. We would work with a patient who actually could oxygenate but couldn't breathe. The patient was automatically given oxygen, thinking that that would help, when in fact what the patient needed was just help in breathing room air. There is a qualitative difference which, if we keep the concept straight, may lead to a more logical management of the patient.

COMMENT: My comment comes a little late but I want to mention one thing. In my country, years ago, we had the problem of having many cases of acute diarrhea in infants. We were worried about the incidence of acute renal failure in dehydration because we were not seeing it. One thing we did was to study a group of 200-250 babies with pre-renal nitrogen retention and check them afterwards in a week or ten days with concentration tests. It was a quite simple but correct way of studying tubular necrosis.

The incidence of tubular necrosis was very, very low, less than 2%. All the other children had very good kidneys and high urea in blood. That was all.

COMMENT: I would like to mention that we have seen, and I wonder if you have looked at this, a renal tubular acidosis after this kind of problem with dehydration. I have the impression that this is a little more commonly seen than a concentrating defect. Clearly, that's a functional residual of an acute pre-renal azotemia.

COMMENT: We have not studied that deeply, but we have the same observations. Aminoaciduria and excess bicarbonate in urine, suggesting proximal tubular damage, are found frequently.Many of our patients were malnourished and some of them had deficiency rickets. It is known that that may increase bicarbonate in urine and also aminoacids. Many had received toxic doses of antibiotics. At that time we were using also tetracycline. It may have been old; we had no way of knowing. What I mean is, I think you are right. There are subtle signs of tubular damage after dehydration but this typical finding of low density in the urine with 3% loss of body weight because of dehydration, was uncommon in this group of patients.

COMMENT: Nevertheless, when there is evidence of functional damage like that it's because we've probably transgressed that thin line between simple diminished blood supply to an acute tubular necrosis.

COMMENT: I think there must be an ample grey zone between functional compensation with dehydration and the beginning of anatomic damage.

QUESTION: In terms of the children that you have seen with acute tubular necrosis, were you able to correlate that with the serum sodium at all? You would expect it to be more common in the hyponatremic children.

RESPONSE: We have not had that experience but I can answer that. One thing that was true was the delay in treatment. I think it is very important in acute diarrhea, to emphasize in poor countries that diarrhea is simple to treat before you get hemodynamic consequences, if you start treatment early. Time is an important aspect of dehydration treatment.

COMMENT: I'm just remembering that in the ASN meeting there was a presentation of a brief paper. What they did was important. They looked at acute renal failure, albeit in rats, and did functional correlation with glucose absorption and with sodium absorption and anatomic correlations. Interestingly, within 48 hours, they were able to show a dissociation between the functional and the anatomic defects. The functional appeared first and then the anatomic. I think this is going to be a help in research if we can look at these functional changes before getting involved with anatomic changes, seeing earlier on what's happening in the pathophysiology of acute renal failure.

QUESTION: One of the things that often is very high is the uric acid. I wonder whether the panelists would comment about it, whether any drug therapy such as intravenous allopurinol is necessary sometimes.

RESPONSE: The hyperuricemia that has been reported in infantile gastroenteritis has resolved just with rehydration. I don't have an answer for the question. I raised this when we talked about uric acid in the hemolytic uremic sydnrome. At what point in acute renal failure do you consider therapies for uric acid? But as was pointed out, we were talking out in the hall, if you've got a uric acid of 15 or 20 or 30 and you happen to have a leukemia, everybody screams at you, "Do something to lower the uric acid." Yet, if you happen to have trauma or the hemolytic uremic syndrome, and a uric acid of 15 or 20 or 25, we sort of say, "well, do the general treatment and it will go away." But maybe indeed it has something to do with how long the reduced renal function lasts, maybe it has something to do with the worsening of the process. At least in my own mind, I add it into the things that say to myself, it's time to dialyze the patient. But I don't know of any data that say it's of value. Some people do treat it.

COMMENT: My problem sometimes is worse than this. In fact, sometimes we are dealing with other adult colleagues whose patients have uric acid in the 35, 36, 37 range. I think this is even more of a problem. I don't know whether we should. I just haven't seen any acute complications of this severe hyperuricacidemia.

COMMENT: Some people say - and there is an article published that says - that if you have a urinary uric acid to creatinine ratio of greater than one, those are the patients who will deposit uric acid and develop acute uric acid nephropathy. Maybe that is another guideline to use. Usually they have no urine, of course. But if they do, you can use the ratio.

COMMENT: Often I have asked myself whether or not there is something about uremic syndrome that somehow makes uric acid more soluble so that we don't run into the problems that one runs into with elevated uric acid under other circumstances. We certainly see large numbers of patients who've got very high,impressively high, uric acid levels. If anybody knows of data on that, I would like to hear it. If not, I think it's something that my colleague here ought to take up as a very simple project. All you have to do is find some way to incubate uremic serum with uric acid and study solubility with normal plasma.

COMMENT: Solubility, I can't answer but I did mention that uremic serum does inhibit the movement of uric acid across the proximal tubular epithelium. This has been demonstrated in isolated, perfused tubule. That's chronic serum. Acute serum, I don't know.

COMMENT: Solubility would be the critical piece of information with regard to development of the complication.

MODERATOR: I wanted to make a point about one of the speaker's absence yesterday. Were you in the bathroom when you were talking about that It happened to me when I first came to this country. I was talking to the Chairman of the Department as he and I were doing different things in the bathroom, went out into the conference room, and he said, "I just talked with José about this, that, and the other..." I thought that what you said in the bathroom didn't count. But this is for your information; in this country, it doesn't matter where you said it, you will be quoted.

COMMENT: The conversation took place in your suite, José.

QUESTION: Basically, the question is whether or not we've had any experience with Naloxone, which is thought to be an endotoxin antagonist. No, we have had no experience with it. I know that there are some intensivists who specialize in the treatment of shock who are working with it at the present time. I really don't know whether that is or will prove to be of value.

QUESTION: I have a question concerning your talk yesterday but it might apply today. Could you expand a little bit, educate us about what you mentioned as the cumulative memory for aminoglycosides, even one year after the initial dose. How does that work and how can we obviate that?

RESPONSE: I have no idea how it works but it has been observed both in rabbits and in people, that what I stated yesterday generally happens. That is, when you restart an aminoglycoside even weeks or months later, you start, as far as toxicity is concerned, on the day that the drug was stopped the first time around. And you can't get around that by using gentamycin the second time when you used Kanamycin the first time. It's cumulative not to specific drugs but to the whole group. I do not know the mechanism. There are some interesting data at the present time - again, they were obtained with rabbits of different genetic background - and regarding toxicity of an aminoglycoside to the rabbit's hearing. What they do is count the hearing cells missing after the drug has been given. Very precise. That is not dependent on serum levels but is dependent on the amount of drug that appears in the endolymph. There is no correlation between that and the serum level. This is determined by genetic factors which explains to some degree another observation, which is that if you have a child who's getting the perfectly accepted, every-one-agrees-on dosage of an aminoglycoside for an appropriate length of time, that there is a small group of these patients who are going to end up deaf. This is not related to anything that we can define except apparently individual susceptibility. Somewhat the same mechanism seems to operate in this memory bit. If you take a rabbit and treat him with aminoglycoside, you get certain levels on the endolymph after a while. Then, you stop for a couple of weeks and you use aminoglycosides again. It's interesting that the second time around, despite the fact that the blood levels are tested to be in the same range that they were the first time, the concentrations in the endolymph are higher. Apparently the mechanism that actively transfers the aminoglycoside from the serum to the endolymph is activated someway. The enzymes are induced or whatever; they are therefore capable of doing this thing. This is highly theoretical but I really know of no other explanation why this may be so.

MODERATOR: Carlos Vaamonde a couple of years ago here at this Seminar presented material showing that gentamycin in the kidneys stays in the tissue for months. Could that play some role or have some relationship with the levels in the endolymph?

RESPONSE: I don't know. I really don't know. I don't think that has been looked at. I'm aware of the observation but somehow I've never connected it in my own mind to whatever happens in patients. I think that somebody ought to really look at that.

MODERATOR: I would like to ask the last question, before we finish. Do you have any thoughts on when do the acute renal failure mineral changes become the changes of chronic renal failure? Are there dramatic differences? Once I had a distinguished visitor who saw a patient (my first dialysis and transplantation patient) who presented with acute glomerulonephritis clinically but had changes in mineral metabolism which led this consultant to conclude that the patient most likely had chronic renal failure preceding the acute glomerulonephritis. Accordingly, he believed that those changes in calcium and phosphorus were due to the chronic character of the disease. What would be your final message on that subject?

RESPONSE: There are analogies but there are also differences between the acute and the chronic circumstances. In general, the concept on which most people would agree today, is that in the context of chronic renal failure slowly progressing, detectable changes in serum phosphorus and calcium are a late event and occur usually below creatinine clearances of 20 ml/min/1.73 m^2. However, there probably are transient changes that are the whole foundation of the "Trade-off hypothesis". On the other hand, more recent data from San Francisco, particularly in children, show that very early in the game there are decreased levels of 1,25 vitamin D in chronic renal failure. Thus, vitamin D deficiency seems to play an important role, also. In acute renal failure, those changes seem to take place within hours. In the experimental model and in the human within one to two days, and in the experimental model within six hours of bilateral nephrectomy, hyperphosphatemia, hypocalcemia, elevated PTH, and low 1,25 vit D levels may develop.

MODERATOR: Thank you very much. I think that we have had rewarding days-heavy at times, but I feel that we are emotionally and scientifically recharged because of these experiences. For all your help, thank you very much. And we hope to see you again next year.

V

WORKSHOP

WORKSHOP: CLINICO-PATHOLOGIC CORRELATIONS

José Strauss, M.D., Moderator

MODERATOR: We are going to start with Dr. McVicar who is prepared to present the first case. Dr. Pardo, Professor of Pathology and also Director of the Electronmicroscopy Laboratory at the VA Hospital here in Miami, is going to help us with the histopathology.

DR. McVICAR: This was a six year old white boy who became acutely ill with vomiting after mild URI. Edema developed over the next 2 days. The following laboratory tests and results were obtained. In urine: urinalysis with protein 4+, 8-10 RBC, 3-7 WBC and 2-3 RBC casts/HPF and 24 hr protein 5.8 g; in blood: albumin 2.1 g/dl, cholesterol 585 mg/dl, BUN 45 mg/dl, creatinine 1.4 mg/dl, total bilirubin 3.9 mg/dl (indirect 3.7 mg/dl), hemoglobin 7.0 g/dl, peripheral blood smear with many distorted and fragmented RBC, platelet count 31,000 mm^3 fibrin split products elevated, C_3 14 mg/dl (Normal 55-120), C_4 23 mg/dl (Normal 20-50). Physical examination revealed petechiae over the abdomen and abdominal tenderness. Arterial B.P. was 140/90 mm Hg.

Two weeks after onset serum creatinine stabilized at 1.8 mg/dl with improved clinical condition and platelets 350,000/mm^3. Three weeks after onset petechiae reappeared and the patient appeared acutely ill again. Platelets again decreased to 23,000/mm^3 and hemoglobin to 6.2 mg/dl. BUN increased to 144 mg/dl and serum creatinine to 6.2 mg/dl. When serum creatinine reached 8.5 mg/dl, hemodialysis was initiated; uremia was controlled and platelet count returned to normal. A renal biopsy was performed and showed vascular thrombosis consistent with hemolytic uremic syndrome. Eight weeks after onset, petechiae reappeared. Platelet count decreased to 19,000/mm^3 and arterial B.P. was 180/100 mm Hg. The patient had restlessness, irritability and mental confusion; his pupils had alternating dilatation. He developed a grand mal seizure with B.P. of 180/90 mm Hg. Lumbar puncture showed elevated pressure with 8,000 RBC/mm^3, no WBC, glucose 70 mg/dl and protein 74 mg/dl; cultures and smear were negative. EEG indicated diffuse bilateral cerebral dysfunction. His condition again stabilized with gradual correction of hematologic abnormalities except for anemia of chronic renal failure. Arterial B.P. was maintained at normal levels with Aldomet 500 mg/day and hydralazine 45 mg/day. GFR increased to 20 ml/min/1.73m^2. After seven months hemodialysis was discontinued. Eight months after onset, hypertension escalated to 200/120 mm Hg (peak 300/180 mm Hg) and was unresponsive to serial dialyses to dry weight. Peripheral renin was 48.4 ng/ml/hr, right renal vein was 52.6 ng/ml/hr, left renal vein was 38.6 ng/ml/hr.

Renal arteriogram showed marked attenuation of the renal cortical arterioles. Arterial B.P. was subsequently controlled with Minoxidil 6 mg/day, propranolol 400 mg/day, Lasix 80 mg/day, alphamethyldopa 1 g/day. Subsequent hypertensive crises were readily and rapidly controlled by acute increase of minoxidil dose on an outpatient basis, at times over the telephone. This boy at this time is seven years old. We used to call him "Little Shaver" because he used to shave. He had that side effect of Minoxodil, a very hirsute appearance. He is like a young man now, and is very eager to become a missionary. He is a very robust boy. His GFR is up to 40% of normal and I think that's also unusual - to recover that much renal function. He still has proteinuria, which makes us very sad and I remember the comments on the first day of this seminar about the prognosis of youngsters like this but I would like to hear the comments of other experts. I know some of you have had HUS cases with recurrences.

In summary, this case history illustrates several points which are instructive about the hemolytic uremic syndrome. Delayed onset of malignant hypertension, sometimes in the recovery phase of the disease, is a serious complication of HUS which can sometimes blemish an otherwise excellent recovery. It would appear that the pathogenesis in our patient is related to the marked attenuation of the renal cortical blood vessels. Remissions and exacerbations of the clinical findings of HUS are known to occur, usually in the early stages of the disease, and do not appear to affect prognosis. Although decreased serum complement is extraordinary in HUS, it has previously been reported. Since renal immune complex deposition is characteristically absent in HUS (as it was in our case), the significance of this finding is unclear. Finally, the use of Minoxidil for control of hypertensive crises, especially in out-patients who cannot immediately receive intravenous therapy, has important implications for the treatment of hypertensive emergencies.

MODERATOR: Dr. Pardo has evaluated the biopsy, and he has nothing to add.

MODERATOR: Thank you, Dr. McVicar. Would the panelists or the audience care to make statements or ask questions?

COMMENT: I wanted to make a few points, if I may. This particular glomerulus has a rather lobulated appearance. Secondly, there is a very foamy appearance that one sees in the mesangium, and thirdly, you don't see it well on this very badly damaged glomerulus, but in the others I'll show you, there is thickening of the capillary wall. Dr. Renée Habib has drawn attention to the foamy appearance of the mesangium in patients with hemolytic uremic syndrome. And some people in Czechoslovakia some years ago stained biopsy specimens of patients with hemolytic uremic syndrome for lipids and demonstrated the presence of lipids in the glomeruli. For anyone who wants that reference, it's quite an interesting but very little known paper, quoted in my reviews. There is heterogeneity with respect to the glomerular abnormalities here.

This glomerulus looks somewhat different, but still somewhat lobulated. I'm looking for a loop where one can see thickening of the wall (which you can appreciate on light microscopy) as indicative of the subendothelial accumulation of various substances and also the fact that the endothelial cells are markedly swollen.

COMMENT: I was going to ask if anyone thought the histopathology might be compatible with anything other than the hemolytic uremic syndrome.

DR. PARDO: Without the clinical history, the age of the patient and so on, there are six or seven syndromes that are associated with intravascular coagulation. One that is seen in adult pathology associated with glomerular thrombosis and also thrombosis of the afferent arterioles is malignant hypertension; it is very similar. As a matter of fact, I received an autopsy of a child from the Bahamas; I called it malignant hypertension. Immediately I realized that it was hemolytic uremic syndrome. I find those two pathologies very similar.

COMMENT: These two pathologies are almost indistinguishable and some people say that if you show a pathologist slides of patients with TTP, HUS, malignant hypertension, or spiradenoma with renal failure and hypertension, the pathologist would have a great deal of difficulty differentiating.

I want to make some comments about a few things I find very interesting about this patient, if I may. This patient presented with nephrotic syndrome which is a somewhat unusual presentation for hemolytic uremic syndrome. And if it were not for the fact that the child had the other features of HUS - if there were only features of nephrotic syndrome plus the low C_3 plus this biopsy appearance leaving aside the thrombi, you would think of a form of MPGN. We have made the point in one of our reviews on the pathology of HUS that indeed many of the cases have an appearance that looks like MPGN, for what that is worth. It's not worth very much. But what I think is fascinating about this child is the fact that the C_3 was low. Was the C_3 low persistently? Because about one-third of cases of HUS have low C_3 and it's usually not a very marked depression of the C_3. It's not as low as your patient's was. It's usually just slightly below the lower limit of normal. And it's usually transient. Then there have been a few cases (we reported one in the Archives of Pathology in about 1976)who had a low C_3 with C_3 nephritic factor, and that particular child had a recurrence of HUS. The interesting thing about his recurrence was that the first episode was just like this child, relatively mild; but the second episode was associated with profound hypertension. He ended up losing his kidneys, being dialyzed and transplanted during his second episode.

Then, there was a report in Spanish from Spain of a woman with C3 nephritic factor associated with HUS. That's what I call a subset. When I looked at recurrent HUS, I found 30 cases in the literature and from communications. Now there are more than 50 cases that people know about. It's a very mixed bag, this recurrent HUS. I think within this mixed bag, there are some cases like the one we are discussing. He fits with cases I have heard about. Dr. Gianantonio, if I could put words in his mouth, would say, "This belongs to the hemolytic uremic syndromes;this is not hemolytic uremic syndrome."

COMMENT: That's semantics. Really, I would agree with you. This is a peculiar patient. We have seen three or four of these during my many, many years in Nephrology - patients with recurrent intravascular coagulation and with abnormal findings like this. We would not call these patients the hemolytic uremic syndrome of Buenos Aires. Practically, I am sure now, we are facing in our place, one special type of hemolytic uremic syndrome that is endemic, epidemic, self-limited, has a certain prognosis. In short, it is a disease, not a syndrome. This is peculiar, and occasionally we go over atypical familial cases with recurrences. I would not know how to call this. It is a syndrome, and belongs to the syndrome. It is not what we described in the literature on the basis of our cases. One thing is important, we have repeated these complement studies in our babies, small infants, and they are normal. We have samples in the first hour after admission in many patients and C_3 and C_4 are normal. Nephritic factor is absent. We have one patient in which we found the same, two or three times, with recurrence of coagulation. Everytime he had a recurrence, he had a drop in C_3, not so low as the patient we are discussing but significantly low.

QUESTION: Did you look at CH_{50}?

RESPONSE: No, we do not run that routinely.

COMMENT: Because I found, and I don't know if it was an artifact or not, that all our patients had low CH_{50}. I think it probably was just an epiphenomenon.

COMMENT: If you have free hemoglobin in the blood and the liberation of so many protein products because of destruction of tissues and blood and so on, I think you may have perhaps some non-specific activation following the classic way of activation of complement. We have not done CH_{50}.

QUESTION: In those cases of the few you have seen that are similar to this, were there fluorescent studies? In our cases the immunofluorescence was negative. Was it also negative in your cases?

RESPONSE: We have only one patient with immunofluorescence; it was negative. Incidentally, all the C_3 patients were older children (pubes) or near puberty and two of them died after weeks of these recurrences. The cause of death in one of them was massive cerebral hemorrhage in the course of a hypertensive crisis.

MODERATOR: Let me ask about the recurrences and the membranoproliferative glomerulonephritis. The case I mentioned in a previous session, the one with the recurrences and the systemic activity that was treated with all those poisons before transplantation, and so on, was an iterative case with membranoproliferative glomerulonephritis. In your concept of the syndromes, does that appearance have any tendency to recur or is it just coincidental that the two are together like in this case.

RESPONSE: We don't have enough cases of this to be able to be certain.

MODERATOR: I should tell you that during the five minutes while you were not here this morning, the subject of genetic characteristics of patients was brought up and I quoted some of your remarks that you made the other night. I am sure I quoted you correctly. The subject did come up in terms of a specific make-up of patients. Perhaps you would like to enlarge on that now or at a later time (response: "later").

QUESTION: About the rash. Was this truly a petechial rash that you see with thrombocytopenia or was it a more extensive rash such as you see with cutaneous vasculitis, periarteritis, or hypersensitivity angiitis?

RESPONSE: These were crops of petechia which appeared and didn't resemble purpura at all or the usual kinds of rashes one sees in collagen vascular disease.

COMMENT: My reason for asking, we've seen a couple of children who have had more extensive rash, who had low complements, who had what looked like a microangiopathic hemolytic process with hypertension where the ultimate diagnosis was thought to be some sort of hypersensitivity angiitis. We had one child who had two or three such episodes.

COMMENT: I think you would expect quite a different histology in that circumstance.

COMMENT: Yes. I would think so.

COMMENT: The skin in the hemolytic uremic syndrome. This has not been done routinely. We have not published our observations, but many years ago we performed some 30 to 40 skin biopsies. One particular type of lesion that our babies show - not all of them - is a subcutaneous, small hematoma, very small, more or less the size of a couple of millimeters. Scattered, three or four of them, with petechia and so on. They may appear when thrombocytopenia is extreme. We biopsied them and we found in over 50% of the cases- we were fortunate enough to get a small vessel here, deep in the dermis, or perhaps in the hypodermis, the same thrombotic lesions as could be shown elsewhere. I think that these are vasculitis or thrombosis or some kind of endothelial damage very different from the average petechia of thrombocytopenia or the extensive areas of ischemia in the skin that you may have in other kinds of vasculitis in pediatrics, especially associated with sepsis.

QUESTION: If that child were 26 instead of 6 years of age, I would have called this TTP. Can you tell me why I couldn't do that? And if that is the case,maybe you should consider using plasma.

RESPONSE: I wanted to call this case TTP because I felt that the cerebral involvement was quite prominent and for me, that started to push me more in the direction of a diagnosis of TTP. I happen to be of the school that considers the two entities a sort of a spectrum of the same disease. That may not be an accurate assessment but it is the way I tend to view hemolytic uremic syndrome with the major target organ being the kidney, and TTP, with the brain being the major target organ. We were quite concerned about that and finally, mainly because clinically the cerebral manifestations quieted, and the renal persisted, we called it hemolytic uremic syndrome. I would have used plasmapheresis if at the time this child was acutely ill, we had known about that. If this child came to me today, I certainly would do that.

COMMENT: It's hard to answer that question, but I think that there are patients who have HUS and they are unequivocally HUS because they are young children, they have the typical hematological features and predominant renal involvement. If the CNS is involved, it's because they are hyponatremic or hypocalcemic or hypertensive or all of those. I think that few would argue that there is a hemolytic uremic syndrome which occurs in children who fit those criteria. On the other hand, there are adults who have predominantly CNS involvement with very minimal renal involvement, fluctuating neurological signs, and they are called TTP. Now, there are patients who overlap, where it becomes very difficult to say whether they are HUS or TTP. Why? Because they are adults who have neurological involvement but also very severe renal involvement or they are children who have very severe renal involvement but also neurological involvement that you can't account for on the basis of some electrolyte disturbance or hypertension. So, it becomes a bit confusing. If you look at this particular child, you say, "you know, this isn't exactly HUS, because right to start off with, the bilirubin was 3.9 which is somewhat unusual in my experience with hemolytic uremic syndrome, suggesting to me that not only was there kidney involvement and physiological involvement, but also hepatic involvement right off the bat. So this child is closer to the category of TTP than to HUS. I would agree. Not only that, but although some people would disagree with me, in my own experience, thrombii such as shown over here, in the glomerular and extra glomerular vessels, are somewhat unusual.

In other people's experience, I know that it is not unusual, but I am just talking about myself. So, as I was saying this morning, it seems to me that this whole discussion of TTP and HUS, it's like looking at all of you; so I look at all of you and say, "well, I am in Miami, the United States, you must all be Americans. You're all men", and (excluding the few women quickly) I say: "All the men are Americans. They are all men and all in the United States. They must all be Americans." But, then someone stands up and starts to talk and says he comes from South America. So he's a little bit different. And that one sounds as though he comes from Georgia. That's a little bit different. There's something going on over here. But, I need a marker to know whether in fact you are different. In HUS and TTP, we have lacked the marker. All we have are these clinical features, the one set described in 1925 in a 16 year old girl, and the other in 1955 in five children who died. Fortunately,we are now perhaps getting the markers. To my way of thinking the markers are as follows (I'm having free liscense here):

1. The thrombii in HUS, when they occur, tend to be predominantly fibrin thrombii and in TTP,they tend to be predominantly platelet thrombii.

2. The multimers, the von Willebrand and Factor VIII multimers, are absent in the recurrent form of TTP <u>during</u> the episode of TTP. In HUS, as I learned from Dr. Byrnes on Monday, the opposite is true. And there is a platelet agglutinating factor in the serum of patients with TTP, but not with HUS.

It seems to me there are beginning to be some differences. Whether these markers will define the whole lot or whether we will find within the group of HUS some who have these and some who don't, and similarly with TTP, I don't know. I firmly believe that we are now in the era with HUS and TTP that people were in with respect to the nephrotic syndrome and nephritis before the era of renal biopsies, immunofluorescence, and electron microscopy. Ellis Type One,Type Two. Do you remember Ellis Type One, Type Two? HUS and TTP to me, are like Ellis Type One and Type Two. We need more sophisticated ways of differentiating. And you know the funny thing about this whole story? When you take Ellis Type One or Ellis Type Two and you treat them with prednisone and cyclophosphamide and azathioprine, whether it's Type One or Type Two , you may get the same. results in both groups. The same with plasma in HUS and TTP, but I am going to shut up now because I'm getting carried away with my analogies.

MODERATOR: That was beautiful!

QUESTION: How often have you seen bilirubins of this level in HUS?

RESPONSE: I have seen high levels, perhaps higher sometimes but only occasionally. In the average patient, what you get is intravascular hemolysis and free hemoglobin plasma levels, low haptoglobins with normal, or very slightly increased, indirect bilirubin because the liver is able to metabolize rapidly the hem molecule freed from the hemoglobin erythrocytes. But, there is a group of hemolytic uremic patients that because of early age, prolonged malnutrition, induced by treatment, or superimposed injection, they have signs of liver compromise but not liver failure. We have other patients with high ammonia levels with low vitamin K dependent coagulation factors, and some of them have high bilirubin. But, I think this is not caused by the syndrome; it is due to other circumstances in a very severely ill baby.

COMMENT: We have one child who has had what looks like recurrent hemolytic uremic syndrome, who was dialyzed either once or twice, who had bilirubins of this level, and low serum complements. Unfortunately, we were not able to get any kidney tissue. He also had irritability, behavior changes. Our neurologists took him away and have tried to work him up for one of the enzyme deficiencies in the ornithine transcarbamylase cycle. I believe there are some scattered reports of deficiencies in that cycle associated with an HUS-like picture. I just don't recall all of the pieces.

COMMENT: In the Journal of Pediatrics in about 1970 or '71, there was a paper on coagulation findings in HUS from your group. What bothered me about that paper, because it didn't agree with my view of the world at the time, was that I wondered whether the coagulation abnormalities that you were describing could not be attributed to malnutrition and liver disease. And I wonder if you would be willing to comment on that with respect to, say, the patients who were middle class, well-nourished, beautiful children who suddenly had HUS. Did any of them have similar pertubations in their coagulation profiles?

RESPONSE: That's important. When all these reports were published, our patients belonged to a special category, when you look at them from the socio-economic point of view. They belonged to medium to high class families. This has changed lately perhaps because our country is poorer now than it used to be some ten years ago. But, also, because we are seeing more infants with the syndrome who are from deprived families. But, none of these patients who were included in this study of coagulation had malnutrition when admitted. What they say is that several of them (at that time we were beginning to use early peritoneal dialysis), were fed a very poor supply of protein and calories for a week to ten days and were having acute malnutrition, or undernutrition, very acute, because of lack of protein, nitrogen and calories. It was in some of these patients that we had these particular findings. As you remember, in the paper there were two kinds of findings, some related to activation of coagulation early. We were finding rebounds in Factor VIII and fibrin degradation products in the blood, early. But, some of them had later on decreasing vitamin K dependent factors. More or less, if I remember correctly, around 35 or 40%. These, I think, do not belong to the coagulation picture of the hemolytic uremic syndrome we see classically in small infants. We study that because we need the information to help us with difficulties in the care of these patients. We are continuously finding the same things: early coagulation, signs of recovery when the patient is admitted to the hospital. An exceptional patient who had two or three bouts, also had consumption of Factor VIII, fibrinogen, and decrease in the number of platelets. This is occasional. So, these findings, I agree with you, are not related the primary process. These are some kind of parasitic findings that do not belong to the picture.

COMMENT: I am very pleased to hear that because it worried me a great deal at the time,as you can imagine, because I was preaching that one shouldn't use heparin. I think one may have to reinterpret high Factor VIII levels in HUS for the following reason. It seems to me that aside from the high FDP which are universally found,the way to study this problem is along the lines of some workers in Holland who are looking at fibrinopeptide A and B, a more sensitive index of intravascular coagulation. They have come up with the notion that there is a low grade coagulopathy occurring, which I accept. But, what I think is another area for research is the high Factor VIII because it's not clear to me whether this Factor VIII - but it may not be clear to me because I may not know enough about it - whether it is the antigen or whether it is biologically active Factor VIII. Because there is widespread endothelial damage in HUS, it may be that what we are seeing is merely a release phenomenon, that the Factor VIII antigen is being released from damaged endothelial cells and that's what we are seeing. I don't know the answer to that. That's something people could look at in the future.

QUESTION: What was the race of this child?

RESPONSE: White, upper middle class.

COMMENT: Because in the last couple of days nobody has mentioned what seems to be the lack of ocurrence of this syndrome in black populations. The patients that we mentioned were in an urban, inner city hospital; not one was black. I am aware of some similar reports.

COMMENT: I drew attention to that. The fact of the matter is that in South Africa where the blacks outnumber the whites about six or seven to one, one hardly ever sees HUS in blacks. In Kenya, there was a report of cases of hemolytic uremic syndrome. Not a single case was in a black child. One of the interesting things is, it has been shown that fibrinolytic activity in blacks in South Africa is much, much more active than in whites. What that has to do with the price of eggs, I don't know, but it is an interesting observation. It is interesting that also in the United Stages, HUS seems to be very uncommon in black children. I'm glad you have corraborated that. It is very interesting.

MODERATOR: We must continue now with the next case. The first was a fascinating case; I'm glad that I needled the Faculty on their little escapades. Thus, they brought up those pearls.

Dr. Gaston Zilleruelo is going to present Case #2.

DR. ZILLERUELO: LT is a 15 year old white female referred to our Medical Center for renal evaluation in August. She was doing well until about 1 month prior to admission when mother noticed progressively increasing lethargy and anorexia. Three weeks prior to admission, patient had a temperature of 104°F and noticed some streaks of blood on coughing approximately two days prior to onset of fever. In addition, she was seen by a private M.D. who found a urinalysis with 2+ protein, 3+ blood and too numerous to count white blood cells and red blood cells in the urine sediment. She was started on treatment with amoxicillin and subsequently with Septra. Fever resolved but pyuria and hematuria persisted. The probable diagnosis at that time was that she was having a urinary tract infection. The amoxicillin was discontinued after five days treatment and Septra was given for 10 days without improvement . On August 12, a blood test was done which showed a BUN of 114 mg/dl and a creatinine of 9.2 mg/dl. Patient was admitted to a local hospital for evaluation. She was normotensive with a blood pressure of 110/70 mm Hg, afebrile, She had right upper quadrant tenderness without rebound and a few palpable posterior cervical lymph nodes.

The laboratory workup done was as follows: hemoglobin 4.8 g/dl, with hematocrit 13.5%, platelet count 223,000/mm^3, reticulocyte count 5.1%, PT and PTT were within normal limits, mono spot was negative, RA latex was negative. The white blood cell count was 7,400/mm^3 with a differential of 53% polys, 29% lymphs, 4% bands, 3% monos, 6% eos. Electrolytes were as follows: sodium 140 mEq/L, potassium 5.2 mEq/L, chloride 115 mEq/L, CO_2 18 mEq/L, BUN 94 mg/dl. Serum creatinine was 8.0 mg/dl, total protein 6 g/dl, albumin 3 g/dl, cholesterol 140 mg/dl, direct Coombs' test was negative. ASO 50 Todd units (normal < 25), ANA titer < 1:24, cryoglobulins negative, phosphorus 5.9 mg/dl, calcium 8.8 mg/dl, uric acid 7.9 mg/dl. Urinalysis: specific gravity 1.010, protein 2+, blood moderate, glucose negative, pH 6, WBC 3-5/HPF, RBC 25-30/HPF, no casts were seen. Urine culture done twice was negative. Renal scan showed normal size kidneys. Chest x-ray and abdominal flat plate were within normal limits. Haptoglobins 160 mg/dl, C_3 118 mg/dl, 24-hour urine collection showed a creatinine clearance of 10 ml/min/1.73m^2. Hepatitis profile and anti-GBM antibodies were negative.

The patient maintained a urine output throughout this hospitalization of between 1300 and 1600 ml/day. She was started on sodium bicarbonate 10 g TID. The diet was restricted to 2 g of sodium, 2 g of potassium and 60 g of protein/day. Subsequently, the patient was admitted to the University of Miami/Jackson Memorial Medical Center on August 19. There was no recent history of sore throat, joint pain, skin rashes or edema. There was no family history of renal disease. At physical examination: temperature was 98.7°F, heart rate 60/min, respiratory rate 20/min, blood pressure 110/70 mm Hg, weight 123 1/2 lbs. Her skin was pale without any rashes or petechia. The fundi were within normal limits. The neck was supple without significant adenopathies. The lungs were clear. The heart had a regular rhythm without any murmur heard. There was minimal pitting edema at the lower extremities.

Additional laboratory work-up done included ANA and anti-double stranded DNA; both were negative. C_3 and C_4 were within normal limits. Circulating immune complexes were negative. PT and PTT were within normal limits. PPD was placed in the right arm which was read as negative 48 hours later. The voiding cystourethrogram was normal without any evidence of reflux. A renal scan showed bilaterally decreased flow and function. A renal biopsy was done on August 24 under local anesthesia, and with ultrasound localization of right kidney.

It was decided to treat the patient with high doses of Solu-Medrol between August 28 and August 30. There were no complications. A repeated creatinine clearance prior to discharge was 8 ml/min with a total protein excretion of 3 g/24 hours.

Upon discharge, medications were: Basaljel 2 tsp. TID, sodium bicarbonate 10 g TID, Kayexalate 1 tsp. po TID, Allopurinol 100 mg QOD, Prednisone 20 mg TID.

Subsequently, her renal function stabilized and she slowly improved. She was treated for two months with prednisone po and never required hemodialysis. Most recent creatinines are stable at 4 mg/dl. Patient is only on phosphate binders.

MODERATOR: Are there any questions on the Clinical History?

QUESTION: Why did you start your patient on Allopurinol?

RESPONSE: The uric acid in the local hospital was 7.9 mg/dl but in a repeat at our hospital, it was 11.6 mg/dl. So, it was definitely going up; that's why we started Allopurinol.

QUESTION: There were a few palpable posterior lymph nodes. What happened to them when she came to you?

RESPONSE: They probably disappeared. Apparently she did have a URI or similar infection which triggered the visit to her doctor and the finding of the urine abnormalities. From then on, everything started to clear up.

QUESTION: She was on amoxicillin before she presented with the high BUN. Is that correct?

RESPONSE: She was on amoxicillin only for a few days.

QUESTION: Did she have eosinophilia?

RESPONSE: No. There was no eosinophilia. In fact, in the previous CBC done at the local hospital when she had the intercurrent illness, she had 6% eosinophils.

QUESTION: Was she on another drug or was she a user or abuser of drugs? A sniffer?

RESPONSE: No, definitely no.

QUESTION: Wasn't she on Septra for 10 days?

RESPONSE: She received Septra (after the amoxicillin) for 10 days, that is correct, but I believe that the question was about the period before or during the amoxicillin treatment. No, she did not.

QUESTION: You show a BUN of 114 on August 12. This was after she was given amoxicillin and Septra. Is that correct?

RESPONSE: That is correct. The patient at that time was thought to have a URI or a UTI. Apart from that, there was no evidence of oliguria or Acute Renal Failure.

QUESTION: Do you have an approximate time course interval between the administration of those two antibiotics and when she was found to be in advanced renal insufficiency?

RESPONSE: I believe that at the end of the 10 days course of Septra, because of the persistent urinalysis abnormalities, the blood was drawn. So, it was shortly after Septra.

MODERATOR: If nobody else has questions about the Clinical History, Dr. Victoriano Pardo will present the histopathology.

DR. PARDO: In this biopsy we had 17 glomeruli studied by light microscopy; in 15 of them we found a crescentic reaction involving about 1/2 of the circumference of the glomerulus. Also, there was collapse of the loops. This could be seen in a PAS stained section. Also there was an increase in fibrous tissue in the interstitium; there was a mild inflammatory infiltrate and there were some atrophic tubules. By electron-microscopy the patient had deposits of dense fibrillar material, probably representing fibrin, in the crescents. By immunofluorescence she had deposits of IgM and C_3 in a diffuse and segmental fashion.

MODERATOR: Any questions or comments for Dr. Pardo?

QUESTION: With all the recent talk about IgM nephropathy, I am not sure in my own mind whether rapidly progressive glomerulonephritis is known to occur with the so-called IgM nephropathy. Could you comment on that?

RESPONSE: I interpret these deposits of IgM and C_3 perhaps as non-specific trapping in some of the lesions.

COMMENT: I would like to respond to that. To my knowledge, you don't get that type of picture in what is being called IgM nephropathy. That is mainly associated with Minimal Change Nephrotic Syndrome, if that is what you are describing. Some individuals have found progression, but I don't think that is a Rapidly Progressive kind of course.

COMMENT: That is my understanding also, but I asked the question.

QUESTION: Did the history state that the patient was coughing up blood? That there was blood streaking in her sputum?

RESPONSE: Yes, she did and there was.

COMMENT-QUESTION: When I heard that, and then the story unfolded, I wondered whether she could have Goodpasture's or Wegener's. Then we learned that the chest x ray revealed normal lungs. So, then, I thought that that couldn't be Wegener's or Goodpasture's. Did anyone look for macrophages loaded with iron in the sputum? Did the coughing of blood continue or was this transient?

MODERATOR: It was transient. We shall come back to this point with another patient who had a much more dramatic pulmonary presentation. This was not remarkable and went away. Any other comments in terms of the diagnosis or the treatment?

COMMENT: I would gather that the diagnosis after the biopsy was thought to be Rapidly Progressive Idiopathic (non-streptococcal related) Glomerulonephritis. This just brings up for discussion the therapy. I see that she had three consecutive days of pulse therapy as opposed to the every other day for a couple of weeks. In a few similar patients we have tended to use every other day prednisone, sometimes, with the addition of some of the other magic drugs such as dipyridamole, cyclophosphamide, etc. I would be interested to know what the other people present here are doing with these patients.

COMMENT: We have used daily prednisone for several weeks, plus azathioprine, and then we switched to alternate day prednisone and continued the azathioprine daily. I don't think that there can be a uniform opinion as to how to treat these patients. What I think is interesting is that when I was a resident about 20 years ago, these patients just went and lost their kidneys. Some form of agressive therapy is making a difference; whether it is the high dose prednisone plus or minus the other drugs, I am not sure.One sees them surviving and not losing their kidneys. But that is completely anecdotal. What we are dealing with here is that we don't have a handle on these patients.

COMMENT: Perhaps the most important effort in this Crescentic Nephritis is to try to find an etiology. Some of them are examples of diseases that have specific treatments such as Lupus Nephritis. We have sent for publication,12 patients with Crescentic Nephritis of different etiologies; some are due to Membrano-Proliferative Glomerulonephritis; others are due to Lupus Nephritis, and others are idiopathic. All of them were treated with pulse therapy and my associates are very happy with the results. But I agree with the previous commentator that what we did before, to treat them with high corticosteroids by mouth associated with cyclophosphamide, yielded similar results; I don't think that this is a tremendous advance. But, since this is an aggressive approach, it may help the doctors more than the patients.

COMMENT: In a paper which I believe was in the Journal of Pediatrics, a comparison was made of two treatments provided to patients with this type of nephropathy: some were treated with pulse methyl-prednisolone and others with oral prednisone. Although in the immediate post-treatment period those with pulse therapy seemed to do better, over long term there really were no differences. I would tend, in a situation like this, today, to use plasmapheresis as well as high dose prednisone, not because there are any data to support that, but because I consider plasmapheresis as safe if not safer than high dose prednisone, at least in our institution and the way it is handled. Because I think we are in a desperate situation, I want to be as aggressive as I think I can safely be. I don't think we are ever going to get a controlled trial in this group of patients because their plight is so difficult that nobody wants to withold therapy to test, and yet nobody knows what we are doing with corticosteroids, plasmapheresis or other modes of treatment.

COMMENT: I must take issue with the last commentator. When we don't know what we are doing, it is probably better to do nothing than to do something. I think that what will happen is that if an important person such as my colleague advocates plasmapheresis, it will become entrenched and it will take us years and years and years to prove that it is of no value (if it is of no value), and we may not. The point that I am trying to make is that if we don't know what we are doing, I don't think we should do it unless somebody starts a collaborative multicenter study, and looks at it carefully. I think that there is a terrible danger in starting a form of therapy without knowing what we are doing.

MODERATOR: Just to defend the poor-quiet-defenseless commentator, what is the difference between not knowing what one does with plasmapheresis and not knowing what one does with prednisone, or pulse therapy, or triple therapy?

COMMENT-RESPONSE: I think that we perhaps should have a symposium on this subject alone. I will submit to you that the fact that we have done wrong in the past is no reason to do wrong in the future. We should have learned from the past. I teach my Residents constantly to beware of what we are doing to our patients. And I am using an example now called the "Gasping Syndrome" - the use of sterile water in nurseries to flush out umbilical artery catheters that contained benzoyl alcohol, poison, which was killing little babies. We laugh at what was done in the 1930's where people were using mercury ointments to treat acrodynia, not knowing that acrodynia was caused by sensitivity to mercury. I think we have to be very, very careful when we start new forms of therapy. And the FDA will not allow us to use moxalactam or Septra or Captopril until there will be an awful lot of studies. But, plasmapheresis we are allowed to use, because it is not controlled. I find that a somewhat strange approach. We may be taking away factors with plasmapheresis which are protecting our patients, we don't know what we are doing. That's all I wish to say.

COMMENT: I saw a paradox in what was just said. I wanted to take issue with the first part of the comment that stated that patients used to die years back and now they don't die because we are doing something aggressive, and now he comes and says exactly what I wanted to say. That is, I think we are lumping concepts together ; maybe our supportive therapy and our better understanding of other aspects of the problem are responsible for the fact that those patients are alive today. I agree entirely with you. I think that safe hemodialysis in those very sick patients is probably as effective as those heroic maneuvers like plasmapheresis.

COMMENT: It's well taken. Thank you.

QUESTION: I would like to ask about this case specifically. Number one, if you found complement in the kidney biopsy, was it in such small amount that it would not account for any decrease in the serum complement, since we have values that are normal? And second, there is right upper quadrant tenderness in this patient; I don't know how to explain this. I don't know whether it is related to the progressive glomerulonephritis or not. How would this process cause pain?

RESPONSE: I find it extremely difficult to interpret deposits of C3 in the glomeruli. One may do a complement fixation test using an in vitro system to see if the complement fixed in a biological manner. But, really, the only thing that one sees by immunofluorescence is that there is complement there, perhaps non-immunologically mediated. I believe that it is very difficult to do correlations with that. I don't think that anybody has hard data on this subject. In general, it is very difficult to do correlations anyway. I believe that the only thing that one determines is if they are there chemically, but they may be biologically inactive. So, the information may have no practical significance, just a non-specific deposition due to the local disturbances, with denudation of the endothelium and massive lesions that you see in the capillary wall.

MODERATOR: We need to go to the next case but we will entertain the last question.

QUESTION: I want to ask a quick question for everybody. In the patients in whom you have been able to turn off the acute process, what has been your experience with the long term outcome or the course up to date in those patients you have been able to follow?

RESPONSE: Our limited experience has revealed two populations. Those who seem to recover their GFR almost to normal, (and all through the years we have followed,they seem to do well), and those who are left with GFR's of 20 or 30 ml/min/1.73 m^2, who tend to have problems as the years go by. I think that maybe what you see at the end is the result of how severe the damage was at the outset. Although I am not a pathologist I like to mention that people comment on how big are the crescents, how large is the volume, and whether they contain fibrin or are all epithelialized. Perhaps all have some sort of prognostic significance.

RESPONSE: I have a lot of difficulty in evaluating the degree and extent of crescents. I believe that, in general, even when you look at biopsies serially, you can see sections that show 20 glomeruli, then you see a section that shows only 3 glomeruli. There is a great deal of variation in the number of glomeruli and in the area of each glomerulus through which the cut was made (the pole, the equator, etc). I think that is a very difficult manner in which to evaluate treatment. If you are going to do clinico-pathological correlations it is clear that a kidney with Crescentic Glomerulonephritis that has 10% of crescents is very different from the one that has 80% but the sampling error is a formidable problem in evaluating the significance of a biopsy.

MODERATOR: Now, we must stop this discussion here and go to the next case.

Patient T.W. is a 10-year-old black boy who was well until December 1st when he presented with fever, headache, vomiting and red urine. He had had a cold three weeks prior to the onset of complaints. A single episode of epistaxis occurred one week prior to admission.

On December 10, he was admitted to the University of Miami/Jackson Memorial Medical Center in severe respiratory distress, with BP 150/90 mm Hg. Edema 2+ was present in legs, abdomen was distended with fluid, and there were decreased breath sounds with occasional rales in lungs, bilaterally.

Chemistries: In blood: BUN 143 mg/dl, Creatinine 9.8 mg/dl, Na 131 mEq/L, K 4.8 mEq/L, CO_2 17 mEq/L, Cl 90 mEq/L, glucose 98 mg/dl. Urinary protein 2.7 g/24 hours. ASO 1:400, sickle prep negative, RPR negative, HB 9.2 g/dl, WBC 18,500/mm^3. C_3, C_4 were normal. Chest x-ray showed bilateral pleural effusions. Culture of pleural fluid was sterile.

Patient underwent peritoneal dialysis and hemodialysis on several occasions, and renal function improved. Pleural effusions resolved. Renal biopsy was performed on December 29 with serum creatinine 1.6 mg/dl and BUN 49 mg/dl.

Within the next 3 months BUN and creatinine fell to normal, and proteinuria subsided to about 300 mg/24 hours. Arterial BP had reverted to normal before discharge. Since then, patient has remained well. There is no hypertension or proteinuria at this time. Microscopic hematuria persists.

This patient needs to be clarified. He had not only epistaxis but during the admission he had red-tinged sputum which was analyzed and was negative for iron-stained cells. Dr. Pardo performed the test on normal kidney looking for anti-basement membrane antibodies. The result was negative. Any questions about the brief history?

QUESTION: When you said his blood pressure reverted to normal, do you happen to know what those numbers were?

RESPONSE: No, I'm sorry. I don't have that information here. But he is a perfectly healthy individual. We were sure that we were dealing with a case of Goodpasture's.

DR. PARDO: The biopsy revealed a diffuse and global proliferative and exhudative glomerulonephritis. There was a marked increase in the number of nuclei. The lumen of the capillaries was practically absent. There were numerous granulocytes also. There were no crescents and the interstitium did not show any chronic changes, but there was some intertubular edema. Looking at the tubules, there was some irregularity in the size and staining characteristics of the nuclei. Here again you could see some areas that showed something like a nuclear drop-out. There was desquamation of epithelial cells. In some portions of the biopsy there was, in addition to the interstitial edema, an interstitial inflammatory infiltrate with some plasma cells and a few eosinophils. To what extent could this be acute interstitial nephritis instead of acute tubular necrosis or vasomotor nephropathy, as was my first diagnosis, can be a subject of discussion. But we know that in ATN you can have interstitial edema and a mild inflammatory infiltrate.

Since the predominance of the tubular or epithelial lesions was quite clear, I would rather call it acute vasomotor nephropathy or acute tubular necrosis. Since I am always worried with these "degenerative" changes, I always try to look for signs of regeneration. We saw two pyknotic nuclei and there were some nuclei which were vesicular with prominent nucleoli that perhaps were regenerating. And finally, there was a mitosis in one of the tubular cells. That is what I like to see, to be relatively sure that this is a process of tubular necrosis. By electronmicroscopy there were subepithelial deposits of the "hump" type. This confirms the diagnosis of post-infectious glomerulonephritis.

MODERATOR: Any immunofluorescence?

DR. PARDO: There was a lumpy-bumpy appearance with IgG and C_3.

COMMENT: I think clinically that the diagnosis of an acute post-infectious nephritis, probably post-strep, fits very well. The clinker in it was what was determined to be hemoptisis. But we know the youngster had epistaxis and right away one wonders if the hemoptisis was not returned swallowed blood. One can be fooled that way, obviously.

MODERATOR: In fact, the history says pleural effusion by x-ray. I had my reservations about that statement; there may have been a component of pulmonary edema. But, the picture was so confusing that, if you were to make the diagnosis of Goodpasture's, you would have been entitled to. Actually, the original description by Goodpasture was simply a pulmonary and renal association. So that if you wanted to be very free, you could call Goodpasture the clinical picture we had here. But, since we have the markers, we looked for the specific anti-basement membrane antibody and they were negative in this qualitative test which Dr. Pardo performed. It is a biologocal test; now, it is commercially available so that one can document more accurately the presence or absence of the antibody.

COMMENT: Years ago we had an endemic problem with acute post-streptococcal nephritis; now they are not seen so often. Some of these children were admitted with acute pulmonary edema and some of them were bleeding very heavily through the respiratory tract. Sometimes people were confusing this with blood coming from the stomach. These patients required very rapid, acute intensive therapy because they could die from the anemia.

QUESTION: I see normal values for C_3 and C_4 and I question this. How often do you see normal complement in post-streptococcal nephritis?

RESPONSE: In most series where the diagnosis is clear - for instance, the series from Dodge's group, and when the patients are seen early, the complement in almost 90%, I would say, is found to be depressed; C_3 in particular. In other instances where the patients are coming in at different time intervals, then we see that the complement is not so often diminished. Kurt Lange, in the heyday of acute post-streptococcal glomerulonephritis that was genuinely the diagnosis in so many patients, published some 450-odd cases. All but a handful had low C_3; it was called hemolytic complement at that time. So, it is a very consistent finding in the acute stages of the disease. One wonders about the fact that it is normal in this case.

COMMENT: I noticed that Dr. Pardo called this Post-Infectious Glomerulonephritis. He didn't call it Post-Streptococcal Glomerulonephritis because he didn't see streptococcal antigen or any signature of streptococcus in the biopsy. All he saw was evidence of Post Infectious GN. It raises the question: are there any other infections that can cause a similar picture? I would start off by saying that the throat culture must have been negative; otherwise, he would have mentioned it. The C_3 was mentioned as normal, and the ASO titer was 1:400. Did the ASO titer rise or fall? Or did it remain static? Because about 10% of the pediatric population can have an increase in ASO titer. I would put it another way. I would say, "Sure this could well be a Post-Streptococcal GN." Who am I to say that it is not? But it could also be GN associated with Strep pneumoniae infection because that has been described. It could be GN associated with micoplasma pneumoniae; that's been described. And I'm certain that there may be a number of other infectious agents that could produce the same picture.

MODERATOR: Let me answer some of those questions. The ASO titer did return to normal. It was a true streptococcal infection at around that time but not documented by culture. There are coincidental infections that are not necessarily causative of the problem that one sees. The reason Dr. Pardo used that term is that here we have had Dr. Habib, Dr. Gordillo, etc. We have kicked this around so much that even Dr. Habib went back and in one Seminar of ours, started using "Post-Streptococcal Glomerulonephritis"; we started correcting her. She wanted to use a term that people would understand in this country but she and we prefer the more general term of "Post-Infectious GN". I said "listen, in the last Seminar we agreed that we are not going to call this 'post streptococcal'." So, in this room, where we have been for nine years now and one year in another hotel, we have agreed that we are going to use "Post-Infectious Glomerulonephritis". We agree that it is a very valid point. Muniere Yuceoglu in New York, she and I trained together, described one of the associations with viruses. Certainly it can be present with other entities.

QUESTION: About the pathology, I am aware of necrotizing arteritis being reported in association with post-streptococcal nephritis but you mentioned the lesions of acute tubular necrosis with regeneration. Assuming that this child was not hypotensive, where did his ATN come from? I know that ATN has been described in children with the Hemolytic Uremic Syndrome but how about Post-Infectious Nephritis?

COMMENT: Somebody wrote a paper in the forties and many of the patients described had ATN and tubular interstitial disease in association with Post-Streptococcal Glomerulonephritis.

MODERATOR: We wrote a paper in 1959 in Pediatrics on the Post-Infectious Glomerulonephritis with Acute Renal Failure. We did not call it ATN at that time. We did not have renal failure indexes and so on but it seemed to follow the general picture. Some people hold the concept or used to hold the concept that it does not happen, that the Post-Infectious Glomerulonephritis patient would not have ATN, but I believe that occasionally we do see that.

COMMENT: Since you are calling this "Post-Infectious", it is nevertheless a little bit peculiar that the complement was normal since in the Post-Infectious GN from other etiologies, the complement is also depressed.

MODERATOR: That point is interesting. I had never seen a patient with Post-Infectious Glomerulonephritis from impetigo. We used to see here a lots of the so-called "Florida sores". In Alabama, they are the "Alabama sores", and so on. Here, especially in the summers, we used to see quite a bit of these patients, and the complement was always low. So, we have a dogma: anytime we see an imcomplete form of Post-Infectious Glomerulonephritis, we biopsy. The incomplete form means, among other items, a normal complement. We recently had an adolescent who was presented and discussed. She actually had the nephrotic component; to make matters even worse, she was an adolescent black girl. I said "This girl does not have acute Post-Infectious Glomerulonephritis unless otherwise proven, and therefore, she must have a biopsy". She did have a biopsy and she had the typical changes of endothelial and mesangial cell proliferation with the lumpy-bumpy deposits and so on and the girl is doing great. It's the first case we've had with a normal complement with that type of presentation. There are exceptions. I think it is very good, for clinical purposes, to use the concept that you will rarely see a normal serum complement with Post-Infectious Glomerulonephritis. Dr. Luis Callis from Barcelona reported at our Seminar in 1975 that C_3 could normalize after 10-15 days of the disease.

COMMENT: We published our findings on C_3 in Acute Post-Streptococcal Glomerulonephritis. We had a group of patients with very high C_3 values, showing us a rebound. When we followed their curves, some patients, let's say around the fourth week, fifth week, reached double the normal value for our standards. So, I think that sometimes you may get a patient in the middle of a recovery with normal or high normal C_3 because of no reason. Perhaps he may have this change rapidly in the first week or so. This patient perhaps had nephritis days before being admitted because he was admitted as an emergency. He needs several days to accumulate such an amount of fluid. That may be the reason for a normal value.

MODERATOR: Yes. Actually one of the speakers gave a figure of, I believe, three weeks. If the patient remains with hypocomplementemia for more than three weeks, would you then call that persistent hypocomplementemia? Is that what you said?

COMMENT: That certainly is arbitrary. I would feel better about waiting for six weeks but most complements have returned to normal by three weeks.

MODERATOR: I thought three weeks was a little too close.

COMMENT: The type of Post-Streptococcal Nephritis we see is rather mild. That's the kind where within two to three weeks, the complement is normal. That's different, I think, from what other people see, and it's different from what we used to see in New York City.

COMMENT: I would like to suggest that we have been brain-washed into believing that there is a particular disease called Post-Streptococcal Glomerulonephritis, which has a particular appearance. I think there is such a disease but several years ago we reported two cases of Post-Streptococcal Glomerulonephritis associated with Henoch Schönlein Purpura. Or if you want to look at it another way, there is another report of a case of Henoch Schönlein associated with Post-Streptococcal Glomerulonephritis. The point was made here that Post-Streptococcal GN can be associated with a necrotizing vasculitis. In the cases reported in adults, I think the mortality was 100%. We have seen an extension of Post-Streptococcal GN into a picture with arthralgia, the typical Henoch-Schönlein Purpura rash and abdominal pain. But, in addition, the renal lesion was not HSP: it was Post-Streptococcal GN. We have this view of acute Post-Streptococcal GN as we think it should be and then, on the outskirts, there have to be outsiders behaving in strange ways.

MODERATOR: We will move now to the next case which will be presented by Dr. Michael Freundlich.

DR. FREUNDLICH: This is a 15 year old white girl with a two-month history of scalp rash, wandering arthralgias, facial edema and progressive asthenia with anorexia. <u>Initial examination</u>, at another hospital, revealed a moderately-sick looking girl, with trace edema. BP 180/120 mm Hg. Knee and ankle arthralgias but no overt arthritis. Oriented, no neurological signs. Heart, lungs, fundi normal.
Laboratory: BUN 101 mg/dl, serum creatinine 3-4 mg/dl, serum albumin 2.3 g/dl, ESR 110 mm/Hr, "active" serological parameters. Urine: hematuria and proteinuria. Daily proteinuria ranged from 2 to 3 g. Initially she was managed with parenteral antihypertensive drugs, diuretics and low sodium diet. Prednisone (80 mg/day) was started as well. After 1 week, she was transferred to our care. Upon arrival to the University of Miami/Jackson Memorial Medical Center, the most relevant findings included: BP 170/110 mm Hg, trace edema; indurated, 3 cm in diameter tender, anular, cellulitis-like lesion in the pre-sacral area.
Laboratory: Hb 6.5 g/dl, WBC 6,300/mm^3, platelet 157,000/mm^3, BUN 158 mg/dl, serum creatinine 4.5 mg/dl, K 4.8 mEq/L, CO_2 16 mEq/L, albumin 2.5 g/dl, ESR 120 mm/Hr, C_3 30 mg/dl, C_4 5 mg/dl, ANA 1:2048 (homogeneous); AuAg and Mono-test, both negative. Urine: ph 5, SG 1017, 3+ protein, large blood. Sediment revealed numerous red cells, 10-15 white cells/HPF, and granular casts. Daily proteinuria averaged around 2.5 g. Management: Antihypertensive agents, diuretics, intermittent hemodialysis, fluid and dietary restrictions, and antibiotics. Prednisone was maintained initially at 80 mg/day.
<u>Subsequent course</u>: BP was brought under control; dialysis frequency was decreased; pre-sacral cellulitis improved with carbenicillin. Laboratory data 1 month later: BUN 82 mg/dl, serum creatinine 2.1 mg/dl, hemoglobin 9.8 g/dl, CO_2 22 mEq/L, K 4.7 mEq/L, platelets 126,000/mm^3, ESR 30 mm/HR, C_3 111 mg/dl, C_4 9 mg/dl, ANA 1:2048, WBC 10,800/mm^3. Creatinine clearance 28 ml/min/1.73 m^2. Current medications: Clonidine 0.2 mg QID, Minipress 1 mg BID, Lasix 40 mg BID, prednisone 20 mg TID, Amphojel 10 cc TID, Folic Acid 1 mg/day, Multivitamin 1 tab/day.

MODERATOR: Any comments or questions? You will have to make the diagnosis. Really, there is no trick. The diagnosis is straight forward. Would you care to make the diagnosis without further information?

COMMENT-QUESTION: Certainly, this young girl fits the criteria for the diagnosis of systemic lupus. She seems to have had a rather fulminant cause to advanced renal insufficiency, that is not terribly unusual. I was just wondering if there was anything here that might have precipitated it. Had she been out in the sunlight? She never had any prodrome and this happened all at once, I gather. She presented as a very acutely ill child who fits the diagnosis of serological parameters and on renal parameters. She did not have a typical photosensitive or facial erythema. We are told that she had arthralgia but not arthritis; that troubles me a little bit, because you would like to see arthritis to actually make the diagnosis. If we are going to count current day criteria, it looks to me like we have three out of four.

COMMENT-RESPONSE: She was a completely healthy girl until all this started. She is a white, blonde girl, middle class American, fully grown, and well nourished.

QUESTION: Did she have a depressed white count or something like that? That could have been helpful.

RESPONSE: The WBC at our hospital was 6,300 /mm^3; we did not see a report from the outlying hospital.

MODERATOR: What about anti-DNA, LE preparation, and similar tests?

RESPONSE: They were positive. They were elevated but I don't recall the titers.

MODERATOR: So, we thought that we had a clear case of Systemic Lupus Erythematosus. What we did not feel we had was a typical presentation. In our experience, this is an extremely rare presentation with Acute Renal Failure, etc, of short duration, with rapid improvement in renal function (hemodialysis had to be discontinued shortly after the initial sessions). The infection may deserve a bit further elaboration.

DR. FREUNDLICH: We were not clear about the diagnosis of that cellulitis-like area. Several needle biopsies were performed and cultures were not very revealing. Finally, a third skin biopsy after several antibiotics (ampicillin, gentamicin, etc), finally grew pseudomonas. Very unusual. She responded after two days of carbenicillin. She has improved and done well since.

COMMENT: Subcutaneous nodules are often seen along the extensor surfaces, but can be seen almost anywhere. And then, secondarily infected after punctures...

RESPONSE: No, it started as a clear-cut infection, a subcutaneous infection which spread under our eyes from day to day. Typical for cellulitis, with sharp margins, progressing over days.

MODERATOR: Let me say that, for me, it was not a typical infection. We have a paper which will appear shortly in the Dermatology literature together with Dr. L. Schachner and his group. That paper describes fat necrosis in a nodular form, with a peculiar infiltrate. So, I called Dr. Schachner and told him that I thought we had the second case of the problem we had described in that paper. I thought it was fat necrosis. To me, it was a very odd type of inflammatory, necrotic, type of lesion that had a center with a black area. I thought it was fat necrosis.

COMMENT: There has been a semi-characteristic rash of pseudomonas cellulitis described that sounds like this; we have seen it a couple of times.

MODERATOR: In lupus patients?

RESPONSE: No, in all types of patients. We have seen it in one of our transplant patients.

MODERATOR: The neonatologists will tell you that that is a problem, and that you make the clinical diagnosis of pseudomonas infection by the appearance of black spots, necrotic looking. But, it was a very slow growing process in this patient; therefore, the initial skin biopsy did not have a positive culture and several days went by before the diagnosis was made on a culture from that first biopsy. A very unusual situation. Dr. Schachner is writing this up since he believes that in the dermatological literature this is not well known.

QUESTION: What do you think about the discrepancy between a BUN of 83 and a creatinine of 2.1?

RESPONSE: We are told that she was moderately sick and had a poor appetite. I would expect a youngster like this to be quite catabolic. That would be one explanation for it. An additional explanation is that she may have some degree of pre-renal azotemia, although I don't see much evidence with what is here to invoke that. Usually these patients have intravascular volume overload rather than volume contraction.

COMMENT: I think she was on steroids. We see this very commonly in adults.

COMMENT: It could have been the effect of the steroids.

MODERATOR: Dr. Pardo, could we go to your material?

DR. PARDO: This patient exhibits a diffuse mesangial and intracapillary proliferation associated with segmental and focal "wire loops" and sclerosis. The arterioles have intimal myofibroblastic proliferation with virtual obliteration of lumina in some areas.

COMMENT: This certainly fits with the cases presented earlier today, with Acute Renal Failure and various etiologies, the six cases that we reported at the American Society of Nephrology. One of those was vasomotor.

COMMENT: I'd like to make a comment about the six cases that were presented earlier today. Four of them were on inhibitors of prostaglandin function. It's quite interesting that there are a number of reports now on the use of PGE to treat NZBW mice with Lupus Nephritis. And it was found that administering PGE improves the renal pathology and prevents progression of the declining renal function that is seen in these animals. This is true not only of NZBB mice but also of rats with Masugi nephritis. What I think I am trying to say is that if an experimental model PGE, and incidentally not PGF but especially PGE, has a beneficial effect on the progression of Lupus Nephritis, then one should be very wary perhaps of using these newer non-steroidal anti-inflammatory agents for the treatment of patients with Lupus. Not only because of the PGE but also because of their propensity to lower GFR and also because of the reported association of tubulo-interstitial disease in patients who have been treated with some of the newer drugs. We have seen 30 cases of Lupus over the years and not a single one has presented with Acute Renal Failure. When I was a resident in adult Nephrology, I reviewed 50 cases of Lupus and I can't remember a single case presenting in Acute Renal Failure. What I am beginning to wonder is, if they do present in Acute Renal Failure, what is the other factor that is involved. Is it that they have been on some other agents or have they been vomiting and have become volume depleted and this has produced Acute Tubular Necrosis? Perhaps the predominant lesion is as you are suggesting, an Acute Tubular disease rather than glomerular disease which is causing the Acute Renal Failure. But this is just speculation on my part.

COMMENT: I think this case is interesting also because, if one has a series of cases and one could treat these cases by any method, one could say that this is the success of the treatment of Diffuse Proliferative Glomerulonephritis in Lupus. I believe that the biopsy control is extremely important.

COMMENT: To give another example, we had a patient who recently had been found to have lupus. She was on a very high dose of prednisone, came to the hospital with oliguria and went into oliguric Acute Renal Failure. Later on she confessed that she had abruptly interrupted treatment and she went into a corticosteroid suppression syndrome. This was perhaps the reason. She went out very nicely and then recovered. She had a pattern of Acute Tubular Necrosis.

COMMENT: A number of the non-steroidal anti-inflammatory agents have been reported to give rise to an interstitial nephritis in Acute Renal Failure in and of themselves, which is a problem with using any of these agents and any of the drugs. We have seen a couple of children given these drugs who have developed Acute Renal Insufficiency.

QUESTION: I wonder if you ever see a patient with Lupus presenting just with renal involvement initially and nothing else, and later on developing involvement of other systems. I was under the impression that that would be a very unlikely occurrence, that you would see just the proteinuria, then a long lag period, and after that other manifestations of Lupus.

COMMENT: It is an unusual presentation but certainly there are cases reported where individuals have presented with renal manifestations and subsequently developed the clinical, systemic manifestations that make the diagnosis. I just wanted to make the comment to emphasize what the authors of that report recommended for patients with the presentation of Acute Tubular Necrosis. They advocated that all patients who present with Acute Renal Failure and the diagnosis of Lupus should be biopsied prior to therapy because, God forbid, they might be given plasmapheresis or something on the assumption that they have a Diffuse Proliferative Lupus Nephritis. I think I would concur with that assessment. We are talking about a very serious disease with important therapeutic implications. Given that perhaps rarely but certainly several individuals have had experience with Acute Renal Failure that is not secondary to the lesion but rather secondary to other causes, one probably should know what one is dealing with before treating aggressively.

COMMENT: In one series in the early seventies in Medicine, 6% of the cases were said to have presented with renal involvement; but in addition to that, there are reports of cases with Idiopathic Epimembranous Glomerulopathy subsequently going on to develop features of Lupus within a year or several years after the presentation of Nephrotic Syndrome. So, rare cases can present with renal disease.

MODERATOR: Thank you very much to all of you for your participation.

PERITONEAL DIALYSIS IN CHILDREN

H. Jorge Baluarte, M.D., Michael B. Grossman, R.N., Martin S. Polinsky, M.D., Abdelaziz Y. Elzouki, M.D., James W. Prebis, M.D., Alan B. Gruskin, M.D.

Hemodialysis and peritoneal dialysis have been successfully used in children with end-stage renal disease (ESRD) (1,2,3,4). While neither form of dialysis is optimal (5), intermittent peritoneal dialysis (IPD) has been shown to be as effective as hemodialysis and offers certain medical and psychosocial advantages. Although simplicity has been the hallmark of peritoneal dialysis since its inception (6,7), the successful employment of arteriovenous shunts followed by the perfection in dialysis techniques and the proliferation of treatment facilities relegated peritoneal dialysis to a secondary role. These developments created a gap in the clinical application and technology between the two treatment modalities.

The turning point in restoring peritoneal dialysis to its current and expanded role in the management of chronic renal failure was the introduction of the permanent peritoneal catheter, originally designed by Palmer, then modified by Tenckhoff and Schechter (8). The Tenckhoff catheter offered a number of advantages: chronic access to the peritoneal cavity became simple and safe, minimized the complications of bowel perforation and reduced considerably the incidence of peritonitis. Finally, the introduction of automated peritoneal dialysis machines including the Lasker automatic cycler (9) which utilizes commercial containers of dialysis solutions, and functions by means of a series of valves which constrict the dialysis tubing at preset intervals permitting gravity to fill and drain the peritoneal cavity, made home peritoneal dialysis possible.

The purpose of this manuscript is to review our early experience with the use of peritoneal dialysis in our pediatric ESRD program and to describe the clinical course of these children. Home peritoneal dialysis has been a suitable alternative to many patients and parents referred to us from long distances from our dialysis center, especially when closer adult-oriented units were unwilling to accept children in their program. Peritoneal dialysis was also indicated in young and small children because of technical difficulties which included mechanics of performing a hemodialysis, because of the inappropriate size of existing dialyzers, and because of the lack of suitable vessels to create an adequate vascular access. This treatment modality also offered an alternative for children in need of "prolonged" dialysis because the presence of a malignant tumor required a period of time to be sure that metastases had not occurred prior to considering them satisfactory transplant candidates, and for children in whom high antibody titers reduced their opportunity to receive a renal graft. Since any form of dialysis can be disruptive to the life style of the family and child (5), we instituted a program of home peritoneal dialysis in an attempt to deal with the above problems and to overcome certain limitations of hemodialysis.

We report here the clinical course of 9 patients on IPD referred to St. Christopher's Hospital for Children for management of end-stage renal disease from June 1977 until December 1979. Five patients were begun on peritoneal dialysis whereas the other four patients were initially maintained on hemodialysis from 2 weeks to 12 months. The distance from the dialysis unit was the main reason for initiating home peritoneal dialysis in 7 patients. Preference for peritoneal dialysis was the reason in patient 6 and the lack of adequate vascular access after 12 months on hemodialysis was the reason for beginning peritoneal dialysis in 1 patient. Access to the peritoneal cavity was established by surgical implantation of a double dacron felt cuff Tenckhoff catheter, under local or general anesthesia. This was followed by intermittent daily dialysis for 3 to 5 days to assure the patency of the catheter. Patients were then maintained on a regular three day a week or an alternate day schedule.

After catheter function was assured, the parents and patients began their home-training which was usually accomplished in 12 dialysis days. Instructions included the following: principles of dialysis, components of dialysis exchange, i.e. dwell times, chemical composition of dialysate and modification of dialysate, catheter care (including aseptic preparation), measurement of vital signs, charting and record keeping, administration of medications, mechanical aspects of automated cycler system; prevention, signs and symptoms of peritonitis, fluid management, causes, signs and symptoms of hyper- and hypovolemia and explanation of the follow-up program by the pediatric nephrologist, primary nurse, nutritionist, social worker and psychologists from the ESRD team.

Commercially available dialysate supplied in 2 liter bottles (McGaw, Irvine, California) was used and the mechanics of the dialysis was performed with an automatic peritoneal cycler LJ300 Series II (American Medical Products Corp., Freehold, N.J.). Each dialysis treatment including set up and take down time lasted an average of 10 hours and used 16 liters of dialysate. Variable dextrose concentrations (1.5 - 4.25%) were used depending on the amount of fluid to be removed. An exchange volume of 40 ml/kg up to 1 liter was used with an inflow and dwell time of 20 minutes, and an outflow time of 10 minutes. A "dry weight" was established during the period of training and the patients were encouraged to attain this weight after dialysis. All patients were instructed in a high protein (2-3 gm/kg) low sodium (800-2000 mg), low potassium (1500 mg) and a low phosphate diet which was modified based on individual needs and degree of residual renal function. The fluid limitation imposed depended upon the existence of hypertension and whether the patient was oliguric or polyuric. Laboratory studies were performed at monthly intervals during clinic visits; blood transfusions were arranged at local hospitals or during visits to our dialysis center.

Clinical data of the 9 patients prior to initiation of peritoneal dialysis are summarized in Table I. Ages ranged from 5 to 13 4/12 years; all of the patients had been hypertensive but blood pressure was controlled in 5; height was below the 3rd percentile in all of the children; two patients were anephric, four had a urinary output below 100 ml/day while urinary output in three ranged from 700 to 2000 ml/day. The BUN concentration ranged from 70 to 200 mg/dl, serum albumin from 2.5 to 4.8 gm/dl; serum calcium was low in 4 patients and normal in 5; 9 patients had an elevated serum phosphorus value, alkaline phosphatase was elevated in 2 of 9, and 7 of 9 had elevated PTH

Table I. Clinical Data Prior to Peritoneal Dialysis

PATIENT	DIAGNOSIS	AGE AT ONSET IPD (yrs)	BLOOD PRESSURE mm Hg	WT. (LB) HT. (IN) AT ONSET	URINE OUTPUT cc/day RESIDUAL GFR (cc/min)	BUN CR (mg/dl)	T.P. ALB (gm/L)	CA PO_4 (mg/dl)	A'Pse PTH (units)	OSTEODYSTROPHY BONE AGE (BA)
1	Wilm's Tumor	6	100-150/60-100	34 42.75	Anephric	70 8.5	5.5 2.9	8.5 6	310 986	Rickets o Osteitis + BA 5 yr
2	CGN	5	100/60	36 39	<100 -	120 9.8	4.4 2.5	6.1 11.2	199 215	Rickets o Osteitis + BA 4 yr
3	CGN	10.5	140/110	51.5 47	<100 -	98 15.3	6.1 3.2	9 8.6	110 1375	Osteoporosis BA 7-8 yr
4	CGN	9	130/90	64.5 50.5	<100 -	150 16	5.2 2.9	8.5 8.3	97 540	Rickets o Osteitis o BA 8.8 yr
5	Medullary Cystic Disease	12.5	120/80	76.5 59.75	1800 6	180 13	7.2 4.3	9.5 9.5	422 820	Rickets o Osteitis + BA 12 yr
6	Hypoplasia	9.5	145/95	44 43	Anephric	108 9	6.6 4.8	10 6.4	365 2900	Rickets o Osteitis + BA 4 yr
7	CGN	10.7	120/66	57.5 53	700 5	200 13.8	5.9 4.1	5.5 14.5	232 797	Rickets o Osteitis o BA 8.8 yr
8	Reflux Nephropathy	13	120/70	79 55	2000 6	155 12.2	6.8 4.8	10.2 6	190 216	Rickets o Osteitis o BA 12.5 yr
9	Hypoplasia	13.3	140/100	77.5 57.5	<100 -	190 18	6.6 3.7	4.2 16	286 530	Rickets o Osteitis + BA 12-13 yr

levels (normal <300 pg/ml). Roentgenographic studies revealed osteoporosis in all of the patients, none had rickets/osteomalacia and 5 of 9 had bone changes consistent with hyperparathyroidism.

Clinical data obtained during the course of home peritoneal dialysis are summarized in Table II. Total time on dialysis averaged 11.2 months and ranged from 3 to 30 months. Eighty-two percent of the dialyses were performed at home, the remaining treatments were done in the hospital either during the training period or during hospitalization for complications and/or renal transplantation. The "dry weight" arbitrarily taken to represent a state of euvolemia was determined for each patient during the course of their home-training period. Their actual weights fluctuated from 0 to 12.5% above their dry weights, requiring various combinations of dextrose concentrations and/or additional treatments depending on the amount of fluid to be removed.

Children maintained on home peritoneal dialysis encountered many of th medical problems of children maintained on hemodialysis: growth failure, hypertension, anemia, and bone disease. Inadequate growth continued to be a significant problem. Three patients underwent dialysis for less than 6 months, a period too short for growth assessment. In five of the remaining six patients height increments were documented but when whole-year velocity standards for height (14) were plotted three patients were below the 3rd percentile, one in the 50th percentile and the other between 10-25th percentile. The combination of anorexia, decreased caloric intake, osteodystrophy, uremia and corticosteroid therapy may have contributed to the chronic growth retardation.

The hypertension observed in dialysis patients is usually a manifestation of fluid over-load and inadequate dialysis, unless a hyper-reninemic state exists. Eight of nine patients required antihypertensive medications. Blood pressure was adequately controlled in 7 of the 8 patients. Two out of the 7 patients with controlled hypertension underwent a bilateral nephrectomy prior to peritoneal dialysis. Hypertension in spite of drug therapy in patient 6 was the reason for nephrectomy while in patient 1 the reason for nephrectomy was the presence of bilateral Wilms tumor. Bilateral nephrectomy for

Table II. Clinical Data on Peritoneal Dialysis

PATIENT	LENGTH ON IPD (MO)	DRY WEIGHT(LB) HEIGHT (IN) AT END IPD	RANGE OF WEIGHT (lb)	BLOOD PRESSURE (range)	TRANSF INTERVAL (WKS)	BUN CR (range)	T.P. ALB (range)	CA PO_4 (range)	OUTCOME
1	30	34 44.5	35–38	110–120 / 75–90	8	70–100 6–7.7	4.8–6 3.3–4	9–10 6–8	Ascitis (Chylous)
2	22	32 40.25	31–33.5	110–140 / 58–112	7	60–90 6–10	6–6.9 3.5–4	10–11 5–5.4	Transplant (C)
3	8	39 47	41–46	140–160 / 90–110	8	70–120 10–12.3	5–6.1 3–3.6	8.2–10 4–7	Pericarditis Seizures (HBP) Transplant (C)
4	3.5	50 50.5	60–67	105–120 / 70–90	7	90–110 8–12	5–5.9 2.3–4	9–10.4 4–6	Transplant(LR)
5	14	79 62.25	79–84	110–120 / 65–75	8	70–100 10–14	5–6.5 3.2–4	9.2–10 4–4.6	Progression of ROD Transplant (C)
6	5	43 43	44–45	110–130 / 70–80	5	60–80 7–9	6–6.2 4–4.3	9–10.7 3.2–5	Transplant (C) Died
7	9	56 53.75	58–61	110–120 / 70–72	8	50–90 9–10	5–6.8 3.2–4	8–10 3–7	Transplant(LR)
8	7	64 55.75	64–72	110–130 / 65–70	14	40–60 5–6	7–8 4–4.5	9–10 4–5	Progression of ROD Transplant(C)
9	3	68 57.25	65–73	110–120 / 65–70	6	80–90 12–16	5.4–6 3–3.5	8–8.5 5–6	Transplant(LR)

renin-dependent hypertension will improve the patient's well-being and eliminate much of the drug therapy required to treat hypertension. Nephrectomy should not be undertaken lightly, since preservation of residual renal function is desirable. Nephrectomy is likely to be associated with a more rapid evolution of bone disease and worsening of anemia (3); in addition the presence of kidneys may permit a larger fluid intake.

Blood transfusions with packed RBC's buffy coat-free were given to the children when their hematocrit values fell to less than 18% or if symptoms developed. The average interval between blood transfusions was 6.8 weeks, which is longer than the transfusion interval for our patients on maintenance hemodialysis. The increased requirement for blood in hemodialysis patients most likely reflects the greater amount of blood loss because of more frequent blood sampling, hemolysis by blood pumps, bleeding from the vascular access, and ruptured or clotted dialyzers.

The BUN concentration ranged from 65 to 93 mg/dl and the serum creatinine values from 8 to 10.7 mg/dl. We recommended a diet containing 2-3 gm/kg/day of protein to compensate for the peritoneal losses of albumin. Although the ingestion of this amount of protein may contribute to greater azotemia, predialysis values for BUN in the range of 80-110 mg/dl are not detrimental according to Tenckhoff (3) if the patient feels well. Total serum protein concentration ranged from 5.5-6.5 mg/dl and serum albumin ranged from 3.2-3.9 gm/dl. Protein losses are not constant throughout dialysis. Protein concentration in the dialysate is highest in the first cycle, dropping rapidly over the next 3 to 4 cycles, followed by stable low levels throughout the rest of the dialysis (15). Protein losses are constant as long as the dialysis technique is constant and a steady state of serum protein is reached by increased synthesis and decreased catabolism.

Serum calcium and phosphorus concentrations were adequately controlled on peritoneal dialysis. Calcium supplement, phosphate binders as well as Vitamin D_3 preparations were generally prescribed. Progression of hyperparathyroidism occurred in 3 of 9 patients but no patient required parathyroidectomy.

In addition to the commonly accepted problems experienced by children undergoing maintenance hemo- or peritoneal dialysis, the problem of peritonitis has been a limiting factor in patients on chronic peritoneal dialysis. Five patients had a total of 8 episodes of peritonitis during 101.5 dialyses-months, an incidence of 1 episode/12.6 patient-month or 0.55% of 1440 dialyses. The incidence of peritonitis was lower than the general experience reported among adults and other children's units (3,4,6). Peritoneal infection occurred 5 times after a documented break in sterility, 2 times associated with an exit site infection; the cause of the other incident was unknown. Despite episodes of peritonitis the catheter survival was satisfactory. Seven out of nine patients retained the original catheter; patients 1 and 2 needed catheter replacement 2 and 3 times respectively. The most common symptom was abdominal pain (8/8) followed by fever (7/8). Most of the episodes of peritonitis were due to Staphylococcus aureus (62.5%); the others involved Staphylococcus epidermidis (25%) and Klebsiella (12.5%). Treatment consisted of 4-5 days of continuous peritoneal lavage supplemented by a systemic priming dose of antibiotics after Gram stain and culture of the fluid were obtained. Adjustment of the nature and concentration of the antibiotics was done within 24-48 hours according to the antimicrobial disk sensitivities. Lavage with an effective antibiotic produced marked improvement within 24 hours. Oral and intraperitoneal antibiotic therapies were continued for 6-8 weeks to reduce the chance of relapse.

In our opinion IPD offered several advantages compared to in-center hemodialysis. It gave the family and patient greater autonomy and control over the treatment of the disease. Successful rehabilitation also became a more realistic goal because of the encouragement in our program of self-care dialysis (10,11). The cost of home peritoneal dialysis was similar to home hemodialysis (12,13), but compared to in-center dialysis it represented less of a financial burden. The family was allowed to remain in their home-town rather than move to another city, also transportation to dialysis center was required less frequently. Overnight dialysis was possible and partially offset the disadvantage of the long dialysis time (30-40 h/week) required with this method. Being at home increased the opportunity for the family and patient to maintain a more normal relationship with peers, relatives and school.

Of the 9 children who have undergone IPD during the study periods, 8 are alive, three remain on peritoneal dialysis and one died following a cadaveric kidney transplant of causes unrelated to dialysis. Three underwent a successful live-related kidney transplant, 5 patients underwent cadaveric kidney transplant, 2 have good functioning grafts at the present time and 3 patients had irreversible acute rejection. Although no form of dialysis is optimal, home IPD can be as effective as hemodialysis and offers certain psychosocial and medical advantages.

ACKNOWLEDGEMENTS

The authors would like to thank the nurses in the Dialysis Unit for their assistance in caring for these patients and gathering the pertinent data. We appreciate the secretarial assistance of Ms. Virginia Rivera, and Eileen Morris.

REFERENCES

1. Potter, D., Larsen, D., Leumann, E., Perin, D., Simmons, J., Piel, C.F., and Holliday, M.A.: Treatment of chronic uremia in childhood. II. Hemodialysis. Pediatr., 46:678, 1970.

2. Jones, J.M.B., Cameron, J.S., Berwick, M., Ogg, C.S., Meadow, S.R. and Ellis, F.G.: Treatment of terminal renal failure in children by home dialysis and transplantation. Arch. Dis. Child. 46:457, 1971.

3. Counts, S., Hickman, R., Garbaccio, A. and Tenckhoff, H.: Chronic home peritoneal dialysis in children. Trans. Am. Soc. Artif. Intern. Organs 19:157, 1973.

4. Brouhard, B.H., Berger, M., Cunningham, R.J., Petrusick, T., Allen, W., Lynch, R.E. and Travis, L.B.: Home peritoneal dialysis in children. Trans. Am. Soc. Artif. Intern. Organs 25:90, 1979.

5. Khan, A.V., Herndon, C.H. and Ahmadian, S.Y.: Social and emotional adaptations of children with transplanted kidneys and chronic hemodialysis. Am. J. Psych. 128:1194, 1971.

6. Tenckhoff, H.: Peritoneal dialysis today: a new look. Nephron. 12:420, 1974.

7. Boen, S.T.: Overview and history of peritoneal dialysis. Dialysis & Transplantation 6(2):12, February, 1977.

8. Tenckhoff, H. and Schaechter, H.: A bacteriologically safe peritoneal access device. Trans. Am. Soc. Artif. Internal Organs 14:181, 1960.

9. Lasker, N.: Chronic peritoneal dialysis. Pa. Med. 74:67, 1971.

10. Grossman, M.B.: Comprehensive follow-up, an essential ingredient to a home training program. Presented at the Realities of Nephrology Patient Care in the New Decade. 11th National AANNT Symposium. New Orleans, April 15-17, 1980.

11. Grossman, M.B.: Self-Care for children and adolescents on dialysis. Presented at the Realities of Nephrology Patient Care in the New Decade. 11th National AANNT Symposium, New Orleans, April 15-17, 1980.

12. Diaz-Buxo, J.A., Chandler, J.T., Farmer, C.D. and Smith, D.L.: Chronic peritoneal dialysis at home - a comparison with hemodialysis. Trans. Am. Soc. Artif. Internal Organs 23:191, 1977.

13. Christopher R. Blagg: Peritoneal dialysis and the Medicare ESRD Program. Dialysis & Transplantation, Vol. 8, Number 11, November, 1979.

14. Tanner, J.M., Whitehouse, R.H., Takaishi, M.: Standards from birth to maturity for height, weight, height velocity and weight velocity; British Children, 1965, Arch. Dis. Child. 51:454-471; 613-635, 1966.

15. Scarpioni, L., Poisetti, P.G., Ballocchi, S., Bergonzi, G.: Follow-up of plasma proteins during long-term peritoneal dialysis. Effect of protein loss (Abst.). The first International Symposium on Peritoneal Dialysis, June 25-08, 1978, Chapala, Mexico. Journal of Dialysis 2(5&5), 421-455, 1978.

Supported in part by NIH General Research Grant RR-75 and Hoechst-Roussel Corporation.

Mailing Address: Section of Nephrology, St. Christopher's Hospital for Children, 5th & Lehigh Avenue, Philadelphia, Pennsylvania 19133

PARTICIPANTS
AND
INDEXES

PARTICIPANTS

Program Chairman

José Strauss, M.D., Professor of Pediatrics; Director, Division of Pediatric Nephrology, University of Miami School of Medicine, Miami, Florida, USA.

Guest Faculty

Heinz F. Eichenwald, M.D., William Buchanan Professor of Pediatrics, University of Texas Health Services Center at Dallas, Dallas, Texas, USA.

Carlos A. Gianantonio, M.D., Chief, Department of Pediatrics, Hospital Italiano, Buenos Aires, Argentina.

Alan Gruskin, M.D., Professor of Pediatrics, Temple University; Chief, Section of Nephrology, St. Christopher's Hospital for Children, Philadelphia, Pennsylvania, USA.

Bernard S. Kaplan, M.B., B.Ch., Director of Nephrology Service, Department of Pediatrics, Montreal Children's Hospital, McGill University, Montreal, Quebec, Canada.

Melinda McVicar, M.D., Director, Children's Kidney Center, North Shore University Hospital, Manhasset, New York, USA.

Local Faculty

Donald M. Buckner, M.D., Associate Professor of Surgery and Pediatrics, Department of Surgery, University of Miami School of Medicine, Miami, Florida, USA.

John J. Byrnes, M.D., Associate Professor of Medicine; Chief, Department of Hematology, Veterans Administration Medical Center, Miami, Florida, USA.

Cherry Charlton, R.N., Head Nurse, Pediatric Dialysis Unit, Jackson Memorial Hospital, Miami, Florida, USA.

Richard Curless, M.D., Associate Professor of Neurology and Pediatrics, Department of Neurology, University of Miami School of Medicine, Miami, Florida, USA.

Jane L. Frank, M.D., Assistant Professor of Radiology and Pediatrics, Division of Diagnostic Radiology, Department of Radiology, University of Miami School of Medicine, Miami, Florida, USA.

Michael Freundlich, M.D., Clinical Assistant Professor of Pediatrics, Division of Pediatric Nephrology, Department of Pediatrics, University of Miami School of Medicine, Miami, Florida, USA.

Ronald Goldberg, M.D., Assistant Professor of Pediatrics, Division of Neonatology, Department of Pediatrics, University of Miami School of Medicine, Miami, Florida, USA.

Bonnie Hazen, R.N., Clinical Educator, Pediatric Intensive Care Unit, Jackson Memorial Hospital, Miami, Florida, USA.

Bernard H. Holzman, M.D., Assistant Professor of Pediatrics; Director, Pediatric Critical Care Medicine, Department of Pediatrics, University of Miami School of Medicine, Miami, Florida, USA.

George K. Kyriakides, M.D., Associate Professor of Surgery, Division of Transplantation, Department of Surgery, University of Miami School of Medicine, Miami, Florida, USA.

Jorge L. Lockhart, M.D., Assistant Professor of Urology, Department of Urology, University of Miami School of Medicine, Miami, Florida, USA.

Charles Lynne, M.D., Associate Professor of Urology, Department of Urology, University of Miami School of Medicine, Miami, Florida, USA.

Berta Morse, M.D., Assistant Professor of Radiology; Chief, Division of Body Ultrasound, Department of Radiology, University of Miami School of Medicine, Miami, Florida, USA.

Victoriano Pardo, M.D., Professor of Pathology; Director, Electron-microscopy Laboratory, Veterans Administration Medical Center. USA.

Guido Perez, M.D., Associate Professor of Medicine; Chief, Dialysis Unit, Veterans Administration Medical Center, Miami, Florida, USA.

Arthur S. Pickoff, M.D., Assistant Professor of Pediatrics, Division of Cardiology, Department of Pediatrics, University of Miami School of Medicine, Miami, Florida, USA.

Lawrence Schachner, M.D., Associate Professor of Dermatology and Pediatrics; Director, Division of Pediatric Dermatology, Department of Dermatology and Cutaneous Surgery, University of Miami School of Medicine, Miami, Florida, USA.

Gwendolyn Scott, M.D., Assistant Professor of Pediatrics; Acting Director, Division of Infectious Diseases, Department of Pediatrics, University of Miami School of Medicine, Miami, Florida, USA.

Emmalee S. Setzer, M.D., Assistant Professor of Pediatrics, Division of Neonatology, Department of Pediatrics, University of Miami School of Medicine, Miami, Florida, USA.

George N. Sfakianakis, M.D., Associate Professor of Radiology and Pediatrics, Division of Nuclear Medicine, Department of Radiology, University of Miami School of Medicine, Miami, Florida, USA.

José Strauss, M.D. Professor of Pediatrics; Director, Division of Pediatric Nephrology, Department of Pediatrics, University of Miami School of Medicine, Miami, Florida, USA.

Akram Tamer, M.D., Associate Professor of Pediatrics, Department of Pediatrics, University of Miami School of Medicine, Miami, Florida, USA.

Stuart R. Toledano, M.D., Assistant Professor of Pediatrics; Acting Director, DIvision of Pediatric Hematology and Oncology, Department of Pediatrics, University of Miami School of Medicine, Miami, Florida, USA.

Gaston Zilleruelo, M.D., Assistant Professor of Pediatrics, Division of Pediatric Nephrology; Director, Comprehensive Children's Kidney Failure Center, Department of Pediatrics, University of Miami School of Medicine, Miami, Florida, USA.

Other Contributors*

H. Jorge Baluarte, M.D., Associate Professor of Pediatrics, Department of Pediatrics, Temple University School of Medicine; Director of Dialysis Unit at St. Christopher's Hospital for Children, Philadelphia, Pennsylvania, USA.

Abdelaziz Y. Elzouki, M.D., Fellow, Pediatric Nephrology, Department of Pediatrics, Temple University School of Medicine and St. Christopher's Hospital for Children, Philadelphia, Pennsylvania, USA.

Jack S.C. Fong, M.D., Assistant Director, Department of Nephrology, Montreal Childrens' Hospital, Montreal, Quebec, Canada.

Paul R. Goodyer, M.D., Researcher, Department of Nephrology, Montreal Childrens' Hospital, Montreal, Quebec, Canada.

M.B. Grossman, R.N., Coordinator, End-Stage Renal Disease Program, St. Christopher's Hospital for Children, Philadelphia, Pennsylvania, USA.

Bruce A. Kaiser, M.D., Assistant Professor of Pediatrics, Department of Pediatrics, Temple University School of Medicine, Philadelphia, Pennsylvania, USA.

Michael Mellon, M.D., Division of Pediatric Nephrology, Department of Pediatrics, Temple University School of Medicine, Philadelphia, Pennsylvania, USA.

Bruce Z. Morgenstern, M.D., Fellow, Division of Pediatric Nephrology, Department of Pediatrics, St. Christopher's Hospital for Children, Philadelphia, Pennsylvania, USA.

Michael Morrison, M.D., Plantation Pediatric Group, P.A., Plantation, Florida, USA.

J. Lawrence Naiman, M.D., Professor of Pediatrics; Chief, Section of Hematology, Department of Pediatrics, Temple University School of Medicine, Philadelphia, Pennsylvania, USA.

Sharon A. Perlman, M.D., Department of Pediatrics, Temple University School of Medicine and St. Christopher's Hospital, Philadelphia, Pennsylvania, USA.

Martin S. Polinsky, M.D., Assistant Professor of Pediatrics, Department of Pediatrics, Temple University School of Medicine and St. Christopher's Hospital for Children, Philadelphia, Pennsylvania, USA.

James W. Prebis, M.D., Assistant Professor of Pediatrics, Department of Pediatrics, Temple University School of Medicine and St. Christopher's Hospital for Children, Philadelphia, Pennsylvania, USA.

Robert K Rhamy M.D., Associate Professor of Clinical Urology, Department of Urology, University of Miami School of Medicine, Miami, Florida, USA.

Gwendolyn Scott, M.D., Assistant Professor of Pediatrics, Head of Division of Infectious Diseases, Department of Pediatrics, University of Miami School of Medicine, Miami, Florida, USA.

David Taplin, Professor, Department of Dermatology and Cutaneous Surgery, University of Miami School of Medicine, Miami, Florida, USA.

Peter D. Thomson, M.D., Univeristy of the Witwatersrand, Johannesburg, South Africa.

*Co-authors

AUTHOR INDEX

SUBJECT INDEX

GPSR Compliance

The European Union's (EU) General Product Safety Regulation (GPSR) is a set of rules that requires consumer products to be safe and our obligations to ensure this.

If you have any concerns about our products, you can contact us on ProductSafety@springernature.com

In case Publisher is established outside the EU, the EU authorized representative is:

Springer Nature Customer Service Center GmbH
Europaplatz 3
69115 Heidelberg, Germany

Batch number: 10761599

Printed by Printforce, the Netherlands